PSYCHOSOCIAL ASPECTS
OF RADIATION THERAPY

PSYCHOSOCIAL ASPECTS OF RADIATION THERAPY

The Patient, the Family, and the Staff

Edited by

Patricia Tretter, Leonard M. Liegner,
Austin H. Kutscher, Richard J. Torpie,
Robert DeBellis, and Margot Tallmer

With the Editorial Assistance of Lillian G. Kutscher

A Volume in The Foundation of Thanatology/
Arno Press Continuing *Series on Thanatology*

ARNO PRESS
A New York Times Company
New York • 1981

Copyright © 1981 by Arno Press Inc.
Manufactured in the United States of America

Library of Congress Cataloging in Publication Data

Main entry under title:

Psychosocial aspects of radiation therapy.

   Bibliography: p.
   1. Radiotherapy--Psychological aspects. 2. Cancer
--Radiotherapy--Psychological aspects. I. Tretter,
Patricia. II. Kutscher, Lillian G. [DNLM: 1. Neo-
plasms--Radiotherapy. 2. Neoplasms--Psychology.
QZ269 P974]
RM849.P79   616.99'40642   80-17583
ISBN 0-405-13096-1

TABLE OF CONTENTS

PROLOGUE

Prolongation of Life
 Pope Pius 1
No Ashes for This Phoenix
 Jay J. Dugan 2

INTRODUCTION

The Enigmas Confronting the Cancer Patient
 Richard J. Torpie 10
Why Be An Oncologist?
 Jan van Eys 13
Reflections of a Self-Consulting Radiologist
 Harry L. Berman 16

APPROACHES TO THE CANCER PATIENT:
Practical, Therapeutic and Psychological

The Radiation Oncology Center as a Therapeutic
 Environment for Patients and Staff
 Arvin S. Glicksman, Glenn W. Mitchell,
  Carl A. Geyer, Curtis Perry and Kenneth Ain 24
Nutrition and the Psychosocial Aspects of Radiation
 James C. Rose 44
Psychosocial Aspects of Radiation Therapy
 Omar M. Salazar, Margaret Dunne, and
  Marjorie Sugarman 59
Patient Reactions to Cancer Diagnosis and Treatment
 Carlos A. Perez, Laurie Braun, Lily A. Hanes, and
  Nell Sedransk 65
The Radiotherapist's Psychological Approach to Cancer
 Sucha O. Asbell 81
Psychological Problems of Patients Receiving Radiotherapy
 Tapan A. Hazra, Carol Rose Martin, and
  Vincent Rose 83
Humanizing the Radiation Therapist
 Leonard M. Liegner 86
Strategies of Psychological Intervention
 L.D. Hankoff and Joseph A. Braun 93

Group Work with Cancer Patients in Radiation Therapy
    Patricia Fobair, Abby Wolfson, Norman L. Mages
    Joan Hall, Irene Harrison, and Julia Vose 99

Patient Group Therapy Sessions
    Joan M. Liaschenko............................ 114

Concepts of Adaptation and Life Change
in Cancer Patients
    Norman L. Mages, Gerald Mendelsohn, and
    Joseph Castro 118

The Male Patient in Cancer Crisis
    Richard O. Lowy............................. 133

The Impact of Pediatric Radiation Therapy
    Giulio J. D'Angio, Nancy Ann Osman, and
    Judith W. Ross.............................. 139

APPROACHES TO MALIGNANT DISEASE
(including Chemotherapy): Disease Entities, Alternative
Modalities, and Patients' Responses

CO^{60} Radiation: Life or Death?
    Isamettin M. Aral 150

The Psychological Impact of Radiation Therapy
Instead of Mastectomy for Early Carcinoma of
the Breast: A Preliminary Report
    Phyllis J. Ager, Jack Terry, Seymour Alpert, and
    Nemetalliah A. Ghossein 153

Pelvic Cancer's Impact on a Woman and Her Family
    William F. Finn.............................. 156

Gynecologic Cancer: A Case Report
    William F. Finn.............................. 164

Are There Miracles?
    Yvonne M. Parnes 167

Management of the Patient with Cancer
    Christie Goeggel and Sigmund Benham Kahn 169

Brain Tumor
    John C.M. Brust 179

Experiences with Cancer Patients in Psychoanalysis
    Selwyn Brody............................... 182

The Effects of Radiation Therapy Upon Psychological
and Behavioral Functioning: A Literature Review
    Gene Kopelson 191

Palliative Radiotherapy in the Patient with
Incurable Cancer
    Antonio Bosch and William L. Caldwell......... 197

Care of the Patient When the Disease Recurs
    A. Daniel Hauser and Richard S. Blacher 201
Palliation Therapy
    A. Daniel Hauser and Richard S. Blacher 205
Dilemma of the Dying—"Why Won't People
Listen to Me?"
    Rae Ellen S. Stager 208

PROFESSIONAL ROLES IN PATIENT CARE

Relegation of Responsibility for Total Patient Care
    A. Daniel Hauser and Richard S. Blacher 218
A Multidisciplinary Approach to Cancer Care
    Gordon A. Braatz and Arnoldus Goudsmit 220
General Principles of Nursing Care
    Jeanne Quint Benoliel 226
The Physician's Role in Catastrophic Disease
    William Regelson 236

TERMINAL CARE AND BEREAVEMENT

Treatment of a Dying Patient
    Charlotte Nadel and Trikante Rajapaksa 244
A Hospice at Work
    Madalon O'Rawe Amenta and Janet Hamnett 248
General Considerations in the Terminal Care
of Patients with Intra-Abdominal Cancer
    Frank Glenn 253
Bereavement Support: An Essential Part
of Comprehensive Cancer Care
    Elizabeth J. Clark 259
Thanatology and The Foundation of Thanatology
    Austin H. Kutscher and Lillian G. Kutscher 263

APPENDIX

Interdisciplinary Dialogue
    C.H. Chang, Austin H. Kutscher, Helen Coutts,
    David Peretz, and others 276
A Medical Student's Viewpoint
    Gene Kopelson 281

Contributor List 284

Prologue

Prologue

THE PROLONGATION OF LIFE

An Adress of Pope Pius XII to an International Congress of Anesthesiologists

Does [the doctor] have the right, or is he bound, in all cases of deep unconsciousness, even in those that are considered to be completely hopeless..., to use modern artificial respiration apparatus...? ... In most cases this situation arises, not at the beginning of resuscitation attempts, but when the patient's condition, after a slight improvement at first, remains stationary and it becomes clear that only automatic artificial respiration is keeping him alive....

The solution to this problem, already difficult in itself, becomes even more difficult when the family — themselves Catholic perhaps — insist that the doctor in charge, especially the anesthesiologist, remove the artificial respiration apparatus in order to allow the patient, who is already virtually dead, to pass away in peace....

... normally one is held to use only ordinary means — according to circumstances of persons, places, times, and culture — that is to say, means that do not involve any grave burden for oneself or another.... On the other hand, one is not forbidden to take more than the strictly necessary steps to preserve life and health, as long as he does not fail in some more serious duty....

The rights and duties of the doctor are correlative to those of the patient. The doctor, in fact, has no separate or independent right where the patient is concerned. In general he can take action only if the patient explicitly or implicitly, directly or indirectly, gives him permission. The technique of resuscitation which concerns us here does not contain anything immoral in itself. Therefore, the patient, if he were capable of making a personal decision, could lawfully use it and, consequently, give the doctor permission to use it. On the other hand, since these forms of treatment go beyond the ordinary means to which one is bound, it cannot be held that there is an obligation to use them nor, consequently, that one is bound to give the doctor permission to use them.

The rights and duties of the family depend in general upon the presumed will of the unconscious patient if he is of age and "sui juris." Where the proper and independent duty of the family is concerned, they are usually bound only to use ordinary means.

Consequently, if it appears that the attempt at resuscitation constitutes in reality such a burden for the family that one cannot in all conscience impose it upon them, they can lawfully insist that the doctor should discontinue these attempts, and the doctor can lawfully comply.

(From *The Pope Speaks,* vol. 4, No. 4, 1958)

NO ASHES FOR THIS PHOENIX

Jay J. Dugan

In the quiet semi-darkness
I lie outstretched, unmoving
on the padded steel table
in my cavernous concrete vault
and I yearn
      desperately
      for Doctor Tulsky's
      silent thunder
      and invisible lightning
Riveted to the massive steel ball,
yoke-hung
inches above my head,
   like a model No., serial No.
   on a Sears refrigerator
     the small metal tag
     announces matter-of-factly:
        ISOTOPES: COBALT 60
        CURIES: 1,727
        DATE OF CALIBRATION: April 1, 1973
What it doesn't say is: **VOLTAGE** — 2,500,000
      (We musn't frighten
      the customers, right?
      ... as if they will ever again
      know a terror
      to match the terror
      they already know.)

He's miserly with his magic
is Doctor Tulsky
eking it out
a few precious rads at a time.

He torments me
with only
65 seconds' worth
a day —
my nuclear 'fix',
    While I crave more,
    shamelessly.
    I covet it,
    hunger for it
    with animal greed.

He's here now,
mirabile dictu,
tall, professorial Dr. Tulsky,
radiologist, physician, physicist.
The collimator's concentric rings
form spiderweb patterns
on his white sleeve
fluttering above my head
in the eerie dimness.
    Wordlessly, he adjusts the aperture setting,
    focuses the slender light beam
    lancing down
    from the mouth
    of his marvelous monster
    on the red targets
    drawn on my naked groin.

He moves behind me,
sets the dosage dial,
trips the delayed action timer
    — and pads noiselessly toward the
    lead-filled door
    with the yellow and black sign—
    DANGER — HIGH VOLTAGE RADIATION
He has just 20 seconds to reach
and close that door
— from the outside.
    On the far away wall
    the green "situation light"
    changes to red —
        CONDITION RED

Alone.
I'm alone
as I've seldom been
in life
   . . . sealed in a lead-lined cube,
   suspended beneath
   ten tons of steel
   and lead.
      Targeted with cold
      scientific precision
      on my bare body
      is a force
      almost beyond
      the power of man
      to contain.
         Utter, impenetrable silence
         for 3 seconds —
         then
         a soft silken swish, as
         heavy tungsten blocks
            in the darkened collimator
            move apart
            and the eye
            of the giant
            opens.

Instantaneously
an unseen cascade
of thousands,
millions,
billions
of avenging
gamma rays
catapult like a crusading
cataclysm
through the aperture
and hurl themselves down,
down deep into my welcoming body
      lancing through flesh,
      cleaving bone,
      ripping through tissue

4

blindly, breathlessly, mercilessly
seeking, seeking, seeking
the loathesome cells
of the detested Phoenix,
impaling them
on barbed shafts,
incinerating,
exploding,
annihilating them
in a mindless
orgy of death
that yields me —
life.
    Seconds slip by —
    ten, fifteen, twenty.
    The awesome carnage goes on.
    The assassin's womb,
    that ponderous metal marble above me,
    slowly, silently courses
    in a great arc
    around and under and over
    my cantilevered bed
    like a benevolent moon
    around a benign sun.
    Now the moon is overhead.
    Into the field of my transfixed eyes
    floats the metal tag:
    ISOTOPES: COBALT 60
$COBALT^{60}$ — "... usually produced in a
nuclear reactor by neutron bombardment
of Co^{59}. Decays to stable isotope nickel 60."
        Burn, babies, burn.
        Slash, stab, skewer.
        Cut a wide, deep swath
        of merciful destruction
        through my troubled loins.
        Obliterate even the ashes
        so that never can that
        spectral bird
        rise
        to haunt my
        sleepless
        pre-dawn hours
        again.

The moon sets on my left,
slips beneath my bed
again
to blast
with its mighty blowtorch
the enemy
from below.
   In 15 seconds
   it will rise on my right —
   another dawning!
   ". . . God separated
   the light from the darkness,
   calling the light day
   and the darkness night.
   And there was evening
   and morning,
   the First day."
  GENESIS of cobalt — (Element No. 27,
  atomic weight 58.94)
  — gestation time: millions of years
  — finally born in a mine pit in Montana
  — separated from its Siamese sulfides
   in Illinois
  — educated, trained, armed in an atomic
   pile in Oak Ridge, Tennessee.

Oh, yes —
OAK RIDGE, TENNESSEE
Many times I flew by it
indolently sipping
a mile high martini
little dreaming
that one day
down there
faceless nuclear alchemists
would brew a steaming bowl
of COBALT^{60}
just for me.
  Rain down,
  knife-edged thunderbolts
  in your uncounted numbers.

       Hurl your lethal charges,
       detonate your mini-bombs,
       self destruct
       in the clasp
       of your mortal enemy
       — and mine.
. . . Too soon
unseen
contacts join,
switches close.
The black moon
halts its transit
across my starless sky,
and metal lids
silently close
over
the eye
of Cyclops.
       On the wall
       the red light
       changes to green
         CONDITION GREEN.

. . . .

"COBALT^{60} has a radioactive 'half-life of 5.26 + .02 years. During that period it dissipates its alpha, beta and gamma rays, reduces to a state of lower energy or ground state. At that point it must be replaced."

    I was waiting in the hospital lobby to be discharged a week after the operation when a large truck drew up outside. Bill-boarded on its front, back and sides was the warning: DANGER – HIGH RADIATION CARGO. The driver asked at the information desk: "Where is your Radiation Department? I have a container of fresh COBALT^{60} aboard."

    That was April 11; I started cobalt treatments April 16. I thought the timing a favorable portent. In two years I will know if indeed it was.

                              — *Jay J. Dugan*

INTRODUCTION

THE ENIGMAS CONFRONTING THE CANCER PATIENT

Richard J. Torpie

One changing reality of contemporary medical care is that much of the care needed for serious and potentially terminal illnesses has become chronic and long-term rather than acute. Medicine has placed a high priority on those efforts which bring diseases into a state of clinical long term *control*. Often, these efforts are massive and may only provide limited advances in this type of control. In the field of cancer, for example, the analogy might be the limited success of early modes of chemotherapy. However, a price has had to be paid as issues of life or death have ceased to be acute ones. Increasingly, the patient must become wed to the institution, the same institution which basically has done little to change its modes and traditions of care—especially its orientation to acute care. More and more, within our hospitals, there are chronically ill patients, stricken with a life-threatening illness, but trapped in an atmosphere which is poorly prepared to cope with their needs for mental comfort and well-being. Failing to meet the expectancy for success as defined by an acute care facility, the patient finds him or herself in a therapeutic limbo, a netherworld of no expectancy. If patients demonstrate progressive symptoms and expectations of dying, they often find themselves in a world of expendability and loss of caring investment. The medical and nursing professions seem to bear the criticism for this, but, perhaps, in a small way they reflect only part of the mosaic which constitutes the attitudes of our society.

My experience is limited to my role as a physician-therapeutic radiologist whose primary practice is in caring for patients with cancer. In studies of serious illnesses with terminal potential cancer seems to be utilized most often as an appropriate model, although similar elements of caregiving can extend to other disease situations as well. But cancer brings its own influence and prejudices which have their effects on the patient and his family. Cancer is most commonly and universally considered to be a fatal disease. In fact, cancer is a thousand diseases, ranging from the virtually incurable to the nearly completely curable, with wide dimensions of cure and control in between. Among the lay population, however, the expectancy is that there is no cure for cancer and that urgings for cure are better translated into an expectation that there might be a "magic bullet" for the cure of all forms of cancer.

The cancer patient finds himself in a rather unique situation. He has a disease which his prejudices indicate is universally fatal, or which basically is denied socially, this is, his friends and family cannot discuss its importance with him nor can they share their concerns with him. He must live a series of convenient white lies, a victim of the so-called "conspiracy of silence." The seeds of relationship that should provide the partial structure of emotional support are damaged from the time of diagnosis, and they may never be properly nurtured. The patient utilizes a great deal of denial and his family perhaps more; but this is often subtly encouraged by the physician. Early boundaries are established for discussion, and later, when these boundaries must be adapted to the needs of the patient, the family and physician are reluctant to make changes. The necessary communication and trust that should develop between all parties concerned with terminal illness are destroyed. In the institutional setting nursing and paramedical personnel are often placed beyond these boundaries. The patient becomes threatened further by a situation that might jeopardize his relationship with physician and family if he ever oversteps these boundaries. In a sense he becomes an inadvertent contributor to the worst realities of dying, that is, isolation and abandonment.

Renascent interest in the field of thanatology has stressed the painful psychosocial experiences of terminal cancer patients and has also pointed to the defects in the institutional care of all cancer patients as well as of other patients with potentially terminal illness. The distorted attitudes of the lay public regarding cancer create barriers in communication, self deceit, and a strong tendency to perpetuate myths regarding this disease. Professionals and others in institutional settings are not immune from these attitudes and their interrelationships with patient and family are often subject to severe deterioration in communication and understanding. The eventual effects on the survivors can be severe in terms of recrimination, guilt, and pathologic depression. Most disturbing is that this failure to foster communication and understanding may cause a breakdown in the support system needed to guide the patient through diagnostic and therapeutic measures that may add to worthwhile prolongation of life.

Patients referred to radiation therapy centers are usually in a tertiary referral situation with a primary physician and surgeon having been previously involved in their case. Few physicians outside this particular specialty have spent time during any part of their medical education appreciating the clinical intricacies of this form of treatment. This lack of firsthand knowledge by referring physicians may prepare the patient poorly for commitment to treatment. Explanations about potential side effects, duration of treatment, and even the value of treatment are not provided in a knowledgeable way. Too often patients with an excellent prognosis may suspect that the need for radiation treatments confirms their worst fears. These fears are often reinforced by side effects of treatment which, despite reassurance to the contrary, are felt to be manifestations of disease. In patients with advanced cancer, manifestations of the disease are believed to be related to radiation treatments not sufficiently cumulative to be effective.

The lay expectations of violent nausea, internal burning, and severe skin burns are rarely confirmed with the use of modern equipment and treatment techniques. It is unique to cancer therapy to see the disease and its treatment subject to the same prejudices and myths. These are reinforced by the mass media which refers to radiation treatment as "painful" and the patient as the "victim." In a family situation where there is a history of unsupported cancer death, there can be complete verification of all cancer myths. One fantasy believed by some patients is that somehow they are radioactive; this may be a substitute for feelings of uncleanliness or the fantasy of cancer contagion. Too often patients with terminal cancer are denied palliative radiation therapy which, while rarely prolonging life, will prevent ulceration, severe pain, bleeding, disfigurement, paralysis and/or loss of certain functions.

The persistence of general misconceptions about cancer and cancer patients may perpetuate delay in initial diagnosis, the prevalence of quackery, and even refusal to accept treatment. In a sense, succeeding generations of cancer patients are condemned to a self-fulfilling prophecy. These are very real day-to-day problems in major cancer centers. More pathetic is the distress of the cancer patient who is often segregated and isolated and whose basic care is given with indifference and whose personhood and dignity are denied by the system and the environment. Add to this patterns of referral which may take the patient many miles from his home as well as simplistic rules that prevent visits from children, and administrative shuffling of papers in the admissions office cause discontinuity of care when repeated hospitalizations place the patient in a different nursing environment.

The impact of all this is not lost on health professionals. Capable caregivers turn away from this oppressive environment in which they must take upon themselves the daily task of caring for the dying and those patients whose severe anxiety relates to the potential for dying. The lack of psychological support, staff education, and inter-communication creates ultimate frustration. Beyond this, the institution has not bothered to provide a suitable milieu, such as a hospice setting, for the care of dying patients. More difficult to believe are the brutalizing traditions and hierarchical attitudes that prevail against solutions.

The present need for care of the terminal patient is based on social recognition and honest perceptivity that will eventually promote higher standards on all levels of patient care. The participation of sensitive and experienced individuals from psychological support services, social work and family therapy, and the health professionals during all stages of disease, including terminal situations, must be forthcoming. What we have achieved medically in terms of adding months or years of life to patients with incurable illnesses does no good if we have not prepared them to *live* emotionally through this period of time. The radiation therapist can then help facilitate measures of support that allow realistic prudence, excellence of care, continuity of truth and comfort—both physical and mental.

WHY BE AN ONCOLOGIST?

Jan van Eys

In any situation where patients seek help from physicians, it is clearly the patient who should benefit from the encounter in terms of physical and mental well-being. It is the motive of the patient to seek cure of the perceived or real ailment. In this encounter the physician supplies knowledge and experience as well as availability. The gain the physician has from this transaction is of course economical. In most instances that is where the transaction ends, because the illness of the patient is either trivial or can indeed be alleviated if not cured. But the physician has also a motive in joining the encounter, and that motive may be beyond the pecuniary.

In cancer patients the quest for cure is more intense, yet the ability of the physician to deliver cure is more problematical. Therefore, the motive of the physician to become an oncologist, especially a radiotherapist or chemotherapist, cannot be the satisfaction of the usually successful outcome. However, it is hardly only the monetary rewards which would keep physicians in a position of failure—if for no other reason than that few physicians have a vulture mentality. Rather, the converse: most physicians have a sincere desire to help their charges and empathize with their patients.

It is then a legitimate question to ask what the motives of nonsurgical oncologists really are. One could approach this question by an in-depth interview of a sufficient number of oncologists, but that would require a time and scope of inquiry that is hardly achievable, since such motives would not be readily discernable from just a questionnaire approach. One might also suggest that the question should be moot since the posture of oncology should not be cure at all cost, but should allow supported but minimally disturbed dying when the disease is incurable. However, even if that is granted as a desirable attitude, the fact remains that the medical profession approaches patients with malignancy, on the whole, with a more therapeutic vigor, and that most patients initially do expect that from a doctor. That more physicians and patients should acknowledge the inevitable and thereby create more gracious ways of death is without dispute. But during the initial physician-patient contact, when the cancer is discovered, it is possible for the patient to refuse referral to an oncologist. Whether such refusal is pragmatically impossible because of societal or familial pressure is beside the point, because that is outside the patient-physician contact. Once the patient accepts the referral the oncologist will be expected to cure, however mistaken that conception.

What then motivates oncologists to allow themselves to be placed in such a position? If one cannot obtain such information from an exhaustive survey, one could approach the question in the reverse way and postulate several broad, even nearly caricatured, alternatives. Broadly, one could envision the following categories of motives for entering the field of oncology:

1. Cancer presents the greatest opportunity to alleviate human suffering.
2. Oncology presents the greatest remaining medical challenge, and thereby the greatest hope of personal advancement.
3. Patients with cancer are expected to die; therefore, oncology offers the greatest opportunity of rewards with the least danger of having to admit failure.

In these caricatures the nature of rewards are not spelled out, and can indeed range from purely selfish and monetary, through social and academic standing, to quiet self-satisfaction. But that does not change the principles.

Hypotheses are tested by their ability to predict the outcome of events which are perturbated in a controlled manner. In other words through experiments. Not all three possible motives need examination in detail. It is clear that almost no person is motivated purely by only one of these three possibilities. Furthermore, everyone will acknowledge the presence of the first two to varying degrees at varying moments in many physicians. The question is really whether the third postulate—oncology is a psychologically safe field, because it is all right to fail—is indeed a possibility. Of course, no one could live with pure and unvarying failure. In oncology, the assertion that we all will die is a truism but it is trivial and therefore does not resolve the dilemma. The question is not indefinite survival; rather, the question is that death should be from unrelated causes. But oncology is in a state of flux. Many patients are indeed cured, but only in pediatric oncology is cure more frequent than death, and even there that is just barely the case. There is great effort expended on improving such statistics. But success can, during such investigational approaches, be measured by an impact on the average course of the disease, and not necessarily by cure rate alone. In other words, significantly prolonged survival, not necessarily cure, is accepted as a goal. This makes the posture of the oncologist potentially even more secure because reward of doing good for people (and having academic advancement) in face of actual failure, as defined by the patient, are all possible.

What would one predict from the hypothesis that the physician's motive is security in expected failure and rejoicing in unexpected rewards? There is indeed a repeated experiment where the hypothesis is put to the test. The postulated attitude is most tenable when the patient outcome is as close to fifty/fifty as possible. That would maximize rewards and yet not threaten the expectation of failure to cure as norm. Such a failure rate needs, of course, to be overcome if all patients are to be helped. Yet, it is a widely observed phenomenon that if one challenges therapeutic strategies through which about 50 percent are cured, one generates opposition. The objections are that it is "unethical" to endanger the outcome of the cured to improve the outcome of the failures. As presented here, that is conceptually irrational at face value. However, the cry of "unethical" is heard with persistent regularity, especially if one group of oncologists suggests a new modality of therapy to the proponents of the more entrenched modes of treatment. Currently, the classical confrontation is the suggestion of chemotherapy replacing radiotherapy. That it is unethical is precisely what one would predict as outcome from the hypothesis.

Again, a caricature is unfair, but all cancer therapists should re-examine their motives. Do we always deeply grieve for every patient lost? Of course not, because we know our limitations, and we cannot morbidly grieve for the inevitable as long as we know we have done our best and not made inadvertent or careless errors. The question is not that that is a wrong attitude, but that we are at ease with that attitude. During a workshop in our department of pediatrics it was very evident that the concept of cure is threatening. All oncologists are to a degree ambivalent, and the hypothesis that we are at ease with not having to account for failure fits the observed behavioral facts uncomfortably well. There are many physicians who say that they could not do what the oncologists are doing. Yet, in no field are the rewards greater. Oncologists do not deal with a patient population of which more than 80 percent will get better in spite of the physician, as the primary practitioner does. Therefore, the few cures can far more often be claimed as personal accomplishment in oncology than in any other branch of medicine when cures are possible. The stimulus is indeed that, but the security may be that failure is not always threatening.

At the present time this motive serves as well as any, because non-cure is still so overwhelmingly the norm that treatment improvements can actively be sought by all oncologists without changing the conceptual view of cancer as a deadly disease. Very few patients suffer from the attitude of the physician, for care is optimal because inherent in the non-threat of failure remains the conviction of having delivered optimal care. But oncology is making great strides and hopefully a new generation of oncologists will take over who will view the care of cancer patients with motives more in harmony with the patients' expectations. It is even possible, if not likely, that oncology will be a routine branch of primary care medicine. But then our current conceptual equating of cancer with death and unpleasant dying will no longer exist. The special motives of physicians need no longer be postulated.

REFLECTIONS OF A SELF-CONSULTING RADIOLOGIST

Harry L. Berman

Radiation therapy is involved with the management of cancer, a disease commonly equated with impending death. Because accurate knowledge about radiation therapy is not sufficiently available, many individuals conclude that its use is a second-best alternative or that its application indicates an ominous prognosis. A presumption usually exists that surgery would have been selected if cure were possible.

However, there are instances when radiation therapy is indicated as the definitive measure of choice. Nevertheless, all too often the beginning of a regimen of radiation therapy is also the start of a chain of events whose course is progressively downhill and whose ultimate outcome is the demise of the patient.

The suggestion that radiation therapy might be required may conjure up in the patient's mind an impression of a serious ailment, a feeling not readily allayed by assurances that reason exists to anticipate a good prognosis. Any disease with a bad, or even an indeterminate, prognosis will be likely to provoke emotional upsets, even in stable, emotionally well-adjusted people. Not inconspicuous in this combination of circumstances surrounding a particular patient with malignant disease is a gamut of emotional reactions by that individual and members of his family, including varying degrees of despair, disbelief, stress, suspicion, distrust, tension, anger, hostility, depression, fear, alarm, hopelessness, and many other affections, which seriously diminish levels of equanimity in the concerned persons.

The therapeutic radiologist enters the scenario of a given disease under unique circumstances. He is rarely selected by the patient, but rather is referred by the physician or surgeon. The initial consultation between the radiologist and the patient is one in which each is a trifle wary of the other. The radiologist at that time may know very little about the patient's condition. Sometimes he has had access to clinical and laboratory records, x-ray films, other imaging records, and a discussion with the referring physician, and the ensuing consultation with the patient and family can proceed in a logical and informative manner, perhaps subject to certain limitations. However, quite frequently, and particularly when patients are seen initially on an out-patient basis, having come from another city or another hospital in the same city, essential information may be lacking, which restricts the ability of the radiologist to answer questions fully and accurately. Patients are naturally upset when this happens. Unfortunately, this situation is not easily corrected.

Those limitations which influence the discussion between patient and radiologist revolve around the fact that vital information is often withheld from patients. As a radiologist involved with cancer, I am aware of this and my discussion with a patient begins somewhat gingerly. The relatives may give me prior notification or frantically signal to me from unobtrusive positions, if I chance to make my initial appearance unexpectedly in the patient's hospital room in their presence, to avoid mentioning that forbidden word. Strong efforts are made to advise me to refrain from saying anything to suggest the actual diagnosis of cancer. "Don't tell Mom or Pop (or wife or husband or whatever relationship) what the diagnosis is," is a common admonition to the radiologist. And so a little game begins that is guaranteed to create a serious psychosocial situation where one might not have existed. Certainly channels of communication become blocked, and the most important method by which mental stress can be dealt with, namely by better communication, has become seriously complicated.

I recall a situation where a woman, whose family consisted of her husband and an adult daughter, was receiving radiation therapy for breast cancer. All three came to me individually, demanding to know all the details of that particular medical problem and requesting that I withhold this information from the others. And so they all knew all the essential information, each one not suspecting that the others knew, each one presumably carrying the main burden for the entire family. How much better would it have been for all three to have shared the common burden together and to lend support each to the other two!

The radiologist must establish a basis for rapport with the patient and the patient's family. His capacity to do so is developed by experience. His training tends to emphasize the scientific aspects rather than the psychosocial side of the specialty. Certain formulas and recipes for the treatment of specific tumors are learned as though a patient is, perhaps, a cancer of the uterus, or of the lung, or of a particular bone, in each instance surrounded by an amorphous mass of protoplasm. It is distressing to learn that patients' reactions are unmindful of the need to follow specific radiobiological principles, that their symptoms and certain objective findings may interfere with the conduct of what on paper looks like such a beautiful plan of treatment, and that their questions may unduly impose on the radiologists' time.

Radiation therapy departments in medical centers and community hospitals are usually busy places, commonly understaffed, complicated by pressures of inflation and the dictates of certain government agencies, all of which affect fiscal matters. Modern radiation therapy is expensive. Equipment is costly, as are the specially built structures that house these machines. Although we should like to think that the cost of medical care does not affect its quality, understaffing and under-budgeting are bound to have their effects since they often lead to improvisations or options not equal to the best. Naturally, this affects the activities of the radiologist and the time he has available for frequent conversations with patients. But radiation therapy is something more than an appointment with a beam of radiation.

Let us return to the matter of that first consultation. The patient will raise a number of questions. Some centers attempt to deal with these by giving the patient a description of what radiation therapy is like, written on one or two sheets of typed phraseology or in a small pamphlet. This is not as good or as personal as the direct confrontation with the radiologist. The patient will ask these questions—not necessarily in this order:

1) Does the treatment hurt?
2) Do I have cancer?
3) I have been assured by my doctor that I do not have cancer. What I have could turn into cancer, unless treated.
4) How frequent are the treatments?
5) Over how long a period must I be treated?
6) How long does each treatment last?
7) Will I be nauseated?
8) Why do you use radiation for treatment when it is supposed to be bad for people?
9) Is the radiation still inside of me when I leave the radiation therapy department?
10) Am I going to be cured?

These questions must be answered. Obviously, most can be answered truthfully and directly. Some answers perhaps might be couched in euphemistic terms, but outright lies and evasions should be avoided. In addition to answering the questions, the radiologist is legally required to provide all information needed for the patient to give an informed consent for the treatment.

Other facts that should be supplied to the patient include the following:

1) Treatment over the head, beard, axilla, or pelvis will cause the hair to fall out and the result may be permanent, although with lesser doses it may be temporary.
2) Radiation causes redness and possibly blistering of the skin in the treated area, resembling a sunburn.
3) Radiation will cause inflammation of the linings of the internal hollow organs, depending on the site of irradiation, with resultant symptoms such as sore throat, esophagitis with difficulty in swallowing, diarrhea, discomfort on urination, cataracts, and so on.
4) Radiation over the ovaries will be likely to result in sterility and amenorrhea.
5) Radiation of bone marrow depresses blood formation.

In some cases appropriate precautions can be taken, but not always. At any rate, one finds it much easier to deal with patients if they have been properly informed. Patients are willing to put up with certain discomforts if they know what to expect. Furthermore, availability of the radiologist to patients to answer their inquiries on subsequent occasions facilitates the interpersonal relationships and fosters a better attitude on the patient's part.

The discussion of prognosis is especially critical since it inevitably arises, if not in the presence of the patient then certainly with other members of the family. It may be very difficult to give an accurate answer. Prognosis in various disease descriptions is generally stated as survival over a certain period of years in terms of a percentage of a certain group studied. To apply this figure to a single patient is obviously impossible. What does it mean to a patient to know that 40 percent of a group of individuals with that particular disease survive five years? Of course, if you could tell a patient that his possible five-year survival is 95 percent, as is true in the case of seminoma of the testis, the patient would recognize that the odds are in his favor, but what would you tell a patient with a disease whose predictable two-year survival is less than 5 percent?

Generally patients referred for radiation therapy can be categorized in one of three groups as far as prognosis is concerned. These are:

Group 1

The prognosis is excellent, with a high cure rate and minimal complications of radiation therapy. This group includes such malignancies as early cancers of the tongue and vocal cords, early cancers of the cervix of the uterus, seminoma of the testis, and many skin cancers. Early diagnosis permits treatment to be instituted at a time when the disease remains localized to its primary site.

Group 2

The prognosis is fair to good. Cure rates of 25-50 percent are possible. The risk of complications secondary to radiation therapy is fairly high. In this group are found some breast cancers, some testis tumors, certain uterine tumors, and some examples of malignant lymphomas.

Group 3

The prognosis is poor. Cure rates are usually of the order of 0-5 percent. Radiation for cure is seldom effective. Examples of this group are lung cancer, any malignancy with widespread metastases, advanced stages of lymphoma, and cancer of the esophagus.

Obviously, psychosocial problems will arise for those patients in Group 2 and Group 3. Generally, these patients will be the ones with the severer symptoms and with complaints that cry out for more attention. For them hospitalization will frequently be necessary. Just as frequently this hospitalization will be for an extended period, a requirement not looked on favorably by the hospital authorities, who would prefer to see the beds occupied by acute cases for a short duration. Very often patients with advanced cancer receiving radiation therapy are not readily transported back and forth between home and hospital because of pain, paralyses, or other disability. Sometimes the wait for a bed is prolonged over a period of weeks. Often the patient is not more comfortable in the hospital than at home, nor is he provided necessarily with better nursing care, but relatives either are unwilling or unable to cope with the complaints, emotional reactions, or other problems posed by the bed-ridden cancer patient at home. For the most part the care of the advanced cancer patient leaves much to be desired in this country. I see no easy path to or a readily available attempt at a solution to this problem. Society is shirking its responsibility, since these patients deserve better care.

The actual progress of patients through their courses of treatment with irradiation does not pose major problems arising just from the exposure to radiation. Overall they are relatively minor compared to the grave psychosocial reactions of those patients to their diseases and the new situations created by the change in their life style. We might consider a few examples here.

Let us consider first the problems of a young woman, the mother of three young boys, giving birth to her fourth child, also a boy. On the day of her delivery in a military hospital—it was at the time of the Korean War—she received a telegram from the Defense Department that her husband had been killed in Korea. At the time of her delivery she was discovered to have a tumor in the pelvis, subsequently proven to be an ovarian cancer with a terrible prognosis. Both she and her husband were orphans.

She was referred to me for postoperative radiation therapy. At my initial visit with her she was pretty much over the initial shock and grief, and she wanted to discuss all the possibilities for her future. She was already informed about her diagnosis and what it meant. She was excellently in control of herself, and she informed me that her principal concern was for her four young boys, although nothing urgent was immediately necessary. Of great help to her were the Catholic chaplain in the hospital and the wife of the Commanding General of the Military District of Washington. They had assured her that, when necessary, the adoption of her boys would be properly taken care of.

As it turned out, she recovered from her surgery rapidly and tolerated her radiation therapy well. She was alive and healthy four years later, the time of my last contact with her, following which I lost track of her.

I cannot say that this patient's specific problems affected her course of radiation therapy, either in the way it was administered or in the manner of the response of her tissues to it. Nevertheless, the patient's concern for her own health and for the welfare of her children constantly projected itself to the forefront during all her treatments. Initially, the prognosis was very bad and was the cause of her concern for her major problems, ones requiring her attention. Her survival for a longer period than was thought probable was appreciated, but the guarded prognosis was a continual threat to her peace of mind.

That patient's psychosocial difficulties had to be dealt with throughout the course of treatment and even thereafter. Sometimes incidents occur that are important events in the lives of patients and are brought to the attention of the radiologist because decisions must be made for which accurate prognostications are desirable, though not necessarily always available.

One such example was the case of a young woman who had been treated for Hodgkin's Disease with irradiation and who came to see me about the problem at hand when she was in remission. Her problem was that she wanted to get married but was not sure that it would be right for her to do so. She was accompanied by the young man who would become her husband. All I could do was to explain all the possibilities of the uncertain future. I could not assure her that her fate was one of total freedom from disease. I could tell them only that whatever their decision they must agree that they would not engage in hindsight. They did marry and moved to the West Coast. I know that several years later she was again receiving radiation therapy. Other than that I had no further word from her.

The question of marriage of patients undergoing radiation therapy is one which radiologists deal with quite frequently. Questions raised include the following:

1) How much longevity can the patient expect?
2) Can future relapses and the need for future radiation therapy be anticipated?
3) What about children? Might they be abnormal? Is the patient sterile?

Again, there are no hard and fast answers, even in the face of terribly ominous prognoses. Many factors have to be considered and the need to seek counsel from other qualified advisors must be recognized. The emotional elements cannot be disregarded. Not uncommonly, I have seen men with cancer, almost moribund, marry women and die within a matter of hours or days, just so those particular women can inherit the insurance or other gratuities.

I recall another instance of a young woman recently married who came down with Hodgkin's Disease after the wedding. She had recently moved from another city, where part of her radiation therapy had been completed. She came to see me for her initial consultation with her parents but without her husband. The parents told me that the young husband did not know the nature of his wife's illness and that I was to withhold information about it from him. I felt that this was a mistake, although I agreed to honor their wishes. I knew that sooner or later the young man would learn of his wife's illness and that he had a right and a responsibility to know about it. He subsequently did learn of it. Whatever disturbance he might have created at home was not apparent since, in my presence, he controlled himself well. But all of these facades to make diseases seem to be something they are not merely result in making the relationship of the patient and family member with the radiologist needlessly complicated and are not particularly guaranteed to relieve psychosocial stress.

As one might suspect, the emotional responses of a patient to his disease and to the biological effects produced by radiation used in his treatment are related to:

1) The basic personality and level of emotional stability of the patient.

2) The interpersonal relationships that the patient has with family, relatives, certain friends, and possibly lovers.
3) The severity of the underlying disease.
4) The severity of the radiation effects.
5) The interrelationships of the various physicians, surgeons, radiologists, and all others who make up the cancer treatment team, including nurses, social workers, psychologists, and ministers.
6) The attitudes of the patient and the family toward the disease and to sickness in general.

Obviously, some patients handle their problems better than do others. It appears that a strong attachment and significant relationship to a spouse or other family member who lends attentive and sympathetic support by continual presence with the patient, taking care of what may seem to be needs of small importance, provide a firm basis for dealing with an emotionally stressful situation.

Perhaps one might ask, "Why should you as a radiologist concern yourself with a patient's problems? Can't you send those patients for help to other suitable counselors?" Yes, I could, but too often these problems project themselves in such a way as to interfere with the treatment schedule, or to require the radiologist to explain certain side effects of treatment as possible complications of irradiation when they are not; and, finally, the patients seek certain answers which only the radiologist can give.

Since the total care of a patient now involves a team effort which is directed towards the physical, social, psychological and spiritual needs of the patient and family, a discussion limited to radiation therapy alone perhaps is unjustified. I have tried to explain how the radiologist is involved in this effort. I can assure you that this role at times may be the dominant one, but, in the final analysis, it is just a part of a larger team effort and at all times is coordinated with the work of many others toward the purpose of directing a patient through a difficult period to ultimate restoration of good health, even for a limited duration when possible, or through a more difficult period toward impending death. That job, as I stated earlier, includes much more than the supervision of patients' exposure to radiation.

APPROACHES TO THE CANCER PATIENT:

Practical, Therapeutic and Psychological

THE RADIATION ONCOLOGY CENTER AS A THERAPEUTIC ENVIRONMENT FOR PATIENTS AND STAFF

Arvin S. Glicksman, Glenn W. Mitchell, Carl A. Geyer, Curtis Perry and Kenneth Ain

PREAMBLE

This report represents our experience in establishing a new Radiation Oncology Center in which technical skill and capability were of the first priority. Just below in importance was the total ambiance of the new center and the attitudes of the personnel who would work there. Three years later we have been measuring the impact this center has had on the patients, their families, and the staff. From two psychological studies what we have learned has importance in our day-to-day ability to meet the needs of these people and may be of interest to others who deal with similar problems.

INTRODUCTION

Few individuals have not been attended by a physician at one time or other in their life. The physician could have been a specialist or general practitioner (of late, a family physician); some contact with pediatricians, gynecologists, surgeons, internists, and even diagnostic radiologists for such mundane ailments as tonsilitis, bronchitis, allergies, ulcers, pregnancy, is part of our life experience. But the patient who is referred for radiotherapy suffers a traumatic experience of previously unparalleled proportion. For 9 out of 10 patients, this means that a neoplastic process exists even if he has not been explicitly informed about it. There is nothing in the reservoir of the patient's past experience to fall back upon in dealing with this new situation.

First of all, he must deal with the knowledge that he has cancer, an incredibly disturbing fact. He must confront his own mortality, something almost impossible to deal with for most people. We are constantly reinforcing the concept that cancer kills, referring to "the victim of cancer." Yet almost half of all cancer patients will be cured of their malignancy. This number is increasing slowly and while it is unlikely that we will wipe out cancer in our lifetime, it is likely that the patient with cancer will have a 50/50 chance of surviving.

Therefore, radiotherapists today treat an ever-increasing number of potentially curable patients. Over 60 percent of the patients seen at the Radiation Oncology Center at the Rhode Island Hospital are potentially curable, and treatment is designed with curative intent. Only one-third of our patients receive palliative radiotherapy. The psychosocial problems in a department of radiotherapy, therefore, are overwhelming in terms of problem-solving for living, rather than adjustment for dying. In a realistic, forthright, and open manner, it is necessary to have most patients and families understand that, for the most part, realistic assessment of the future entails living with the prospect of having been cured of a formerly fatal illness. For other patients and their families, the realities of an incurable situation must be faced and discussed openly and appropriately according to the patient's needs. Both groups are of concern to us.

In a Department of Radiation Oncology a unique opportunity and a challenge exist for delivering technical assistance for the eradication of disease or for the eradication of symptoms for which palliation is indicated, and, equally, for dealing with the psychosocial problems affecting patients and families when they come to a radiotherapy facility for the management of a neoplastic process. The organization of the department in terms of its physical facilities, its staff and orientation, can all become instruments of policy in these regards.

FACILITIES

In January, 1973, we had the opportunity to plan a new center for radiation oncology at the Rhode Island Hospital. The department opened in July, 1974. Our first consideration was to establish a center of unquestioned technical capabilities. A great deal of effort was directed toward the selection of the linear accelerators, simulator and transverse axial tomograph unit and computers. Similar consideration was given to assure that the design and atmosphere of the new center would be warm and friendly, adding comfort for the patient and family. The facility is entirely underground as are most radiotherapy departments. However, the corridors are wide and high. The lighting is bright: "warm white" bulbs are used, not "blue daylight," which can be somewhat harsh. Carpeting is used throughout; a vinyl fabric covers the walls and an acoustic ceiling keeps the noise level low.

An internal audio system throughout the corridors, waiting areas, and treatment rooms provides soft background music. After much deliberation "shopping center Muzak" was replaced by our own tapes of predominantly Baroque music. We now have 24 3-hour programs that are played randomly to provide variation from day to day.

The Radiation Oncology Center also maintains a permanent art gallery. The corridors of the department are used to display the work of local artists. Up to 200 linear feet of wall space is available for this. Each show is hung for six to eight weeks. The local newspapers, the hospital bulletin, and the University bulletin list these shows as an ongoing event. During a six-week course of treatment, a patient and his family generally see two shows. These can include abstract art, impressionist, realism, graphics, photography, lithography, collage, Chinese art, and early American quilts and wall hangings. *ANYART Journal,* the publication of a local contemporary arts center, reviewed one of our shows and commented on the concept:

> Never having been in a "Radiation Oncology Gallery" before, I descended into the clinical environment, down, down with a great deal of trepidation. I opened the final door and walked into the tunnel-like corridors. As I passed through the halls, I realized how foreboding the space would have been without the beautifully colored distractions on the walls. After a few moments I settled in and became aware of staff and patients stopping to look and to become involved enough to make decisions and comments on the works.

The commentary in one of the local columns described the center as follows:

> The new center is not a place filled only with sterile machines and paper-spitting computers. As much thought and preparation has gone into the human side of the therapy from the dedicated specialists chosen to work there to the warm, friendly furnishings which surround them. It is evident that every effort has been made to reduce the trauma and apprehension associated with cancer. The center is pleasant, stereo music fills the air. Soft wallpaper and carpeting, an abundance of plants, and a huge fishtank make the waiting rooms much more like a home than a hospital. And best of all, everyone who works there tries to make everything seem much easier, not smoothed over in an attempt to avoid reality, but honest, reassuring, friendly. They are handpicked specialists from all over the country brought together to make the center the best anywhere, dedicated people who understand and have great empathy for the patients.

PERSONNEL

An understanding staff is basic for dealing with the patient's anxiety in all its manifestations. The physicians have been selected as much for their humanitarian qualities as for their technical skill. It was our belief that they must be at ease in discussing the patient's problems with the family, explaining the treatment program to the patient, in addition to being excellent clinicians and technically superb in the delivery of radiotherapy. We believe that they should approach each patient and his family with patience and understanding.

Frequently, patients will ask relatively simple questions concerning their illness, their treatment, or prospects for cure. Often, they do not hear the detailed explanations given, and patients may go home to express a feeling of not being informed. This can occur for two reasons. First, the mode of explanation may be unintelligible to the patient. He may not have the necessary frame of reference, background information, or understanding to absorb the explanation. Alternatively, this new and unfamiliar setting may be so anxiety provoking that the patient does not hear the explanation that is being given. Finally, there is another problem: More information may be given to him than he really wants to have, more than he can cope with in any one sitting. He cannot say, "Stop, I don't want to hear any more!" and thus be free to terminate the interview. Therefore, it is the responsibility of the staff to assess what a patient really wants to know.

This does not mean that a jejune, condescending approach to patient information is appropriate. The physician must listen carefully and determine what the patient really wants to know, what the patient is prepared to understand, and at what point the patient will just stop listening and reasoning because he cannot cope with so much information. If denial is the patient's coping mechanism, it must be respected and dealt with as a real phenomenon. If hostility and antagonism are his coping mechanisms, the staff must understand that they are only "the whipping boy" for an intolerable situation that the patient cannot deal with in any other way. If dependence is the mechanism for dealing with the new problems created by disease, the staff should give all possible support. Infrequently, patients will use displacement as a coping mechanism, that is, concern for how the rest of his family will deal with the situation rather than how he should cope with it becomes the major preoccupation and this must be respected as "real."

The fundamental attitude of the entire staff must be toward problem-solving for living, rather than adjustment and resignation in anticipation of death. Sixty to seventy percent of the patients receiving radiotherapy at the Radiation Oncology Center in Rhode Island are receiving curative radiotherapy. Palliation makes up an important segment of our work, but it is not the sole end of radiotherapy. In dealing with the patient's illness, the concept of cure is paramount, and all of our technical skills are marshalled for that purpose. The psychological problems associated with that treatment must also be oriented towards cure and lead directly into active programs of continuing care and rehabilitation. We are hopeful and optimistic above all, supportive to the needs of the patient and his family.

It is clearly recognized that it is not physicians alone who must deal with the patient's problems. Highly skilled technologists spend more time with the patients than the physicians do, and they are frequently the ones to whom patients will turn for information and support. There are rarely any expressions of dissatisfaction with the technologists; however, the group of technologists currently in the Department of Radiation Oncology are unusual in the degree to which they empathize with patients and extend themselves to support patients' needs. The nursing staff also has played an increasingly important role in dealing with patients' reactions to treatment advice on skin care, mouth care, and dietary regimes, as well as general support for the patient. Unfortunately, there are no social workers or behavioral scientists in the department. We believe that their addition to our staff would enrich the scope of our support of the patient and his family during the course of radiotherapy.

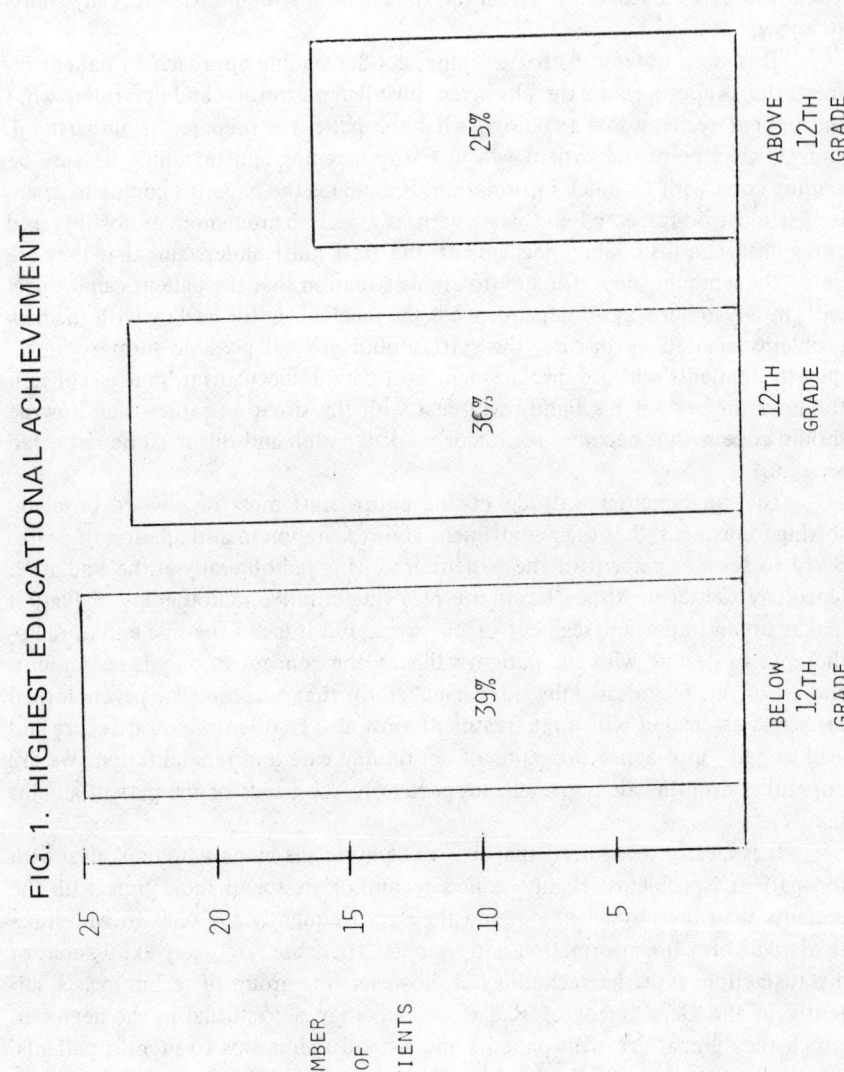

FIG. 1. HIGHEST EDUCATIONAL ACHIEVEMENT

OBSERVATIONS

Having created the physical environment to relieve anxieties, having paid a great deal of attention to concerns of ambiance with decoration, music, and changing art shows, and having assembled a staff of some 30 individuals who are dedicated to the concept of good patient support, we have now turned our attention to evaluating the impact of these concepts on the patient and their family. What do they see? What do they hear? How do they respond to the staff? These are the kinds of questions that we felt we could investigate and try to quantitate in this environment.

In the first study, 64 patients undergoing radiotherapy were interviewed. Each interview was loosely structured and lasted approximately 30 minutes. A random sample was generated by choosing patients whose birthday fell in an even month on one day and on an odd month the following day. In addition, 20 relatives were also interviewed so that we might learn about their reaction to the center.

DEMOGRAPHIC PROFILE OF THE SAMPLE

The mean age of the patient population was 53-years-old, and that of the relatives was 55 years. Generally, these individuals were married and were native residents of Rhode Island. Seventy-five percent of those interviewed had 12 years of education or less, and 39 percent of the population had not graduated from high school. (Figure 1) Consequently, 77 percent worked in a semi-professional or a non-professional capacity.

The predominant religion in Rhode Island is Roman Catholic (78 percent) and 66 percent of the interviewed population attended church regularly. Eighty-three percent of those interviewed found their religious beliefs to be supportive during this illness. One patient remarked, "I can't talk with anyone about my disease, I can only talk in my prayers." Another young patient with Hodgkin's disease related, "Everyone in my prayer class is aware of my condition. I can talk as openly to them as to any patient in the waiting room."

The patients were categorized according to the stage of their disease: 1) localized disease (20 patients) if they were Stage I or II (T1 T2 NO MO); 2) regional (23 patients) if they were Stage II or Stage III (T3's, NO or T2 N1, MO); 3) distant spread (21 patients) with metastases, categorized as Stage IV. On the Karnofsky performance status scale, over 70 percent were 80 to 100 and less than 10 percent were below 50 (Table 1).

WHAT THE PATIENT NOTICES

The patients were strikingly perceptive of their environment. Those with distant spread and with the lower Karnofsky performance status scale noticed the art work most frequently (80.9 percent). A majority of the patients could describe individual paintings or their general impressions of the display. Patients with localized disease were somewhat less aware of the art. Only 60 percent of

TABLE 1

PERFORMANCE STATUS (KARNOFSKY)

		All Patients Percent		Localized	Regional	Distant
100	No Evidence of Disease	6.3		20.0	0	0
90	Minor Signs/Symptoms	31.2		65.0	26.0	4.8
80	Some Signs/Symptoms	34.3	(71.8)	10.0	56.5	33.3
70	Normal Activity Impaired	4.7		5.0	8.6	0
60	Requires Assistance	14.0			4.3	38.0
50	Frequent Medical Care	4.7	(23.4)		0	14.3
40	Disabled, Special Care	4.7	(4.7)		4.3	9.6

TABLE 2

WHAT THE PATIENT NOTICES

	Patients Percent	Relatives Percent	Patients' Disease Status		
			Localized Percent	Regional Percent	Distant Percent
Paintings	73.4	95.0	60.0	78.3	80.9
In General	31.3	40.0	25.0	30.5	38.1
Individual	42.1	55.0	35.0	47.8	42.8
Remembering					
Present Display	48.5	65.0	55.0	43.5	42.8
Last Exhibit	26.0	30.0	5.0	34.0	38.1
None At All	26.6	5.0	40.0	21.5	19.1

these patients could describe the exhibit, while only 48 percent of the patients with regional disease remembered any individual painting (Table 2).

The majority of patients in all three categories (89 percent) were aware of the background music. Their responses to this question usually evolved into a discussion of the kind of music being played, and some patients asked for a more diverse repertoire. In general, however, they observed that it frequently created a happy and cheerful mood (Table 3). The selections of Baroque music included works by such composers as Vivaldi, Telemann, Haydn, and Mozart. One selection—E. Power Biggs performing on the great organs of European cathedrals— was considered too "depressing" by many of the patients. That tape has been withdrawn.

TABLE 3

WHAT THE PATIENT NOTICES

	Patients Percent	Relatives Percent	Patients' Disease Status		
			Localized Percent	Regional Percent	Distant Percent
Music	89.2	100.0	90.0	95.7	81.0
Plants	98.4	95.0	100.0	95.7	100.0
Fishtank	98.4	95.0	100.0	95.7	100.0
No Smoking	86.0	100.0	90.0	87.0	80.9
Machines					
Frightened	6.3	0	0	13.0	4.8
Not Frightened	93.7		100.0	87.0	95.2

TABLE 4

WHAT PATIENTS ENJOY

	Patients Percent	Relatives Percent	Patients' Disease Status		
			Localized Percent	Regional Percent	Distant Percent
Staff	100.0	100.0	100.0	100.0	100.0
Environment	89.0	100.0	90.0	95.7	81.0
Paintings	73.4	95.0	60.0	78.3	80.9
Music	89.2	100.0	90.0	95.7	81.0
Plants	98.4	95.0	100.0	95.7	100.0
Fish	98.4	95.0	100.0	95.7	100.0
No Smoking	86.0	100.0	90.0	87.0	80.9

Almost everyone (98.4 percent) noticed the plants and fishtank in the waiting area. Often, the patients joked about them, "I thought the plants were artificial until the attendant came around to water them one day." The fishtank serves as the main focal point in one waiting area. It fascinates the children and allows patients to "break the ice" when talking with other patients.

As a rule, if the patients noticed something, they generally liked it. "The sophisticated machinery reminds me of Star Trek," commented a middle-aged lady with cancer of the cervix. The looming arms of the transverse axial tomograph and the massive bulk of the linear accelerators did not seem to bother the patients (only 6.3 percent of the patients were frightened by the equipment). Fears about radiation burns were quickly dispelled by the technicians and the self-assurance of the staff. "You know, I feel like I am part of a family. Every day I look forward to the visit because of the people here. I love it," a patient with lymphoma confided enthusiastically. In addition, the general consensus about the atmosphere of the center was extremely favorable (89.2 percent of the patients commented positively about the center) (Table 4).

WHAT THE PATIENTS DO WHILE WAITING FOR TREATMENT

The patients generally spoke to each other or just sat and watched the other people. They were not reluctant to speak to one another (67 percent of the patients). Otherwise, they spoke with their relatives who had accompanied them (66 percent of the patients). Many patients (50 percent) were content to just watch the people come and go. Generally, they did not read (only 30 percent of them did), and very few watched television. When asked how long they spent waiting, most of the patients thought that they waited between 10 and 30 minutes. Thus, patients in the waiting area were generally perceptive of their surroundings and sociable to each other. They are not readers or television watchers, and above all, they appear to be relaxed and comfortable in this environment (Table 5).

KNOWLEDGE AND ATTITUDE

In recent years, there has been a considerable change in our attitude about telling or not telling patients the true nature of their illness. Patients have become much more sophisticated and knowledgeable about diagnostic techniques and therapeutic modalities used in the management of cancer. Thus, they generally expect to discuss the treatment recommended for their disease soon after the diagnosis has been established. What to tell the person about the treatment, instead of whether or not to tell him about the nature of his disease, has become the psychological question of the day.

When should the patient be told, by whom, what reactions are likely, and how should these emotionally based problems be handled? There are little published data on patient attitudes toward treatment systems and their perceptions or interaction with these. In the field of radiation oncology the data are nonexistent. It was the purpose of our second study to provide information on which

TABLE 5

WHAT PATIENTS DO IN THE WAITING ROOM

	All Patients Percent	Relatives Percent	Patients' Disease Status		
			Localized Percent	Regional Percent	Distant Percent
Talk with Patients	67.2	95.0	75.0	69.5	57.1
Who Read	29.7	40.0	15.0	47.8	23.8
Who Talk	56.3	60.0	75.0	34.7	61.9
Who Watch People	49.9	40.0	65.0	39.1	47.6
Who Watch Fishtank	4.7	0	0	13.0	0
Who Do Nothing	17.1	10.0	15.0	17.4	19.0

to base more rational methods of dealing with patients' problems of living in other than the medical sense.

Fifty patients undergoing treatment at the Radiation Oncology Center at Rhode Island Hospital were interviewed. Forty-seven were ambulatory, and 3 were inpatients. They were chosen at random by the chief technologist according to the following criteria: 1) 30 years of age or older and 2) after the completion of 10 or more treatment days. The first 50 patients available to be interviewed were accepted. The two criteria assured that the patients were likely to perceive themselves as individuals separate from their parents and that entirely palliative cases (usually receiving 10 treatments or less) were minimized. Interviewees were told that the study of the experiences of patients undergoing radiation therapy was in progress. They were asked to see a doctor to be interviewed either immediately before or after treatment. One patient refused to be seen.

Each patient was interviewed by Glenn W. Mitchell who identified himself as a doctor interested in the problems of patients undergoing radiation therapy. Each was told that no information about any individual's specific medical condition or treatment was known to the interviewer. The point that information was being obtained in an effort to improve services for future patients was emphasized. It was also stated that no one had been chosen because of a presumed need for specific psychiatric assessment or treatment.

The interviews took about an hour. They were conducted in a somewhat controlled manner so that all questions were answered, although not necessarily in a specific order. The patients were allowed to volunteer information, to ask questions, to offer opinions, and to make suggestions. Information about past medical history, family history, and developmental psychiatric history was not

TABLE 6

ILLNESS

What Problem Are You Being Treated For?

Who Informed You of This?

Are You Getting Better?

Because of the Treatments?

What is Going to Happen to You in the Next Weeks and Months?

TABLE 7

TREATMENT

What Are You Expecting From This Treatment?

What Do You Think of All This Machinery?

Are You Frightened By It All?

What Kind of Problems Are You Having During Your Radiation Therapy?

Do You Think They Are Due to the Treatments?

What Do You Think of the Markings for the Treatment?

Do Other People Remark About Them?

Who Is Your Primary Source of Information about Your Treatments? Your Problems?

TABLE 8

DOCTORS

What Did Your Regular Doctor Tell You About Your Treatments?

Did This Prepare You for What Is Happening To You?

Did the Therapy Doctor Help?

How Often Do You See Your Therapy Doctor? What Is His Name?

What Does He Do for You Exactly?

Is This What You Expect?

Is He Treating You or Does Your Regular Doctor Tell Him What To Do For You?

What Kinds of Problems Does Your Therapy Doctor Help You With? Personal or Family Problems?

Are There Things He Cannot Help You With? Which? Who Does Help With Them?

TABLE 9

STAFF

What Do the People Who Run These Machines Do For You?

Are They the Same People Each Time?

What Do You Feel About That?

What Do You Talk to Them About?

Is This What You Want?

What Do the Nurses Do?

What Kind of Problems Do They Help You With?

Is This What You Expect?

Are There Problems They Cannot Help? Which? Why?

TABLE 10

PEERS

Do You Spend Much Time Talking to Other Patients? What About?

How Do You Feel About Talking to Them?

Do You Think It Would Be Helpful to Spend More Time Talking with Other Patients? Say in Group Meetings? What Would You Discuss?

Who Comes with You to These Treatments Each Day?

requested. The areas covered during the interview were the patient's concept of and attitude toward his disease, his perception of the treatment facility and its staff and his interactions with fellow patients. Individual questions were asked in the same manner of each patient, unless the required information had been given in earlier conversations (see Tables 6, 7, 8, 9, 10, for specific questions).

MATERIAL

Table 11 summarizes the patients interviewed in this study by diagnosis, and Table 12 illustrates the age and sex distribution. Scheduled treatment duration varied from three to nine weeks with 78 percent of the patients having five to seven weeks of planned treatment. At the time of the interview, the patients were 40-100 percent through their course of treatment. More than two-thirds had completed 75 percent of the sessions.

TABLE 11

DIAGNOSES BY LOCATION OF PRIMARY TUMOR

Primary Site	Males	Females	Total
Head & Neck	8	4	12
Lung	3	1	4
GI Tract	5	7	12
GU/GYN	3	11	14
Lymphatics	2	2	4
Other	1	3	4
Total	22	28	50

TABLE 12

PATIENT AGES BY DECADE OF LIFE

Ages	Males	Females	Total
30-39	2	0	2
40-49	2	6	8
50-59	7	6	13
60-69	4	7	11
70-79	5	7	12
80-89	2	2	4
Total	22	28	50

RESULTS

Thirty of the 50 patients used the word *cancer* to describe the reason for being treated. An additional 17 patients used the word *tumor* or *malignancy* in the same context. The remaining three patients said that they were being treated for "a little swelling"; "some condition, my doctor knows what it is"; and "none of your business." All of the patients said that they were told their diagnosis by the physician who referred them for therapy (Table 13).

Forty-three patients remembered coming to the department with positive feelings about the outcome of their treatment. Seven were pessimistic. There was no significant correlation between age, sex, diagnosis, or treatment schedule and the feelings of pessimism.

TABLE 13

REASON FOR TREATMENT

Cancer	30 patients
Tumor, Malignancy	17 patients
A Little Swelling	1 patient
My Doctor Knows	1 patient
None of Your Business	1 patient

TREATMENT

Thirty patients felt improved because of their therapy, 16 perceived no change, and 4 felt that they had become worse. Nineteen persons remembered feeling "frightened" by the equipment at first, especially during the protracted simulation phase prior to their first actual treatment. All had a lessening of anxiety about the treatment with time, and none were frightened of the equipment at the time of the interview. Ten patients expressed the desire to have received more counseling and explanation prior to treatment and/or during the initial simulation.

The following were perceived as side effects of the radiation treatments: tiredness, 62 percent, GI disturbances, 32 percent; other symptoms, including dry skin, alopecia, and loss of appetite, 40 percent. Only one patient who was not receiving abdominal radiation complained of nausea. That person was among the head and neck cases (Table 14). All but two of the patients complaining of general GI upset also complained of tiredness after treatments.

Five patients felt that their markings applied to their skin to delineate the radiation field were socially bothersome to them. The fields involved were on the head and neck above the collarline. Those complaining comprised one-third of the head and neck carcinoma cases interviewed. There was no correlation with age or sex, and all were in the final half of their scheduled treatment course. An

TABLE 14

SIDE EFFECTS OF RADIATION

Tiredness	62%
GI Disturbances	32%
Others:	
Dry Skin, Alopecia	40%
None	24%

TABLE 15

PERCEPTION OF STAFF

Technologists

Role – To Run Machines	100%
Compositional Stability	86%
"Pleasant People"	98%

additional 17 patients, however, complained of the personal hygiene problems caused by the markings, that is bathing without tub or shower.

STAFF

All persons interviewed felt that the role of the *radiation technologist* was that of operating treatment machines. All patients spoke with the technologists about trivialities such as sports and the weather. Seven, however, asked questions such as care of markings and limitation of sun exposure to treatment areas. Four of these seven asked about their general progress or the number of remaining treatments. Forty-three patients noted the relative compositional stability of the team, and 20 of these derived positive feelings from the daily contact with familiar team members. Forty-eight persons noted spontaneously that the technologists were pleasant people and felt that this contributed to their overall sense of ease with their treatments. No patient expressed the desire to obtain more information or to seek more contact time with the technologists (Table 15).

All patients perceived that the staff *nurses* were present to run the examining area and to help the doctor. Thirteen had received treatments and medications such as dressing changes and dietary suggestions from them and 11 had asked about side effects such as nausea and diarrhea. Twenty-three remembered being asked by the nurses for complaints when seen prior to weekly checkups by the radiation therapists during treatments. All those interviews offered variations on a theme, "Medical problems are for the doctor " (Table 16).

TABLE 16

PERCEPTION OF STAFF

Nurses

Role – Help Doctor	100%
Meds and Treatments	26%

The *radiation therapist* was felt to be responsible for the treatment plan during the present phase of the patient's total program by 37 patients, to share equal responsibility with the referring physician by 8 patients, and to be supervised by the referring physician by 5 patients. Forty-seven of the 50 patients interviewed were able to identify by name the radiotherapist responsible for their treatment (Table 17). Forty patients felt that he gave them satisfactory information about their treatment before commencing therapy even though 11 of them

TABLE 17

PERCEPTION OF STAFF

Radiotherapist	
Responsible for Treatment	74%
Shared Responsibility with Referring Physician	16%
Supervised by Referring Physician	10%

remembered being frightened initially. On the other hand, the referring physician was thought to have given satisfactory information about the experience of radiation therapy by only 8 patients, partial information by 16, and was considered to have been of no help in this matter by 26 patients (52 percent of those interviewed). Of the 19 patients who expressed initial fright during therapy, 63 percent were among those who felt that they had received no information about radiation therapy from their referring physicians (Table 18).

When asked about their emotional reactions to therapy and to their underlying disease, 14 patients denied having any personal problems (although by the end of the interview one-half of these had spontaneously talked about problems that they were experiencing). An additional 26 patients discussed openly the fact that they were having problems concerning internal thoughts and/or interpersonal reactions. Of these, 21 percent mentioned depressed mood, 12 percent

TABLE 18

PERCEPTION OF INFORMATION

	Radiotherapist	Referring Physician
Satisfactory	80%	16%
Partial	20	32
No Help	0	52

had family difficulties, 22 percent wished to discuss their situation more fully, and 2 percent said that they had had thoughts of suicide during this illness.

Only 22 patients could identify a resource with whom they could discuss emotional difficulties. Six identified a physician as such a resource, two of these named their radiation therapist. Others noted were clergy, family members, nurses, and in one instance, her horse. Forty-one patients expressed the opinion that both the referring physician and the therapists were "not the people to bring emotional problems to." Thirty-two of these felt that the physician was "too busy with medical problems" to bother with personal troubles. Nine patients expressed the opinion that "the doctor should spend his time on medical problems" since time spent on personal problems would compromise that available for medical consideration. (Table 19).

TABLE 19
RESOURCE FOR EMOTIONAL SUPPORT

Could Identify	44%
Physician	12%
Other	32%
Could Not Identify	50%

82 percent expressed opinion that both the referring physician and the radiotherapist were *not the people to bring emotional problems to.*

PEER RELATIONS

Thirty-two patients said that they spent time talking to other patients during the waiting period before treatment. Nearly one-half of these persons spoke only of "trivial subjects," but 18 discussed their treatments and/or illnesses with other patients. Thirteen patients expressed the desire to spend additional time with other patients in order to discuss common problems, and all of these were among those who discussed their problems openly in the waiting area. Thirty-seven patients, however, felt specifically that additional time spent with other patients was undesirable.

DISCUSSION

For the most part, patients coming to the Radiation Oncology Center of the Rhode Island Hospital generally feel well and show minor signs of symptoms of their disease. Characteristically, a patient's mood is unchanged while waiting for treatment. Only the patients with more advanced disease, particularly those who have had to return for a second or third course of treatment, indicated that they were depressed, frustrated, or frightened. But even these patients were not withdrawn. It was interesting to note that they were more aware than were other patients of their external environment. Other observers have also noted that patients with advanced disease who have accepted their disease become hypersensitive to their external environment. This fact is well corroborated by patient observations concerning the artwork in the radiotherapy center; they heard the music and reacted to it; the plants, the fishtank, the homelike furnishings were all perceived positively by the patients and their relatives.

A point of particular importance which came from the study was the realization that three out of four of the patients interviewed had a high school education or less. Explanations and discussions of their disease must be structured so that these patients and others like them will understand what is being told to them. This cannot be done in a pedantic, condescending manner. The vocabulary, the analogies, and the logic must be easily understood and appropriate if we are to truly inform the patient and gain his cooperation during the treatment situation.

Despite their lack of formal education, virtually all patients were able to identify their condition either as a malignant tumor or cancer. This presumably reflects an increasing consumer awareness and lay sophistication of patients, as well as increasing candor on the part of physicians in dealing with this disease. In 1972, 80 percent of the patients at Mt. Sinai Hospital were able to verbalize these terms. Eighty-six percent of the patients in Rhode Island came to the Radiation Oncology Center with a "positive" attitude towards recovery. This positive attitude is useful in masking prognostic anxiety while allowing conscious awareness of the diagnosis itself.

Concern and dissatisfaction were expressed by a majority of the patients over the manner in which radiotherapy was explained to them by their referring physicians. Twenty-six (52 percent) said that they remembered receiving no helpful information about their upcoming treatment. Sixteen said that it was partial but somewhat helpful, and 8 felt satisfied with it. Of the 19 patients expressing fright at the first treatment, 12 (63 percent) were among those who had been ill-prepared for radiotherapy by their referring physicians and surgeons. This lack of preparation may reflect a lack of understanding of what radiotherapy is all about on the part of the referring physicians and surgeons rather than gross carelessness. Clearly, there is a need for these doctors to understand the procedures of radiation therapy better, and it is incumbent upon the radiotherapy community to develop that understanding. Janice and Levanthal in 1964 emphasized the importance of keeping patients as informed as possible about what to expect since fantasies and conjectures often add to fear and discomfort in new situations. Even more pragmatically, Egbert et al. (1972) showed that somatic symptoms perceived as side effects, such as nausea and vomiting, can be significantly reduced by advance information and counseling.

CONCLUSIONS

Eighty percent of the patients said that the radiotherapist gave them satisfactory information before starting treatment. They did not look to the technologists as a source of this information. All of those interviewed felt that the radiation technologists were people with whom trivialities were exchanged. The nurses were perceived as there to run the examining area and to help the doctor. But the general theme that ran through all of these interviews was "medical problems are for the doctor." Accessibility to the radiation therapist is of major importance, as these findings indicate, and our time must be structured to make accessibility even easier for the patient.

About two-thirds of the patients spent time talking with other patients, and of these the majority discussed their illnesses or treatments. Many patients felt that relief came from knowing that another person was having a similar difficulty. They were able to share remedies and compensatory behaviors for common physical complaints. The proportion of patients stating the desire for further interaction was considerable, and the benefits of patient comfort and education suggest that group sessions (on a voluntary basis) could be a useful adjunct to other support efforts. A skillful and experienced group leader could diminish the problems of misinformation and of treatment failure while at the same time enhancing the information exchange and emotional support that would be given to patients who did join the group.

Less than half of the patients could identify a resource for emotional support although 86 percent wished that they did have someone with whom they could "discuss the situation more fully." Only 6 patients identified a physician as a resource, and two of these named their radiotherapist. Over 80 percent of the patients expressed the opinion that the referring physician and radiotherapist were not "the people to bring emotional problems to." In fact, almost 20 percent of the samples said that they would not tell their doctors about emotional problems. These patients will not tell even the most empathetic, understanding radiotherapist of their problems although they could not, at this time, identify any other resource for emotional help. *Clearly, mental health professionals—psychiatrists, psychologists, trained nurses, and social workers—could make a major contribution in the total program if they were involved in the day-to-day care of patients receiving radiotherapy.* The treatment team requires the assistance of mental health professionals to serve the needs of these patients. The radiotherapists, nurses, and technologists are not perceived by the patient as individuals to whom emotional problems can be brought. Mental health professionals would be regarded as a new resource, not detracting from their cancer care, but adding to their emotional stability and reinforcing their coping mechanisms.

The emphasis must be on problem-solving for living rather than adjustment to dying. There is a reasonable prospect that patients will survive. More than 60 percent of these patients are being treated with cure as the intent, and for well over half of the patients, a five-year survival or better can be anticipated. This is the time for emotional support as part of that long-range intent of cure. If the patient looks to someone outside the radiotherapy team for this support, we must recognize this and add a mental health professional to deal with these problems.

REFERENCES

Egbert L. et al. 1964. "Reduction of Post-operative Pain by Encouragement and Instruction of Patients." *New England Journal of Medicine,* 270:825-827.
Janis, I. and H. Leventhal. 1964. "Psychological Aspects of Physical Illness and Hospital Care." In B. Walman, ed., *Handbook of Clinical Psychology.* New York: McGraw-Hill, pp. 1-43.

NUTRITION AND THE PSYCHOSOCIAL ASPECTS OF RADIATION

James C. Rose

Nutritional problems are often a major concern in the treatment and rehabilitation of the cancer patient. Improved nutritional status may increase treatment response and strength for rehabilitation, thus markedly improving the quality of life available for the cancer patient (Simon, 1975). To provide optimal nutritional care, the registered dietitian must be cognizant of the psychological basis of food behavior patterns, the physiological basis of the cancer-nutrition continuum, how patient interaction may be best effected, and the role of nutrition in cancer care.

CANCER, RADIOTHERAPY, AND PSYCHOLOGICAL STRESS

The patient with a diagnosis of cancer may be preoccupied with thoughts of death, because the high mortality rate of cancer is well known and death from cancer is often associated with pain and physical debilitation (Meinhart, 1968). Further, in some segments of our society cancer bears a stigma, which results in social isolation for the patient. Medical professionals as well as laymen may cease patient interactions that stimulate their own personal identification with serious illnesses, and patient loneliness may result (Quint, 1965). The fear of unacceptability and isolation can present a greater psychological depression than fears of recurrence of the disease (Meinhart, 1968). Such emotional depression interferes significantly with the eating behavior of the patient (Anderson, 1974). Emotional support from concerned professionals and nonprofessionals, as well as antidepressive drugs may engender an improvement of the food-intake patterns (*The Cancer Letter,* 1975).

Of all therapies for neoplasia, radiation therapy is surrounded with the greatest mystique; nothing is seen, heard, or felt during the treatment. The greatest psychological distress is experienced at three different times: at the beginning of treatment, during treatment whenever therapy changes are made because of side reactions and/or extensions of the disease, and at the end of treatment when the final results of the therapy are still undetermined (Schmale, 1974). Detachment and anxiety also may be apparent in the patient. More than other stress factors, psychological stresses may affect food-intake patterns and thus nutritional status, which in turn negatively affects the individual's capacity to cope with stress (Coffey, 1975; Casper, 1975). Further, conditioned aversion to food intake may occur during radiotherapy—that is, if a patient experiences nausea and vomiting, abdominal distress, epigastric fullness, or other gastrointestinal symptoms, he may avoid eating even after the physical symptoms of distress have diminished (Mayer, 1971; *The Cancer Letter,* 1975).

Changes in physical appearance or function may complicate further the psychosocial aspects of nutritional care. As a patient experiences changes in his body image, he may respond with an imagined loss of self-esteem, power, and prestige (Meinhart, 1968) and may, from time to time, express depression, apathy, agitation, and bitterness. During this stage, he may manifest physical symptoms as emotional outlets—for example, crying, anorexia, aching, or nausea.

PHYSIOLOGICAL PERSPECTIVE

Knowledge of the role of nutrition in the development of cancer in man is meager (Shils, 1972). Currently, some areas of research lend considerable importance to diet as an etiological factor in the development of cancer. Diet composition and practices in food preparation are thought to be possible environmental factors influencing tumor development (Goodhart and Shils, 1973).

Nutrition is impaired through multiple routes of interference by the disease state. For instance, tumors may interfere mechanically with the mobility functions of the gastrointestinal tract. Thus, tumors of the oral cavity, pharynx, esophagus, and stomach may severely restrict or eliminate the oral route as a means of feeding. Intestinal obstruction is a common consequence of tumors. Malabsorption syndromes secondary to the infiltration of the intestine by cancer, particularly lymphomas, have been well described (Costa, 1973). Admittedly, therefore, the maintenance of optimal nutritional status in patients with extensive cancer is difficult.

While the disease state may thus cause malnutrition of various etiologies in the cancer patient, nutritional problems may also arise as a result of the specific treatment given to control the neoplastic disease. Shils (1972) reports that radiation treatment of the oropharyngeal area may cause destruction of the sense of taste and thus impair intake. Radiation of the abdomen and pelvic area may cause bowel damage, acute and chronic, with diarrhea, malabsorption, and anatomic complications. The small bowel is especially susceptible to ionizing radiation, which can cause edema and congestion as well as modified peristalsis. Intestinal irradiation may also produce endarteritis in the small vessels. The intestinal wall may show fibrosis, stenosis, necrosis, and ulceration, which over an extended period may result in hemorrhage, obstructive fistula, diarrhea, and malabsorption. Necrosis may become generalized, with fibrous tissue surrounding the indurated bowel (Mayer, 1971). Chemotherapy used in conjunction with radiotherapy as well as infection complications may cause painful ulceration of the oropharynx and esophagus, rendering swallowing difficult. Abnormal intestinal structure and function may lead to malabsorption of carbohydrates, fats, and vitamins. A normal dietary intake of vitamins is inadequate to meet the needs of some of these patients (Bodey, 1970).

Patients who undergo radiotherapy treatment in the areas of the vocal chord, the thyroid, or the ear have few eating problems. However, patients being treated in the tonsillar region, the palate, the tongue, and especially the nasopharynx area experience the most severe therapy reactions and the greatest loss of weight (Polunsky and Pelham, 1973). (In considering weight loss, one must differentiate from mere loss of weight and the overall depletion of all or most of the labile body compartments in constant ratios, from selective depletion or retention of either fat, protein, water, or minerals.)

As the treatment progresses, reactions may become more severe. The patient may have extreme difficulty in swallowing or may stop eating unless consistently encouraged by the family and the dietitian (Polunsky and Pelham, 1973). If the patient has pain at meals, his intake may diminish (Meinhart, 1968). Further, head and neck patients may experience reduction or cessation of salivary secretions, as well as generalized fatigue, loss of appetite, nausea, and vomiting by the third week of therapy (Anderson, 1974). The fact must be recognized that many head and neck patients have preexisting nutritional deficits from age, inadequate intake, or alcoholism, which may have contributed to the production of negative nitrogen balance and hypoproteinemia (Noone and Graham, 1973; Hickey, 1974). Head and neck patients also exhibit increased susceptibility to dental deterioration, for which the use of one percent sodium fluoride gel and adjusting the sucrose content of the diet may be advantageous (Hegedus and Pelham, 1975). Postoperative head and neck patients receiving radiation therapy may have compounded nutrition problems; not only will they often experience reactions to the radiation, but they also must contend with any combination of complications, such as tube feeding dependency, gastric stasis, fistulas, and functional defects in speech, chewing, swallowing, and salivary control (Anderson, 1974).

Diarrhea induced by pelvic area irradiation is self-limiting and responds well to opiates such as paregoric. A low-residue diet may assist in controlling diarrhea. When large volumes of tissues are treated, as in Hodgkin's disease or ovarian carcinoma, nausea, vomiting, and generalized fatigue are common. This reaction, which can be controlled by drugs, occurs shortly after treatment for a few hours and then recedes (Anderson, 1974).

Malnutrition in neoplastic disease is often characterized by decreased caloric intake, hypermetabolism relative to the patient's state of nutrition, anorexia, negative nitrogen balance, and clinically apparent edema (Mayer, 1971; Bodey, 1970).

Anorexia may be defined as diminished appetite or aversion to food (Stedman's Dictionary, 1972). As one of the classic vegetative sequelae of depression, psychogenic anorexia may occur as a reaction to the disease and its prognosis, although clinically apparent anorexia commonly results from the altered effect of physiological conditions on the physiological mechanisms regulating food intake (Maxwell, 1963). Its severity may almost completely suppress spontaneous ingestion of food. Though the pathogenesis of anorexia is unclear, it does not appear simply correlated to cancer type but is frequently one of the initial signs of cancer and may appear before any obvious contributing cause, such as intestinal obstruction, endocrine disorder, anatomic lesions, or sepsis with accompanying fever. Anorexia is frequently associated with mental depression, often with fear and guilt feelings, which may further complicate treatment (Mayer, 1971; Latham, 1975).

Cachexia includes general lack of nutrition and wasting of body tissues. Though "cachexia of cancer" is probably not unique to neoplastic disease, its contribution to overall morbidity may be overwhelming (Costa, 1973). Cachexia is a clinocopathologic syndrome of varying severity characterized by marked asthenia, anorexia, anemia, depletion and redistribution of host components, water and electrolyte abnormalities, hormonal aberrations, increased metabolic rate despite reduced intake and activity, and progressive fading of vital functions, to which local organ involvement may contribute (DeWys; Theologides, 1972; Costa, 1973). Various possible mechanisms to explain the routes through which the tumor may exert its effect on the host must be clarified. The catabolic loss of amino acids from muscle (through altered amino acid metabolism) may be responsible for much of the weakness of cachexia of malignancy (DeWys, 1972; O'Brien, 1975). These derangements may elicit a decline in motor activity attributed to ingestion (DeWys, 1972); the patient may insist that he experiences fatigue during eating (DeWys, 1972). Under normal physiological conditions, increased energy demands are met by increased intake. However, in cachexia, food intake often declines: in six cases of uterine carcinoma, the voluntary intake ranged from 300 to 1200 kilocalories (Maxwell, 1963), indicative of a marked caloric deficit.

Quality treatment demands that the cachexia of malignancy be reversed. Total parenteral hyperalimentation has been reported to increase muscle mass and reverse cachexia (Gailani et al., 1973). However, the preferred route of administration of nutrients is oral. The possibility exists that if anorexia and the associated cachexia were the result of conditioned aversion, this might be reversed by suitable conditioning experiences. Metabolic interfaces, however, may limit this approach.

Efforts must be exerted to prevent cachexia. The major factor in preventing loss of cell mass of muscle and organs is a sustained diet that matches energy expenditure and meets protein needs (Blackburn, 1975). Metabolism may be low, normal, or elevated (Mayer, 1971; Bodey, 1970). Massive food intake is not necessary merely to meet the 10 to 20 percent increase in basal metabolism (Blackburn, 1975). However, assimilation of nutrients across the gastrointestinal tract in the cachectic patient is depressed and much of the administered caloric load is lost in the stool (Dudrick and Copeland, 1974). Simple anthropometric and laboratory tests (transferrin, albumin, urine creatinine) provide an objective assessment of calorie and protein requirements (Blackburn, 1975).

The greatest effort should be directed to motivating the patient to consume adequate calories and protein. The value of forced feeding is under study (Gailani et al., 1973; Pareire et al., 1955).

Thus, it is apparent that little is actually known about anorexia and cachexia of neoplasia. A more complete understanding of normal food intake control mechanisms would be valuable. Neuroanatomic and neurophysiologic research on appetite control has emphasized the role of hypothalamic areas in appetite control. The hypothalamic areas interact with the cerebral cortex, sensory stimuli, and internal chemical and physical factors. In one animal study, lesions of the lateral hypothalamus caused loss of drive for eating and drinking, from which the animals recovered. In the later stages of the recovery sequence, the animal is observed to eat certain foods but avoid others. This may parallel the eating behavior of the anorectic patient. As an example of internal chemical influence on appetite, the onset of loss of appetite within a few days of fasting coincides with the appearance of ketosis; experimental infusion of beta-hydroxbutyrate is known to produce decreased eating in experimental animals. As a possible example of cortical factors, animal studies have shown conditioned aversion to the smell and taste of food induced by drugs, toxins, and x-rays administered hours after eating. Study of sensory stimuli may elucidate the clinical observation of aversion to protein by the cancer patient.

Some researchers contend that the majority of cancer patients who lose interest in food do so largely because of a deterioration in taste perception (Rubin, 1974). The taste of food substantially dictates dietary habits and new food acceptances. Studies (DeWys, 1974) indicate that abnormalities of taste may be significant physiological determinants of anorexia. A positive taste stimulus triggers multiple physiological reflexes, many of which contribute to the intake and digestion of food. For instance, the nature of taste sensation may modify the volume and character of saliva. Appealing foods result in copious gastric secretions. Positive orogastric stimulation also causes a variety of physiological changes conducive to food-intake behavior, including alterations in respiratory quotient and blood glucose. Patients with elevated taste thresholds may not receive a sufficiently positive taste stimulus and thus may not satisfactorily trigger the physiological reflexes; this may explain etiological undetermined swallowing difficulty. Inadequate gastric secretions may account for a sense of early fullness. Inadequate pancreatic secretions may contribute to slow digestion of the first meal of the day, thus elucidating the decreased eating of meals later in the day frequently described by patients. A general reduction in pleasures of taste perception was noted by twenty-five patients in one study. Sixty-four percent noted an aversion to meat, including thirteen who had indicated a general reduction in taste sensation (DeWys, 1974). Hypogeusia with dysgeusia prompted patients to alter their normal dietary habits, refusing to eat meat, fish, poultry, eggs, any foods fried in oil or fat, tomatoes, and tomato products. Diets were self-limited to bland cheeses (such as cottage cheese), lettuce, and fresh fruits. An abhorrent taste quality was associated with the nontolerated foods—food was reported as tasting rancid or spoiled. A persistent sour, salty, bitter, or metallic taste was reported. Those patients with hypogeusia without dysgeusia described their food as tasteless; eating was likened to chewing and swallowing flour paste or sawdust (Henkin et al., 1971). Those patients with abnormalities in taste sensation may improve their caloric intake by increasing the seasoning of food. It should also be noted that the protein aversion is selective and progressive; the greatest dislike is for beef or pork; then poultry and fish, and then cheese or eggs. Pain relief and antiemetics may be beneficial.

FOOD HABITS

Food habits, the products of many personal cultural, social, and psychological influences, are among the oldest and most entrenched aspects of many cultures and may exert marked influences on a patient's behavior (Williams, 1973). Food often represents the crossroads of emotion, religion, tradition, and habit (Schafer and Yetley, 1975), and may symbolize interpersonal acceptance, friendliness, sociability and warmth (Manning, 1965). The cultural psychosocial factors which are based on availability, economics, or symbolism of the individual patient prove most influential in the development of the nutrition behavior complex (Williams, 1973).

The main determinants of food-seeking behavior are hunger, appetite, and custom. Positive and negative components exist for each determinant. Most significantly, appetite may be depressed by worry, fear, and preoccupation with difficulties; but appetite may be stimulated by a situation of calm contentedness, by mild elation, and by conditions of egostimulation (Manning, 1965). Thus, people use food to express their emotions and feelings, and numerous foods may have connotations of symbolic rather than rational meanings (Casper and Wakefield, 1975). Each culture may determine the symbolic meaning of food, and items prized in one culture may be excluded in another. Further, within the same culture, foods may be acceptable for one meal and rejected at another.

However, for the average man, eating is more or less a mechanical, day-to-day experience, and he often does not become aware of its importance until he is asked to change his habits. He may then experience exclusion from comfortable symbolic or social associations. This may result in negative psychological reactions (Kranholdt, 1974).

The registered dietitian who must assist the patient in shaping food habits must be aware of the component of food-directed behavior that includes appetites, remote goals, and aesthetic enjoyments that extend over the whole range of human motivation. He must become attuned to the cultural, social, personal, and situational factors that motivate or encourage patients to eat and that are intertwined with food habits. Specifically, he must develop an environment and a rapport with the patient to ensure optimal motivation and perception by the patient, both of which are particularly pertinent to the molding of food habits. Realizing that people accept food and advice about their food habits more readily from those viewed as friends or allies, the dietitian must cultivate this trust with the patient and the patient's family, utilizing the strength of family influences to motivate patients.

THE DIETITIAN-PATIENT CONTINUUM

In radiotherapy, the dietitian is principally involved in guiding the patient in adjusting his eating habits to prevent weight loss with its resulting complications. To effect this, the dietitian must recognize basic needs, establish rapport, utilize effective interviewing tools, and provide specific recommendations.

The role of a dietitian has been defined (a) as a specialist who can translate for the patient the prescribed regimen into exact amounts and kinds of foods prepared in specific ways; (b) as a specialist in the relationship between intake, food, and physiological need who can guide the patient in making a selection of foods that will produce or maintain a given bodily state; (c) as a specialist in problems of patient adjustment, including consumption, budgetary problems, and conditions of food preparation; and (d) as a member of a team of therapists who are oriented not only to the physical needs of the patient but to his whole personality in a health-care setting. Each of these roles must be clearly apparent to the patient and his family. Patient interaction cannot be truly successful unless there is a clear definition of why the dietitian is there, what the referring specialist has asked him to do, and what the patient may or may not expect (Mead, 1970).

Four general patient-interaction tools are utilized by registered dietitians to obtain pertinent information. The personal interview is normally the first tool utilized. This is an attempt to gain some measure of insight into the patient's personality, including his reactions to his diagnosis and his perception of his illness, the value he places on normality, how he has adapted to stress and previous illnesses, his typical behavior routine (Murray, 1972), what motives may be invoked in changing food habits, and what resistances or prejudices exist; the intelligence and emotional attitudes, financial and living arrangements, cultural background, and previous dietary restrictions are also determined (Mead, 1970). Open-ended statements are more productive than leading questions (Kaufman, 1970). The atmosphere during the interview must be relaxed and unhurried.

Twenty-four-hour "typical" food intake recall records are commonly used (Kaufman, 1970). From memory, the patient lists the food intake. This method is not generally recommended during therapy because of the possibility of skewed or unreliable results due to patient confusion or a conflict in goals. If valid, however, the record allows ease in computation of calorie and protein ingestion for planning and assessing dietary needs.

The food-intake diary may prove valuable. The diary consists of the patient's written record of intake noted at the time of each meal or snack. It has the following advantages: (a) the patient is forced to contemplate intake; (b) memory and recall are not particularly limiting components; (c) more accuracy is possible. The diary, however, may not be valid if the patient is not a reliable historian.

The food-preference questionnaire may provide significant information to the dietitian, who must continually make food suggestions consistent with need. The questionnaire consists of a list of common foods; the patient merely indicates a like or dislike for the foods. Upon its completion, the responses are reviewed by the dietitian with the patient to allow them an opportunity to discuss and amplify responses. Those patients unwilling to complete the questionnaire should not be urged to use it. Unwillingness may, in fact, be a significant clue concerning the attitudes toward diagnosis, dietary restriction, or the authority of those involved in the dietary treatment. For such patients, the more personal approach of the dietary interview is preferable.

Since eating is more frequently psychological and social than intellectual, the dietitian must establish patient trust and rapport (Anderson, 1974a). It must be recognized that the most important psychological factors will be the significance the individual attaches to the diagnosis and treatment, his level of emotional maturity, and the present state of his interpersonal relationships, the relationships he established with the professional staff, his development experiences and adaptive defense, and his culture. It is noted that only those professionals whom the patient accepts can significantly influence a change in his food habits. Further, advice about food is accepted from persons who are considered authorities and who exhibit genuine concern. Good rapport may be more easily achieved if the dietitian is relaxed and an educated listener, interruption should be minimized. An awareness of personal feelings and reactions conveyed to the patient through movements as well as through words and facial expression is essential in establishing rapport.

The dietitian must in practically every instance persuade the patient to attend from a new point of view to the details of diet. This may be psychologically painful for the patient; the conscious application of thought—especially measuring, counting, and so on—to an aspect of life that is ordinarily associated with the gratification of the senses is regarded as reducing pleasure, and is likely to be resisted. Admittedly, since it is difficult for most patients to change firmly-rooted food habits, changes should not be suggested unless they are necessary. The recommended changes should also be consistent with the patient's age, cultural and religious background, financial situation, present living situation, daily routine, and individual food preference. Kaufman (1970) has suggested the use of several questions to ascertain how the patient may respond to change and to determine possible areas of motivation. It cannot be overemphasized that changes are not instantaneous; the dietitian must guard against criticizing beliefs or practices; criticizing may lead to alienation and distrust by the patient.

A patient may express his anxiety via food and by the attempted manipulation of the person providing food. For example, some people may fear rejection if they antagonize authority figures. These patients may feign comprehension of dietary instructions or refuse to select their own food. However, the person who is rebelling against his position as a dependent patient may demand food that is inappropriate or unavailable (Tobias and Goodman, 1972). Those patients who may relate the dietary regimen to social isolation may live in a conflict situation, realizing the need for change but offering excuses and reasons for not following the prescribed diet. The dietitian's patience, tact, kindness, understanding, and firmness may increase patient acceptance and attentiveness.

The dietitian must guard against creating psychological barriers and conflicts. The dietitian may confuse biological necessity with his own cultural patterning; he may remain unperceptive of the uniqueness of the patient's needs and persist in the plan that projects only the dietitian's cultural values. When this plan fails, the dietitian is likely to label the patient "uncooperative." When the dietitian is confronted with angry, bitter remarks, he should aid the person in dispelling anger by remaining calm and listening to the patient without becoming defensive. The dietitian must also recognize that a patient may express a pessimistic attitude to provide protection against disappointment (Schmale, 1974). Each age, each sex has its special problems to which the dietitian must be attuned. For old age, it is important to realize that the patient needs to be treated with the respect due to age and experience of life—yet protected, by written advice, for instance—from a growing forgetfulness. The dietitian must also realize that during illness some degree of regression or fear of it usually manifests itself. This may appear as special patient requests, such as desires for foods preferred when younger or before becoming ill. For instance, ulcer patients on a prolonged regimen may find in such a routine a socially accepted form of symbolic regression, whereas the patient who is emotionally insecure of his adult status may refuse milk and pureed foods, which may symbolize infant foods. This may be particularly evident in those patients fearing intubation.

Especially during recurrence and retreatment of cancer, patients and their families may be skeptical and hesitant in believing what they are told concerning the therapy and support care. During this time, patients are often attracted to treatment claims by charlatans capitalizing on those looking for miracles. A patient searching for a belief with which he may identify may tenaciously adhere to self-treatment protocols that are not scientifically sound and that may present complications. For instance, some patients or their families who adhere to self-imposed dietary restrictions may be unwilling to serve or even purchase a basic food because of their belief that this food will have undesirable effects on their health. This is especially evident in those adhering to the food-faddist regimen, who claim that certain foods may cause or cure cancer. It must be emphasized that illness may be seen as a threat to the ego because illness raises the question of self-worth; thus, for the miracle seeker, selection of miracle foods may be an attempt to offset this threat to the ego, as well as a course of action to return the organism to a healthful state. That is, the food an individual chooses to eat must not only satisfy his hunger but must also be congruent with himself as a certain kind of person. These behavior patterns and attitudes allow a patient to give positive expression to his values and his self-concept. Therefore, an awareness of the patterning and self-needs of the patient will be helpful to the dietitian in understanding the appeal of food fads and the rejection of sound nutritional information. If the dietitian develops this awareness of how food fads may be used by individuals for patterning and self-needs, he may then attempt to alter food attitudes and food selections by faddists by suggesting food substitutions which may optimally contribute to nutritional needs but which also continue to support the social and psychologic needs of the faddist (Schafer and Yetley, 1975). Thus, serving nonrational motives and rational needs simultaneously may increase the acceptance of dietary recommendations, whatever their nature.

CHARACTERISTICS OF THE DIETARY PLAN

As the initial step in planning for the patient's dietary care program, it is essential to read the medical record carefully. Note should be made of the planned radiotherapy treatment period, the area of treatment, and the schedule of treatment. Utilizing this information, the dietitian must set realistic and measurable dietary goals for the patient, assuring that the suggested foods be not only palatable but ones for which the subject has an appetite, if at all possible (O'Brien, 1975). The plan must strive to reflect the strengths of the individual's own eating pattern, modifying past eating habits to meet the therapeutic needs. When drastic changes must be made, however, they should be explained to the patient, who should be involved in the decision about how best to handle the changes. The dietitian must realize that people generally learn only that which they feel will be useful to them, and they retain only that which they believe they need or shall need. The more immediately a patient can utilize the learning, the more readily he grasps it; the more it satisfies his immediate goals, the more effective the learning will be. Therefore, to effect a practical design, three areas must be considered: the reason for dietary regimen, the ready availability of necessary foods, and the subject's psychological need and basis for necessary motivation to make the suggested changes. The overall dietary plan must be assessed; reinforcement of the treatment regimen should be made as the need arises to ensure patient comprehension of the plan to assure him of the professional concern of the dietitian.

Obviously, at the beginning of a six-week course of treatment, the patient has little discomfort from the therapy and follows his normal eating pattern. However, it is essential that this be the period when the dietitian should first contact the patient. His family should also be advised of the planned regimen, for as a result of the mental stress it may be difficult for the patient to absorb the dietitian's advice. It is essential for the dietitian to establish rapport with the patient and his family, in order to maintain their confidence in the dietitian's assistance later as complications arise. Kranholdt (1974) insists that dietary counseling is dependent on the dietitian thoroughly becoming acquainted with the social, vocational, and family constraints of the patient. Then and only then can a meaningful instruction be given, explaining the reasons for and desired results of the diet. The dietitian also may discuss possible side reactions. This will be reassuring to most patients, although it will cause some to become anxious. The possibility of psychological invalidism may necessitate treating the physical symptoms in a matter-of-fact manner, as expediently as possible—that is, to consider them as unavoidable inconveniences that must be resolved by positive action.

On the basis of the initial nutritional assessment and interview, goals should be formulated for each patient during team conferences. Brief follow-up visits for each patient should be scheduled for each time the patient returns to the clinic (Simon, 1975). During these visits, the dietary plan should be reviewed and adjusted, based on the patient's progress; the dietitian must continually encourage the patient to adhere to the dietary program.

In addition to discussions with the patient about his diet, individualized written plans should be provided. The dietitian must, in preparing these plans, be cognizant of the language skills and reading level of the patient and his family. Little success is to be gained from the practice of distributing a diet sheet and instructing the patient to eat accordingly. Further, if the instructions are limited to allowed and forbidden foods, the ratio of success will be small. It is imperative that the dietitian do concrete teaching about foods, the nature of the diet and how the recommended amounts and proportions may be obtained within the framework of the patient's food habits. Instructions must be repeated frequently, patiently, and consistently, in order to enhance learning (Murray, 1972). Since the housewife will only eventually recognize some of the technical problems that may confront her, the dietitian may be of help in assisting the housewife in menu planning—at least in the beginning.

IMPLICATIONS

THERAPEUTIC

Nutrition can significantly support radiation therapy and decrease morbidity and mortality, and improve the quality of life of patients in the various stages of their disease. To be most useful, the registered dietitian must be aware of the possible specific complications of therapy.

Numerous positive suggestions may be made to the patient to increase nutritional intake. Because of the increasing anorexia as the day progresses, nutritious breakfasts and morning snacks before treatment are important (Simon, 1975; Hegedus and Pelham, 1975). A program of between-meal supplemental feedings should be initiated at the beginning of the treatment period; this will develop a "cushion" and training for later problems. Specific behaviors which may stimulate mealtime and snack eating should be discussed with the patient. The patient should be encouraged to maintain an adequate supply of nutritious snack foods in his home; foods could be stored in attractive see-through containers to provide visual stimulus. Patients should be encouraged to suggest items for the family shopping list and, if possible, to participate in food shopping. Meals should be associated with pleasantries; family members should be discouraged from attempting to coerce the patient into eating, since this may result in an unpleasant mealtime milieu and may further interfere with the patient's eating behavior. Meals should appear as normal as possible (McCarthy and Leventhal, 1959), especially for those patients who have high social needs. Anderson (1974) contends that the patient should choose the food, and then the texture modifications should be made. Further, association with others with similar problems may increase intake through encouragement, empathy, support, and observation (Knisely, 1975; Hegedus and Pelham, 1975).

The variety proffered in a cafeteria or restaurant may enhance nutritional intake. Patients, especially those with disfigurement, may not wish to appear in public. They may be observed attempting to hide their disfigurement, or even their treatment markings, with scarves, turtleneck sweaters, and so on. These patients should be given psychological support and be encouraged to function as normally as possible; this will probably increase their self-sufficiency and their intake.

For those patients experiencing hypogeusia or dysgeusia, the use of cold snacks high in protein may be beneficial. Examples are ice cream, gelatin salad with cottage cheese or cream cheese, and nuts and nut butters. The use of fruits may increase the visual, flavor, and texture appeal of such protein-rich desserts as ice cream milkshakes, puddings, and custards. Those patients being treated with monoamine oxidase inhibitors, however, should be cautioned against the use of foods high in tyramine and other pressor amines (Mayer, 1971a). Odors also may be used to stimulate appetite in some patients (DeWys, 1972; McCarthy-Leventhal, 1959; Shils, 1972), especially when severe hypogeusia is evident. However, some odors may nauseate patients, effecting an aversion to food.

If weight loss continues during therapy, commercial supplements with added vitamins and minerals or with elemental properties may be encouraged. The patient's financial and living arrangements must be recognized before any recommendations are made. If this program is ineffective in preventing further weight loss, intubation may be necessary. It must be recognized that intubation interrupts the normal process of food intake with its social and emotional satisfactions; Polunsky (1973) contends that service that includes some identifiable foods, such as juices or coffee, in addition to the tube-feeding formula, may engender positive psychological reactions in some patients. It cannot be overemphasized that the dietitian must be flexible not only in his approaches but also in his recommendations; that is, the psychological need for simultaneous oral intake while intubated may over a short period outweigh the possible negative physical results; also, an occasional salty cracker eaten by a patient on a low sodium regimen may do less harm than insistence against its ingestion. Encouragement and sincere professional concern must be evident to both the patient and his family.

When the patient has completed the treatment course, the dietitian should explain the anticipated progress and possible complications; texture modification may be necessary. Since the home situation will constantly change, patients should be encouraged to contact the dietitian as the need arises.

Further, with the passage of time and the accumulation of data, the dietitian should begin to observe patterns of food preference. For the individual patient, a list of foods tolerated during treatment may prove helpful in subsequent treatment courses. Food-preference responses recorded at various stages of treatment may statistically afford the dietitian insight into possible causative mechanisms or patterns and may offer useful information in later interviews. It is especially important to observe possible metabolic interfaces that may coincide with poor eating behavior. Only when such data are available can positive and accurate organized attempts be made to systematize the analysis of the aberrations of patient ingestion.

ORGANIZATIONAL

One of the most stressful aspects of radiation therapy is the waiting room experience. Here the patient is faced with other patients of varying ages, stages of disease, and degrees of disability. In general, the concept of a separate area for the severely ill and scheduling them at the end of the day when the facility is least congested may be desirable. The sensitivity of the professional staff to the needs of the waiting patients and their families is important to morale.

A separate area should be provided for the dietitian for his interviews with patients and for his storage of teaching tools and records. During scheduled interviews, in a relaxed atmosphere free from the constant activity of the clinic waiting rooms, the patient will discuss his problems more freely. Availability and continuity of nutritional care is essential. Optimally, the same dietitian should provide the necessary care during the in-patient and out-patient periods. Not only will this engender a higher quality of specialized care, but the patient will be more able to identify with a particular person as his dietitian. Once rapport is established with one registered dietitian, it is logical to reinforce and continue the association if at all possible. Patients should be interviewed repeatedly and their progress discussed with them to gain optimal patient participation in his nutritional support (Schwartz, 1975).

The dietitian also must actively participate in planning clinics and conferences; unrecognized needs may be identified early. Adequate exposure of physicians, nurses, and caseworkers to the role of the dietitian and the information utilized by the dietitian may assist, through interaction, in the assessment of the patient's emotional and physical capabilities and needs. With increasingly good working relationships with the dietitian, the physician and other professionals will come to appreciate the importance of conveying to the dietitian clues about the personality of the patient, clues that it may have demanded many hours of patient contact to discover. Further, it devolves upon the registered dietitian to develop the working relationship with the physician so that instead of saying, "Stop in and see Mr. Jones, the dietitian, and he will give you your diet," the physician will realize the psychological impact and importance of the interpretative referral and say, "Now, you will need some help in assuring that you will meet your dietary needs. Mr. Jones, the dietitian, is a specialist in helping people adjust their meals to meet their health needs and will help you work out the details" (Mead, 1970). Only when this type of relationship exists can the registered dietitian provide optimal nutrition care to the cancer patient.

REFERENCES

Anderson, J.R. 1974. "Nutrition of a Cancer Patient (unpublished report)," M.D. Anderson Hospital, The Annex and Rehabilitation Center, Houston, Texas.

————. 1974a. "Psychosocial and Vocational Aspects of the Cancer Patient (an unpublished report)." M.D. Anderson Hospital, The Annex and Rehabilitation Center, Houston, Texas.

Blackburn, G.L. 1975. "Nitrogen(Protein) Metabolism in Advanced Cancer." From a paper presented at the 58th Annual Meeting of the American Dietetic Association, San Antonio, Texas (October).

Bodey, G.P. 1970. "Supportive Care of the Cancer Patient." *Postgraduate Medicine*, 48(5): 203 (November).

Coffey, K.R. 1975. "Body Stress: Pediatric Development and Physical Disabilities and Food Intake Patterns." From a paper presented at the 58th Annual Meeting of the American Dietetic Association, San Antonio, Texas (October).

Cosper, B.A. 1975. "Interrelationship Between Stress and Food Intake Patterns." From a paper presented at the 58th Annual Meeting of the American Dietetic Association, San Antonio, Texas (October).

Coster, B.A. and L.M. Wakefield. 1975. "Food Choices of Women." *Journal of the American Dietetic Association*, 66(2):152+ (February).

Costa, G. 1973. "Cachexia and the Systemic Effects of Tumors." In F. James and E. Frei (eds.), *Cancer Medicine*, Philadelphia: Lea and Febiger, 1035-1044.

DeWys, W.D. 1974. "Abnormalities of Taste As a Remote Effect of a Neoplasm." *Annals of the New York Academy of Sciences*, 230:427+ (March 18).

————. Undated. "Cachexia-anorexia." Unpublished report. Northwestern Medical School, Chicago, Illinois.

————. 1972. "Working Conference on Anorexia and Cachexia of Neoplastic Disease." In *Nutrition and Cancer*. American Cancer Society, 36-40.

Dudrick, S.J. and E.M. Copeland. 1974. "Nutritional Concepts in Head and Neck Cancer." In *Neoplasia of Head and Neck*, Chicago: Year Book Medical Publishers, Inc., 329.

Gailani, S. et al. 1973. "Nutritional Approaches to Cancer Therapy." In F. James and E. Frei (eds.). *Cancer Medicine*, Philadelphia: Lea and Febiger, 872-888.

Goodhart, R.S. and M.E. Shils. 1973. *Modern Nutrition in Health and Disease*, 5th edition. Philadelphia: Lea and Febiger, 984.

Hegedus, S. and M. Pelham. 1975. "Dietetics in a Cancer Hospital." *Journal of the American Dietetic Association*, 67(3):235+ (September).

Henkin, R.I. et al. 1971. "Idiopathic Hypogeusia with Dysgeusia, Hyposmia, and Dysosmia." *Journal of the American Medical Association*, 217(4):434+ (July 26).

Hickey, R.C. 1974. In *Neoplasia of Head and Neck*, Chicago: Year Book Medical Publishers, Inc., 312.

Kaufman, M. 1970. "Expanding Opportunities in the Practice of Diet Therapy." In D. Turner, *Handbook of Diet Therapy*, 5th ed., Chicago: The University of Chicago Press, 141-152.

Knisely, W.H. 1975. "The Food Patterns of Friends." From a paper presented at the 58th Annual Meeting of The American Dietetic Association, San Antonio, Texas (October).

Kranholdt, U. 1974. "Psychologische Aspekte der Diatberatung." *Praxis*, 63(9):1172+.

Latham, M.C. 1975. "Nutrition and Infection in National Development." *Science*, 188(4188): 561+ (May 9).

Manning, M.S. 1965. "The Psychodynamics of Dietetics." *Nursing Outlook*, 13:57.

Maxwell, A. 1963. "Cachexia of Malignancy—Some Possible Factors." *The New Physician*, 12:452-456.

May, R. 1975. "Values, Myths, and Symbols." *American Journal of Psychiatry*, 132(7): 703-706 (July).

Mayer, J. 1971. "Nutrition and Cancer. 1. Problems Due Directly to Tumors and Associated Diseases." *Postgraduate Medicine,* 50:65-67 (October).

———————. 1971a. "Nutrition and Cancer. 2. Problems Caused by Drugs, Radiation, and Surgery." *Postgraduate Medicine,* 50:57-59 (November).

Mead, M. 1970. "Interviewing the Patient." In D. Turner, *Handbook of Diet Therapy,* 5th ed., Chicago: The University of Chicago Press, 127+.

Meinhart, N. 1968. "The Cancer Patient: Living in the Here and Now." *Nursing Outlook,* 16:64-69.

McCarthy-Levanthal, E.M. 1959. "Post-radiation Mouth Blindness." *Lancet,* 2:1138+.

Murray, R.L.E. 1972. "Principles of Nursing Intervention for the Adult Patient with Image Changes." *Nursing Clinics of North America,* 7(4):697+ (December).

Noone, R.B. and W.P. Graham. 1973. "Nutritional Care After Head and Neck Surgery." *Postgraduate Medicine,* 53(7):80+ (June).

Nutrition Program Starts to Zero in on Mass of Data, Plan Contract and Grant Project Areas. *The Cancer Letter,* 1(35):6 (August 1).

O'Brien, M.S. 1975. "Prejudice and Dietary Counseling." *Aviation Space Environmental Medicine,* 46(2):209 (February).

Pareira, M.D. et al. 1955. "Clinical Response and Changes in Nitrogen Balance, Body Weight, Plasma Proteins, and Hemoglobin Following Tube Feeding in Cancer Cachexia." *Cancer,* 8:803+.

Polunsky, B. and M. Pelham. 1973. "Feeding Head and Neck Patients Undergoing Radiation Therapy." In G.H. Fletcher, *Textbook of Radiotherapy,* 2nd ed., Philadelphia: Lea and Febiger, 152-156.

Quint, J.C. 1965. "Institutionalized Practices of Information Control." *Psychiatry,* 28:119-132.

Research Opportunities in Diet, Nutrition Program Outlined. *The Cancer Letter,* 1(28):3+ (July 11).

Rubini, M.S. 1974. "Flavor." *American Journal of Clinical Nutrition,* 27:233+.

Sallan, S.E. et al. 1975. "Antiemetic Effect of Delta-9-tetrahydrocannabinol in Patients Receiving Cancer Chemotherapy." *New England Journal of Medicine,* 293(16):795+ (October 16).

Schafer, R. and E.A. Yetley. 1975. "Social Psychology of Food Faddism."*Journal of the American Dietetic Association,* 66(2):129 (February).

Schmale, A.H. "Principles of Psychosocial Oncology." In P. Rubin (ed.), *Clinical Oncology for Medical Students and Physicians,* 4th ed., Rochester, New York: The University of Rochester School of Medicine and the American Cancer Society, 109-118.

Schwartz, I.S. 1975. "Dietary Management of Advanced Cancer Patients Undergoing Treatment: A Preliminary Report." From a paper presented at the 58th Annual Meeting of The American Dietetic Association, San Antonio, Texas (October).

Shils, M.S. 1972. "Nutritional and Dietary Factors in Neoplastic Development." In *Nutrition and Cancer.* American Cancer Society, 1-9; 10-17.

Simon, J. et al. 1975. "Nutritional Aspects of Cancer Rehabilitation." *Cancer Rehabilitation Newsletter,* 1(2):1 (March).

———————. Undated. "Recommendations for Providing an Appealing, Adequate Diet for the Cancer Patient Receiving 5-fluorouracil." Based on a research project at the University of Wisconsin Center for Health Sciences, Madison, Wisconsin.

Stedman's Medical Dictionary, 22nd ed. 1972. Baltimore: William and Wilkins, Co., 76, 188.

Theologides, A. 1972. "Pathogenesis of Cachexia in Cancer." *Cancer,* 29(2):484+ (February).

Tobias, A. and J. Goodman. 1972. "Psychosocial Seminar for Dietitians." *Journal of the American Dietetic Association,* 61(6):675 (December).

Walike, B.C. 1975. "Nasogastric Tube Feedings: The Nursing Perspective." *Dietetic Current,* (Ross Labs), 2(5): 1-4 (November-December).

Williams, S.R. 1973. *Nutrition and Diet Therapy,* 2nd edition. St. Louis: C.V. Mosby Co., 251-265.

PSYCHOSOCIAL ASPECTS OF RADIATION THERAPY

Omar M. Salazar, Margaret Dunne, and
Marjorie Sugarman

Radiotherapy is one of three basic methods used in treating cancer. It is used both by itself and in combination with the other two leading treatments: surgery and chemotherapy. The technical aspects of radiation are quite complex and extensively reported in the numerous scientific journals. Equally important, but not as well reported, are the psychosocial aspects of radiation therapy: how a person reacts to receiving this treatment for a malignancy and how this therapy affects the members of his family. The individual's attitude during treatment is of critical importance to the outcome of that treatment. It is therefore the purpose of this chapter to examine this very important but often neglected aspect of radiation therapy.

How a person reacts to radiation therapy is dependent upon a number of factors:

1) present emotional status
2) preconceived ideas concerning this modality of treatment
3) doctor-patient and staff-patient relationships
4) the reactions of the family members and close friends
5) the patient's own perceptions during therapy

The mere mention of radiation (cancer) therapy implies both to the patient and his family that there is a serious medical condition that is of greater concern than any ordinary illness. It also implies for the patient the reality of his condition. When a patient's tumor is first diagnosed, he often goes through a period of denial; when therapy for his condition is discussed, he suddenly confronts the full impact of his illness. The patient, therefore, begins his treatments in a state of extreme anxiety and stress. Simultaneously, he has to deal with the knowledge of his disease and the unfamiliarity and uncertainty of the treatment process.

The words "radiation" and "radioactivity" are beyond the ordinary individual's experience and understanding. The only exposure that the average patient has had to the terms in radiotherapy is from such sources as science fiction, the press reports concerning the aftermath of Hiroshima and Nagasaki, or the environmentalists' attacks on the dangers of nuclear reactors. Most available information concerns the harmful rather than the beneficial aspects of radiation. Some patients learn of what the process entails from friends and family members who have known someone treated by radiation. These second- and third-hand reports can be misleading and misinformative for the patient. Until some type of public education program to explain the radiotherapy process and its benefits is instituted, it becomes the duty of the physician, nurses, and social workers to untangle preconceived erroneous ideas and begin the journey toward a proper understanding of the condition, its treatment, and its prognosis.

A person's preconceived ideas and present psychosocial state can dramatically affect the way he perceives the initial treatment procedure. Sidney Page wrote about his views as a radiotherapy patient; he described his first exposure as follows:

> I was struck by the extreme bareness of the chamber. Its one feature was an enormous bomber-like object, of which my rotable couch formed the propeller. . . . A high-pitched noise penetrated my brain as the light intensity increased. I felt a glowing warmth inside my head. It was worse than pain, this manifestation of unfamiliar power (Page, 1970).

The actual treatment does not hurt, but the anticipation can be unbearable. The mystery of the treatment is accentuated by the fact that there is nothing to see, hear or feel to indicate what is happening (Schmale, 1974). Page (1970) emphasized the importance of a preparatory talk between the patient and the doctor before treatments begin so as to allay any misconceptions that may have formed. This indeed becomes a moral duty for the doctor and staff and is, in fact, no more than the knowledge one would like to have before entering any unfamiliar and unknown situation. It must be clearly understood that at the onset of therapy, the cancer patient not only is directly confronted with the reality of his disease but is also scared by the possibility of its spread, the effect of treatment, and the final outcome.

These fears and misconceptions concerning radiation therapy can interfere with the patient's progress during treatment. In a study based on 152 patients, only two improved despite negative attitudes; in the remaining 150 patients their condition correlated with their degree of participation and attitudes toward treatment (Bolen, 1973). Bolen proposed the use of meditation and psychotherapy as a means of improving the individual's attitude; his method combined relaxation exercises and visualization of peaceful scenes. The effectiveness of supportive hypnotherapy during radiation treatments has been emphasized by others (Dempster et al., 1976). Hypnosis was found useful both in alleviating the discomforts that may result as side effects of radiation and in providing a nonthreatening environment in which to deal with issues posed by the disease.

The relationship between the doctor and the patient is another factor influencing the patient's psychological state. As mentioned earlier, the patient is generally extremely apprehensive and worried when he begins treatment for his disease. It is important for the doctor-patient relationship to be one in which the patient feels free to communicate his feelings. "A warm, protective relationship between doctor and patient minimizes many emotional problems and therapeutic management is expedited when the doctor is aware of possible sources of anxiety impinging upon the patient" (Cobb, 1959).

Because of his skill and knowledge, the doctor becomes an authority figure for the patient. Because the doctor holds this trusted position, he is the best one to dispel misconceptions concerning radiotherapy. He must be sensitive to the patient's fears and work to counteract them. Many people regard radiotherapy as a "last resort only to be tried when all else has failed and having little or nothing to offer of a curative nature" (Harper, 1973). If time is taken to explain to the patient what can be accomplished by radiotherapy and why it is important to the patient's particular case, feelings of hopelessness can be dispelled. The doctor must, however, also prepare the patient for adverse side effects likely to be encountered. When a patient has completed his first treatment session, he is often relieved and even encouraged because the treatment was relatively painless. Even though it is tempting to let the patient remain in this optimistic state, it is important for the doctor to inform the patient as to what side effects he might experience eventually and how to cope with them. If the patient is not prepared and suddenly begins to feel ill, he is likely to become resentful and bitter toward the doctor and the treatment (Harper, 1973). Ashbury (1973) mentions three basic models of doctor-patient relationship appropriate for patients undergoing radiation therapy:

1) activity-passivity
2) guidance-compliance
3) mutual participation

The first model, activity-passivity, implies that the doctor is the active force and the patient is the passive recipient. This model generally applies in cases involving intracavitary or interstitial radiation, during which radioactive elements are implanted while the patient is anesthetized. The patient is completely dependent on the physician for his well-being; he has no control over his situation. The second model, guidance-compliance, calls for the doctor to act as an authority figure, telling the patient what to do. The patient will follow the doctor's advice if he wishes to improve. This model is commonly utilized with patients who come for frequent radiation treatments. Instructions and advice that can affect numerous areas of the patient's life and condition are given. Mutual-participation is the third model which postulates that the doctor will help the patient to help himself.

> The woman who has undergone a radiologic menopause or received a lasting skin reaction may need more than hasty reassurance or tranquilizing pills to

adapt to her body image. The patient with Hodgkin's disease, leukemia or recurrent metastases will have an indefinite need of palliative radiation therapy and a sound relationship with his doctor. These, and many others, are the people who need and profit from mutual-participation (Ashbury, 1973).

Ashbury emphasized the importance of a doctor's being aware of all three models and being able to adapt the appropriate one according to the specific needs of the individual. Regardless of which model is used, the doctor and his medical team should give the patient as much support, encouragement, and practical help as possible.

The patient's relationship with his family during this crisis period is another factor influencing his response to radiotherapy. Patients undergoing radiotherapy often perceive their family life to be disrupted. First of all, they are often removed from their productive life and either placed or brought daily into the unaccustomed world of the hospital and radiation center. Separation from family and normal routine can result in feelings of isolation and uselessness. This is a period of frustration and boredom for men who are accustomed to daily work. They begin to worry that they will not be able to continue to provide financially for their family. This worry can become a source of great anxiety. Women worry that they cannot care for their families as they should. If a woman is receiving treatment with radioactive implants, she must go through long periods of time without seeing her children (Harper, 1973). This prolonged separation tends to increase her anxiety and concern. Both men and women feel they are unable to cope with their responsibilities and thus feel guilty about their inadequacies.

Patients who are treated with radium insertions have more restricted visiting regulations. These restrictions often convey, to the patient and the visitor, a possibility of dangerous exposure if one gets too close to the radiated patient. The patient wants to see her family but at the same time fears exposing them to possibly harmful radiation. The family also wishes to visit the patient but has some fears of radiation. Wolfgang (1973) observed this approach-avoidance behavior toward radiated persons in 14 formerly irradiated cancer patients and 14 nonradiated controls. He found that both the formerly irradiated subjects and the nonradiated control projected more social distance between themselves and a radiated patient than between themselves and a normal patient. Questioning these subjects revealed that they avoided the radiated patient because they were uncertain concerning radiation effects and feared danger from contact. This avoidance behavior can have a serious psychological impact on the patient and the family. The patient begins to feel rejected, and the family feels guilty over their desire to avoid contact. Members of the family perceive their behavior to be selfish—being more concerned with their own well-being—thus increasing their guilt reaction. At times such as this, the doctor must intervene and explain to the patient and the family exactly what dangers are involved and what precautions are necessary.

The patient needs support and encouragement from the family during this period in his life. How much he will receive depends largely on the degree of homeostasis found in the family nucleus during this period of diagnosis and treatment. Applying casework skills, the social worker can offer the patient and the family the opportunity to handle critical issues in a beneficial way. As in any major illness, there are necessary role adaptions to be made within the family structure itself. The social worker must help the members remain involved with the patient while helping each person maintain his individuality in facing the realities of the disease.

Family members often become overprotective and overattentive, and this overprotection may hasten regression in a way antithetical to treatment. Dependence is difficult to adjust to for a person who is accustomed to self-sufficiency and caring for others. The patient often becomes depressed and hostile over this need for dependency. Often the most effective rehabilitation of the patient is through the restoration of some degree of self-sufficiency. The patient's attitude will improve significantly if he feels that he is an active force in his treatment. In summary, a delicate balance in the patient's family relationship must be achieved whereby the family provide the needed support and encouragement without becoming overprotective and overattentive.

The patient needs extra support—from the doctor, staff and family—toward the end of his radiotherapy. The results of the therapy are usually unknown and the future is uncertain. "As the patient nears the end of his course of therapy, he again becomes apprehensive and begins wondering what is going to happen to him now. Sometimes, he believes this is the beginning of the end" (Yonke, 1967). A patient has to wait for a period of five to ten years before he can consider himself to be cured and capable of living a normal life. This can be a tense period for the patient and his family. The doctor and his team must continue to keep close watch on the patient. The after-care is as important as the diagnostic tests or the treatment itself.

Complications may be expected in some instances. These can be mild side effects such as epilation and tanning of the skin, diarrhea, or difficulty in swallowing; moderate, such as pneumonitis, cystitis, and nephritis; and severe such as myelopathy, fibrosis, and necrosis. These complications depend on the size of the field, the total dose given, and the location and accuracy of the previous treatments delivered. Unless the patient and his family were warned beforehand of the possible occurrence of such symptoms, they may be misinterpreted then as being signs of recurrent disease. The anxiety builds up until the next follow-up visit. When symptoms are labelled as radiation complications, the anxiety connected with the fear of recurrence may be converted into bitterness and lack of confidence in the physician and the staff. A complete disruption of the doctor-patient and staff-patient and family relationship may occur, which will endanger the adequate follow-up of the patient.

If signs of recurrence do occur at some point during the follow-up period, the patient will experience a new set of psychological reactions, often more distressing than those evident when the cancer was first diagnosed. The situation looks more hopeless than ever for the patient as he considers the virulence of the disease and the inadequacies of the previous treatment and the decreased likelihood of being cured.

Therapy first aims to produce remission; in later stages it is redirected to the relief of pain. "Most patients are biologically aware of the irreversible and progressive nature of their disease when it reaches this stage, whether it has been discussed and explained to them or not" (Schmale, 1974). Thinking of death in the unknown future may not impose any great stress; when that threat is imminent, great stress is evident. The physician and family must help the individual to deal with his prognosis. Patients who have to receive palliative treatment will gradually accept their dependence on the radiotherapist. The radiotherapist must concentrate on the patient's immediate needs and problems. The here and now becomes the important issue. The radiation therapy is aimed at keeping the patient as free of pain as possible during his last days.

The psychosocial impact of radiotherapy is intense from beginning to end. Unfamiliarity, uncertainty, and misunderstandings act to enhance the patient's anxiety as he starts therapy. During the treatment, the patient often experiences unpleasant side effects. He must learn to cope with the disruption that the treatment poses in his life style and that of his family. At the end of the treatment phase, he is uncertain and apprehensive about his future. Each person reacts differently to radiotherapy, and it is the duty of the physician and staff to be sensitive to his patient's feelings. The staff must work to make the patient feel as relaxed and confident about the treatment as possible so that the treatment will have its maximum effect.

REFERENCES

Ashbury, H.H. 1973. "Psychiatric Problems in Patients Undergoing Radiation Therapy." *American Journal of Roentgenology,* 83:571-574.
Bolen, J. 1973. "Meditation and Psychotherapy in the Treatment of Cancer." *Psychic,* 4: 19-22.
Cobb, B. 1959. "Emotional Problems of Adult Cancer Patients." *Journal of the American Geriatric Society,* 7:274.
Dempster, C.P., P. Balson, and B. Whalen. 1976. "Supportive Hypnotherapy During the Radical Treatment of Malignancies." *International Journal of Clinical Experimental Hypnosis,* 24:1-9.
Harper, P.M. 1973. "Radiotherapy and the Patient." *Radiography,* 39:257-261.
Page, S. 1970. "A Patient's View of Radiotherapy." *Radiography,* 36:277.
Schmale, A. 1974. "Principles of Psychosocial Oncology." In P. Rubin, ed., *Clinical Oncology for Medical Students: A Multidisciplinary Approach,* New York: American Cancer Society, IVth edition, pp. 109-118.
Wolfgang, A. 1973. "Projected Social Distances as a Measure of Approach-Avoidance Behavior Toward Radiated Figures." *Journal of Community Psychology,* 1:226-228.
Yonke, G. 1967. "Emotional Response to Radiotherapy." *Hospital Topics,* 45:107-108.

PATIENT REACTIONS TO CANCER DIAGNOSIS AND TREATMENT

Carlos A. Perez, Laurie Braun, Lily A. Hanes, and Nell Sedransk

The interrelationship of cancer and the patient is complex, involving a variety of factors (Figure 1). Whether therapy consists of surgery, irradiation, chemotherapy, or combinations, the outcome is influenced by the patient's psychological and behavioral attitudes, as well as the biological history of the tumor, and the effectiveness of the therapeutic strategy. For a long time attempts have been made to link psychological disorders and stressful situations in life with the appearance and biological behavior of cancer (Brown, 1966; Goldfarb et al., 1967). Galen is reported to have noted that "cancer was more frequent in melancholic than in sanguine women," and in the eighteenth and nineteenth centuries some physicians maintained that depression and life stresses played a role in the etiology of cancer (LeShan and Worthington, 1956). Some authors have reported a significant correlation between unstable or depressed personalities and the appearance of malignant tumors (Blumberg et al., 1954; Brown, 1966; LeShan and Worthington, 1956). Some prognostic factors could be neurovegetative mechanisms linked to the nervous and psychic spheres of the patient. Parkes (1974) stated that "the invisible psychological wounds of cancer are a key to the successful treatment of patients afflicted with the disease." These often silent sources of suffering, derived from a host of determinants, influence the entire course of the illness and often present the clinician with frustrating problems in management (Bard, 1966). Thus, it is conceivable that the psychological and behavioral attitudes of a patient may have repercussions on the biological behavior of the tumor and the response to therapy.

However, the main emphasis of our paper is not on this concept, but on the reactions of the patient to the diagnosis and treatment of cancer. Blumberg et al. (1954) suggested that there is a correlation between the psychological characteristics of the patient and the prognosis; they stated that patients with

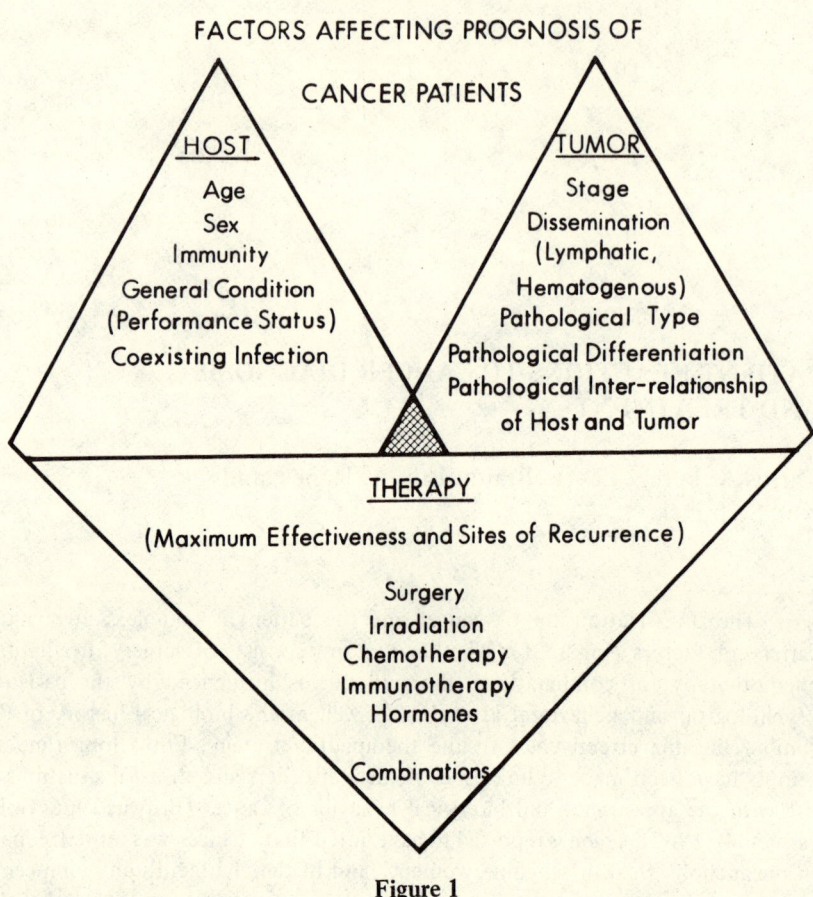

Figure 1

rapid tumor growth are consistently serious, overcooperative, overanxious, and painfully sensitive, had a dependent personality, and found it extremely difficult to release anxiety and tension. Theoretically, this would support, on a scientific, as well as on a psychological and humanitarian basis, the need for intensified behavioral intervention in the case of cancer patients, to assist them in coping with the diagnosis, adjusting to the therapy and reducing their anxiety about the prognosis and fear of death.

REACTION TO DIAGNOSIS AND NEED FOR THERAPY

Perennially the word "cancer" has wakened an unjustified attitude of terror and despair in many patients on whom the diagnosis is made and in others who have had unsavory experiences with relatives or associates who have suffered from the disease. Unfortunately, this fear has interfered not only with early diagnosis but also with the prompt treatment that could yield a higher probability of cure. At the present time, with improved anticancer therapeutic strategies involving surgery, radiation therapy, chemotherapy, or combinations of these modalities, it is critical that we modify these attitudes, so that patients will seek advice and treatment at early phases of tumor development, when prognosis in many instances is excellent.

It is unfortunate that many physicians still have a defeatist attitude toward cancer therapy and fail to instill an optimistic outlook in patients when cancer is diagnosed. Also, physicians very often tend to approach a patient as a medical entity rather than as a person with a myriad of psychological reactions and needs. Although physicians do receive some training in psychology or psychiatry, they generally fail to perceive the need for active involvement with the emotional necessities of the patients and their relatives because of an excessive clinical load or ingrained attitudes. Often, too, lacking the methodology to cope with the patient's anxiety and fear, they may be unable to provide the psychological support that the patients and family will require throughout the treatment and later in the posttherapy phases of rehabilitation.

With the present emphasis on the patient's rights and informed consent, the practice of not informing the patient of the diagnosis is disappearing. A physician's honestly concerned and sincerely optimistic outlook regarding the proposed therapy and the prognosis will enhance the patient's ability to cope with the situation; such an attitude is certainly far more helpful than if the physician seems indifferent, unsure, or frankly pessimistic (Clark, 1976).

When the diagnosis of cancer is disclosed to the patient, there is a natural reaction of disbelief and sometimes anger and denial, frequently followed by depression. However, in most instances there is a gradual acceptance of reality, with progressive adaptation to the demands of the therapy and hope for a successful outcome. Patients are often referred to specialized centers, remotely situated from their home and familiar environment; this increases their psychological stress and feeling of abandonment and of loneliness.

According to Peck (1972) the most frequent response to the diagnosis of cancer is anxiety. Depression is also common, the patients feeling sad and losing interest in their usual pursuits. Guilt was evident in 18 of 50 patients interviewed (36 percent); these patients felt that their own actions had caused the cancer to develop. The behavior they believed to be causative was not related to health care abuse such as smoking, but rather to the deaths of parents or to sexual acts. Overt anger at having cancer was observed in 22 patients (44 percent), who frequently directed their reaction to the doctors, hospital, and relatives. Fourteen of the most angry patients included 10 who were also the most anxious. Findings of aggressiveness and paranoid reaction with complex emotions surrounding the fear of death as well as simple defense mechanisms such as denial and repression, were found in more than half the patients studied by Achte and Vauhkonen (1970). Parkes (1974) described the preliminary results of a randomized study, assessing the impact of emotional and psychological support on patients with cancer and their relatives. Nineteen family members received support and were compared with 22 who received no such support. Twenty months after bereavement those who received support experienced less depression, had fewer psychosomatic symptoms and anxiety, and were less inclined to increase their consumption of alcohol, tobacco, and tranquilizers than the control group.

Although there are a number of papers on this subject, many of them fail to describe completely the methodology used for the studies, or they lack the depth to provide us with a good understanding of the interrelationships of demographic, psychological, social, and medical factors associated with cancer and psychological behavior. It is extremely important that we approach these problems methodically and separately analyze the following areas:

1. behavioral factors involving screening and early diagnosis of cancer
2. initial reaction of patient and relatives to diagnosis of cancer and therapy (shock)
3. adjustment of the patient and the physician to the therapy, immediate side effects, and post-treatment sequelae (assimilation and integration)
4. adaptation of the patient to the consequences of therapy and a realistic expectation of survival, including quality of life (redefinition of goals)
5. methods to deal with incurable disease and the terminal stages of cancer with impending death
6. interaction of the primary physician, oncologist, psychiatrist, psychologist, social worker, and nurses in dealing with the above problems of the patients.

We will try to address ourselves to the present status of the psychological management of the cancer patient in radiation therapy and what can be done to strengthen it in the future. Peck (1972) reported on 50 patients interviewed by a psychiatrist at the time of initiation of radiation therapy. All the patients had a diagnosis of cancer but only 40 (80 percent) gave their correct diagnosis. More important, these 40 patients had not been told of the diagnosis by their own physicians. Peck concluded that physicians must be in touch with their own feelings about patients, their reactions to the disease, to treatment, and to the role of physicians in the treatment of patients with cancer. A physician who is anxious and frustrated in working with cancer patients will be unable to perceive and deal with his own emotional reactions to the disease; the physician may then defend himself by unconscious aloofness or by a rigid technical management of the patient. At times, this anxiety leads the physician to empty words, circumlocution, omissions, and untruths when trying to talk to the cancer patient (Hayes, 1976). As stated by Stehlin and Beach (1966), the relationship of oncologists with their patients should be open and honest and "sustained by hope within the framework of reality." At the time of diagnosis of cancer the physician should be careful in relating this to the patient and explaining the procedures necessary for workup, the type of therapy that is planned, the sequelae of the treatment, and the anticipated prognosis. The physician should appear sympathetic, sure of the diagnosis and the therapy, and must always maintain a note of optimism.

Because of the multidisciplinary framework of cancer therapy, specialists in other oncological disciplines should be consulted, and they should follow the same general psychological approach to the patient. The unknown forthcoming events facing the cancer patient are manifold, and may cause anxieties, ranging from the fear of dying, disfigurement or pain to other facts such as fear of unemployment, loss of income and financial threat, the possibility of losing family support and social status, and apprehension about the inability to recover and achieve complete rehabilitation with return to full time work after the treatment. The social worker and properly trained nurses will be invaluable in assisting the medical staff in establishing a successful relationship with patients and their relatives.

Even though it is accepted that the primary physician should assume a major role in dealing with the psychological aspects of the cancer patient, the radiation oncologist should become a major source of assurance and confidence for the patient because of the length of their interaction and the patient's anxiety concerning radiation therapy and its side effects. Parents of ill children many times react with an even greater degree of anxiety than the patient and often exhibit extreme grief. At the same time a sympathetic parent can provide immeasurable emotional support to a child requiring treatment for cancer.

Fedor (1966) published a short review summarizing some of the reactions of patients referred for radiation therapy and their understanding of the diagnosis and the radiation treatments. He advocates telling the patient the truth about the disease and prognosis and points out the need to prevent patients from developing a feeling of isolation or rejection.

Radiation therapy is generally not a familiar therapeutic modality to most patients and is poorly understood by many physicians. Patients assume that it is used only for cancer treatment, and their experience with it often is that it was used for somebody they knew who eventually died of the disease. The complex and massive pieces of therapy equipment make the initial experience even more frightening. The fact that the patient is placed on the treatment couch and left unattended in the treatment room while treatment is being delivered increases anxiety. Contributing to the psychological unrest of the patient is the revelation or expectation that side effects may result from the therapy and that, in a certain proportion of the cases, some injury to normal tissues must be expected.

It is extremely important to familiarize patients with the new environment, technical personnel, and equipment. They should be carefully informed of all therapy procedures and ramifications. Planning and delivery of radiation therapy is a complicated operation requiring multiple steps (Figure 2). All these procedures should be described so that the patient will know what to expect. In general, reassuring words and the explanation that little physical trauma or pain is involved help greatly to diminish apprehension.

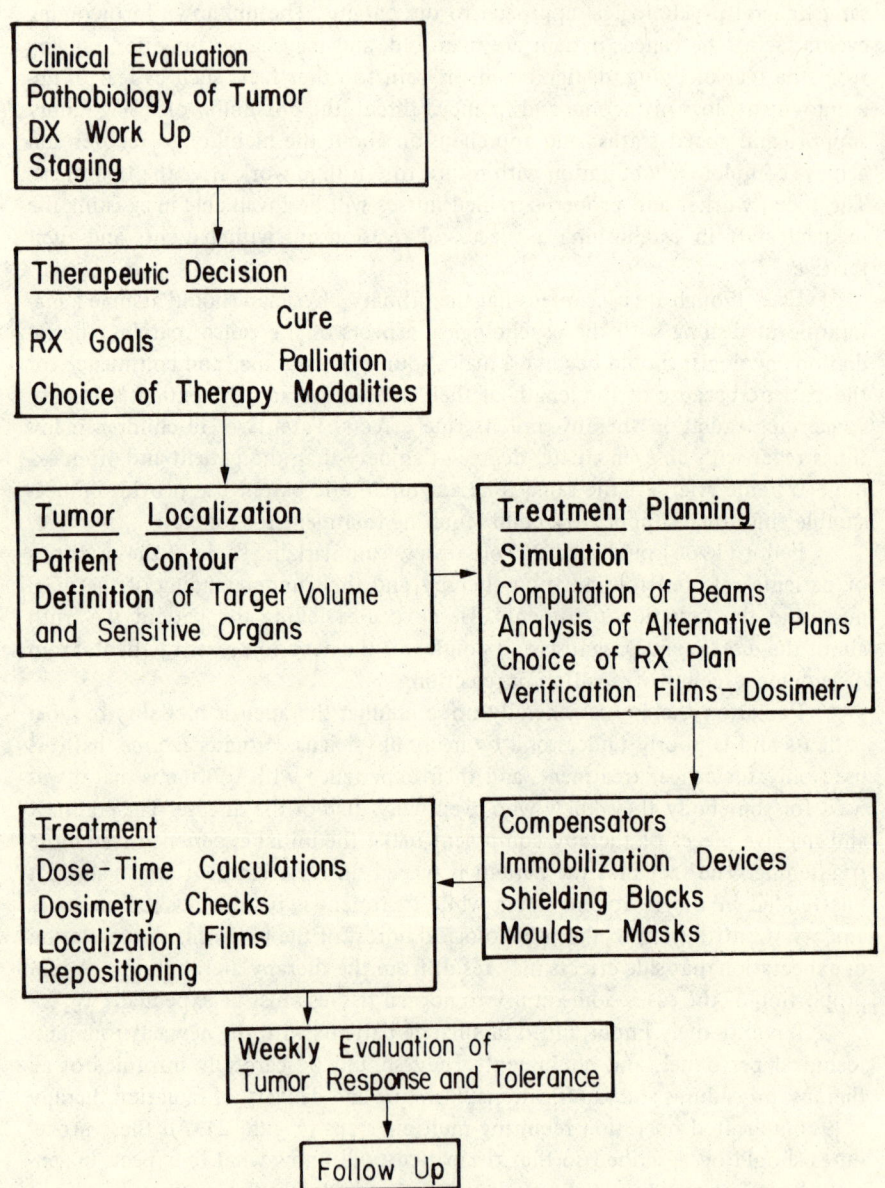

Figure 2
STEPS IN RADIATION THERAPY

During the radiation therapy the technologists and nurses should be extremely understanding and empathetic with patients, conveying to them concern for their welfare as individuals, in addition to interest in them as patients.

MATERIAL AND METHODS

In order to assess the awareness and concern of physicians or specially trained personnel such as the social worker in the area of psychosocial aspects of cancer and radiation therapy, a review of randomly chosen radiation therapy records was carried out. We carefully reviewed 125 records of patients with malignant tumors of the head and neck, lung, breast, cervix or endometrium, urinary bladder or prostate and Hodgkin's disease to identify the proportion of charts containing specific comments regarding a variety of parameters dealing with psychosocial reactions and background of the patients. At the same time, 100 records of patients who had been interviewed during the same period of time by a social worker were reviewed in the same manner. The patients were treated between January 1 and October 30, 1976, at the Division of Radiation Oncology, Mallinckrodt Institute of Radiology and St. John's Mercy Medical Center, St. Louis, Missouri.

In addition, 60 patients treated between December 1, 1976 and January 15, 1977 at the same institution were asked to fill out a detailed internally controlled questionnaire to evaluate the following parameters:

1. preconceived notions about cancer and radiation therapy
2. understanding of diagnosis, plan of treatment and prognosis
3. attitude toward technical aspects of irradiation
4. expectation of relationship with referring physician and radiation therapist
5. social and self-concept, including specific questions about anxiety, depression, and
6. family constellation and social adjustment

RESULTS

Table 1 summarizes the results of the retrospective review of randomly chosen charts. Although there was a slight variation in the concern of physicians toward some of the psychosocial aspects of the patients, the notations on the charts are significantly less frequent than those of the social worker. The social worker entered substantially more notations concerning the family environment and emotional status of the patient (95 percent vs. 5.6 percent for physicians), attitude toward other patients, diagnosis and therapy, and financial problems of the patients. The only area in which entries by the physician were found in all charts was the discussion of side effects and prognosis (100 percent), whereas this was a matter of concern to the social worker in only 24 percent of the patients.

The questionnaires to 60 patients at the initiation of radiation therapy showed that 20 admitted being nervous, sad and tearful, or frankly depressed

TABLE 1. Psychological Reaction of Patients to Radiation Therapy and Cancer

Comparison of Entries in Radiation Oncology Records

Subject	Physicians (125 Charts)		Social Worker (100 Charts)	
Family Emotional Relationship	7	5.6%	95	95%
Patient Reaction to Diagnosis	14	11.0	43	43
Attitude Toward Therapy	20	16.0	54	54
Attitude Toward Prognosis	0	0	37	37
Discussion of Side Effects and Prognosis	125	100.0	24	24
Financial Problems	2	1.6	39	39
Problems Related to Work/School	3	2.4	10	10
Medication-Psychotropic Drugs	2	1.6	3	3

TABLE 2. Psychological Reaction of Patients to Radiation Therapy and Cancer

(60 Responses

My referring doctor provided me with all the information I wanted about my illness.

	Number of Responses	%
Agree	36	60.0
Undecided	13	21.7
Disagree	10	16.7
No Response	1	1.7

My radiation therapist and/or assistant answered my questions about radiation therapy.

	Number of Responses	%
Agree	50	83.0
Undecided	3	5.0
Disagree	6	10.0
No Response	1	1.7

(33 percent) and eight stated that they were not sure about their feelings (13.3 percent). The other 53 percent of the patients definitely rejected the idea of anxiety or depression.

To the question of whether the referring physician provided adequate information concerning their diagnosis of cancer, 60 percent of the patients responded affirmatively and 21 percent were undecided. Ten patients (16.7 percent) definitely felt that they had not been properly briefed about their illness. In contrast, 50 of the patients (83 percent) felt that the radiation therapists and their staff had satisfactorily answered their questions concerning radiation therapy and the side effects and three were undecided. Only six (10 percent) thought that adequate information had not been provided (Table 2).

Fifty-five patients (91.7 percent) felt that their radiation therapist was genuinely concerned with their welfare and prognosis. Approximately half of the patients were disturbed by the disclosure of side effects of therapy and found it somewhat troubling to sign the informed consent that is routinely obtained prior to initiation of treatment at our institution (Table 3). Perhaps more detailed explanations of the complications of therapy or stressing that they happen infrequently will significantly diminish this fear of the patients.

TABLE 3. Psychological Reaction of Patients to Radiation Therapy and Cancer

(60 Responses)

Signing the treatment permit was difficult for me because it was disturbing to learn of possible side effects.

	Number of Responses	%
Agree	28	46.7
Undecided	9	15.0
Disagree	21	35.0
No Response	2	3.0

It was of interest to observe that there was some correlation between the mental status of the patient and a positive attitude toward radiation therapy. Of 17 patients who felt depressed, only 10 (58 percent) answered that they felt radiation therapy would be helpful, and the rest (41 percent) were undecided. In contrast, 24 of 28 patients (85.7 percent) who did not feel depressed were optimistic about the results to be obtained from the radiation (Table 4). This difference cannot be explained on the basis of lack of communication or poor understanding of the treatment offered, since approximately the same proportion of the patients in the depressed or not depressed group (about 70 percent) stated that they had a good idea of what could be achieved with the planned irradiation. Therefore, it appears that the mental status of a patient substantially conditions his attitude toward treatment. Also, age at the time of diagnosis seems to show some correlation, the older patients having less understanding and hope of what could be achieved with the radiation therapy (Table 5).

TABLE 4. Psychological Reaction of Patients to Radiation Therapy and Cancer
Radiation Therapy Will Be Helpful to Me.

		Agree	Undecided
I FEEL DEPRESSED	No Response	3	–
	Disagree	24/28 (85.7%)	4/29 (14%)
	Undecided	11/11 (100%)	–
	Agree	10/17 (58.8%)	7/17 (41%)

TABLE 5. Psychological Reaction of Patients to Radiation Therapy and Cancer
I Have a Good Idea of What Can Be Achieved with Radiation Therapy.

	Age–Less Than 40 (7)		Age– 40-59 (23)		Age–60+ (31)	
	Number of Responses	%	Number of Responses	%	Number of Responses	%
Agree	7	100	20	7.0	18	58.0
Undecided	–	–	2	8.7	9	29.0
Disagree	–	–	–	–	3	9.7
No Response	–	–	–	–	–	–
Other	–	–	–	–	–	–

This parameter may be related not only to the general condition of the patient, but also to the type of tumors that are more prevalent in older patients as well as to possibly a more advanced stage.

Also, 15 of 24 men (62.5 percent) felt that radiation therapy would be helpful and eight were undecided (33 percent). In contrast, 30 out of 36 women (83 percent) felt radiation therapy would be helpful to them and six (16.7 percent) were undecided. Again, this could be related to the type of illness and age at the time of diagnosis, and this difference will be further evaluated.

We realize that the results of this questionnaire are preliminary and, in most instances, the differences have no statistical validity. However, they point toward a definite attitude of the patients and some areas in which the radiation therapist and the staff can provide great support at the initiation and during the treatment.

PRESCRIPTION FOR THE FUTURE

It is extremely important that physicians be truthful to patients and reveal as much information as they feel a patient can cope with regarding the nature of the disease and prognosis. Cancer is not only a fascinating biological process and a threatening personal disease, but also it has a very interesting cluster of behavioral and psychosocial ramifications that need to be carefully incorporated into the management programs of this disease.

The physician must be careful to restrain feelings of anger or frustration because, for example, the patient did not seek therapy sooner or was antagonistic at the time of the interview. An effort must be made to avoid a cold, impersonal professional interaction with the patient or, in the case of advanced disease, a progressive abandonment of the patient, as the physician shifts his efforts to patients who can benefit more from his skills (Clark, 1976). As Stehlin and Beach (1966) point out, the relationship of the oncologist and the patient should be open, hopeful and realistic. The authors stress that "incurability is a state of the body and hopelessness is a state of the mind" and that one can always display a hopeful attitude to the cancer patient, regardless of the ultimate prognosis.

Hayes (1976) stated that the inescapable conclusion seems to be that physicians possess and frequently demonstrate an attitude that is suboptimal in the management of cancer patients. Since it would be extremely difficult to train only those individuals who have attributes necessary for ideal cancer care, it is critical that we identify these characteristics and attempt to incorporate them in the training of all individuals concerned with cancer care. This implies that the attitude of the faculty may have to be drastically overhauled in order to encompass this prospective problem-solving approach. Also, this will require some changes in the general education of medical students, including exposure to psychology and behavioral sciences in college for applicants to medical schools, the offering of behavioral science courses or electives in the medical school curriculum, early exposure of students to patient contact, and emphasis on the psychosocial aspects of medicine. It is crucial that we help students understand their reactions toward the patients, that we assist the students and the faculty in interrelating with patients, and that we stress to the hospital and medical school administrators the need for adequate staff to deal with psychosocial aspects of medicine. In particular, oncology training programs, regardless of the discipline, should have special courses dealing with these areas and, in addition, should give the trainees the necessary resources and teaching to cope with the emotional needs of the dying patient as well as the relatives who must face this desperate situation. Besides verbal communication and informative sessions, which can be aided by audiovisual presentations, it is helpful to provide patients with written material that contains simple explanations of many of the subjects described above.

There is no question that social workers or other behavioral professional staff can be most valuable in teaching the physician how to attend to the psychoemotional and behavioral needs of the cancer patients. These counselors should

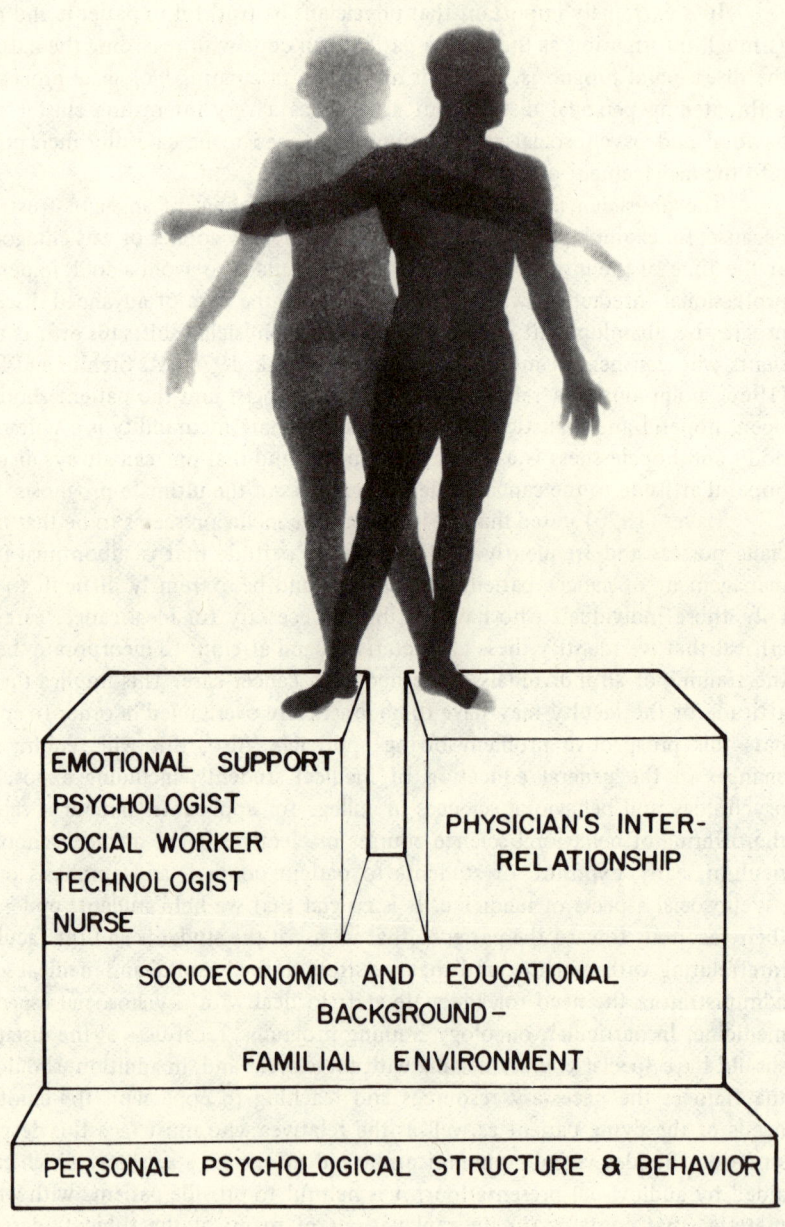

Figure 3

be familiar with some of the technical aspects of cancer and radiation therapy, so that they may provide logical and appropriate answers to some of the queries or concerns of the patients. They should also be able to advise the rest of the staff in the radiation therapy center about their relationship with the patients and some of the methods useful in dealing with day-to-day emotional support (Figure 3).

One of the best ways to familiarize the patient with possible developments is counseling by volunteers who have themselves been treated successfully for the disease and who may have some resulting anatomical or physiologic handicap. This is particularly true in patients who must have a laryngectomy, mastectomy, ileostomy, colostomy, or an amputation of an extremity.

Although it is not the specific subject of this presentation, we would like to underscore the significance of rehabilitative techniques to enhance the quality of life as an integral part of the overall management of the cancer patient. The return of the patients following treatment to a normal family, social and working life is important to rehabilitation. By definition this means the restoration of the individual to a sound state of physical, mental, and moral health through treatment and training, but technically it has numerous implications. In the rehabilitation process the following general areas must be considered:

1. the repercussions of the anatomical or physiological deficit caused by the tumor or the treatment (disfigurement or loss of function)
2. type of orthotic and prosthetic appliances or reconstructive procedures necessary to reestablish anatomical and functional integrity
3. specific rehabilitation programs (physical therapy, occupational therapy)
4. counseling and/or psychotherapy by specially trained professionals, including psychiatrists, social workers, psychologists, and nurses
5. special cooperative programs with volunteers, some of whom have previously suffered from cancer (Reach for Recovery, "ostomy" training, etc.)

Because of the individuality of the patients, the multiplicity of anatomical areas involved, and the numerous procedures and techniques involved in rehabilitation, this is an intricate area requiring a great deal of team effort, coordination, and multifaceted resources and professional support (Figure 4).

Children or old patients constitute a distinct problem population, since parents of a sick child can feel a great deal of strain stemming from the demands of their other children; stress among relatives of elderly patients who require intensive attention, care, transportation assistance, and help in every day activities also requires interventive measures. In these situations the physician's intensified counseling and stronger efforts to improve the understanding of the situation and the relationship of the parties involved are valuable.

The establishment of integrated rehabilitation programs including training for the staff and physicians is important in a cancer treatment center. Such a group should include psychiatrists, psychologists, sociologists, oncologists, social workers, nurses, rehabilitation specialists, physical therapists, and occupational

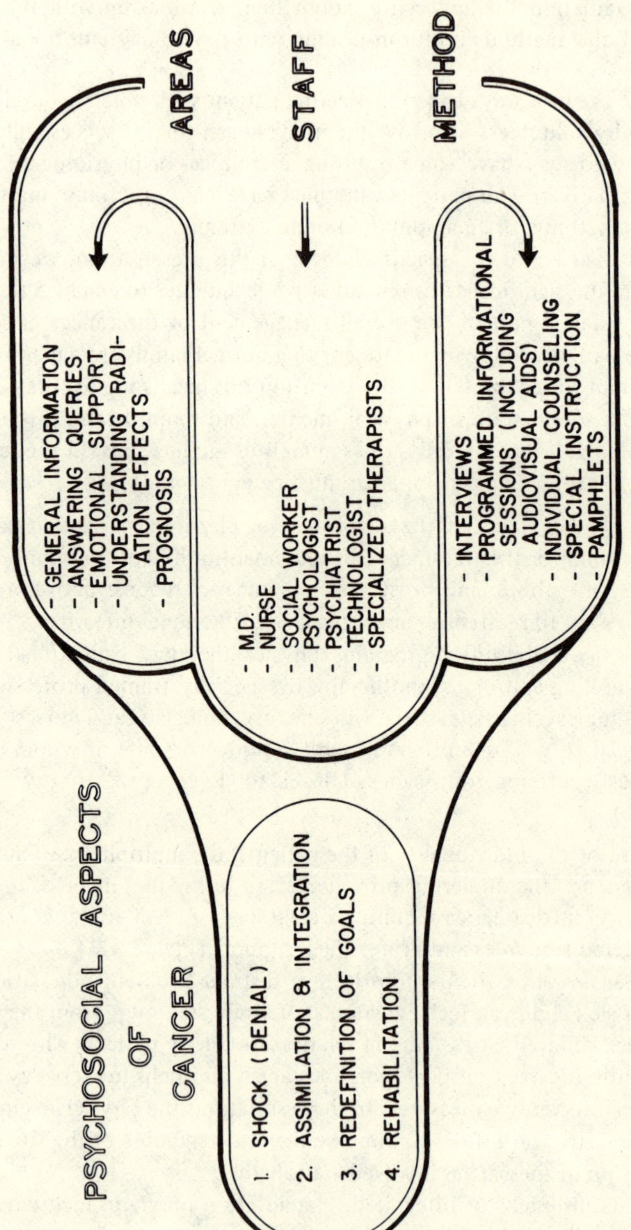

PSYCHOSOCIAL ASPECTS OF CANCER

1. SHOCK (DENIAL)
2. ASSIMILATION & INTEGRATION
3. REDEFINITION OF GOALS
4. REHABILITATION

AREAS
- GENERAL INFORMATION
- ANSWERING QUERIES
- EMOTIONAL SUPPORT
- UNDERSTANDING RADIATION EFFECTS
- PROGNOSIS

STAFF
- M.D.
- NURSE
- SOCIAL WORKER
- PSYCHOLOGIST
- PSYCHIATRIST
- TECHNOLOGIST
- SPECIALIZED THERAPISTS

METHOD
- INTERVIEWS
- PROGRAMMED INFORMATIONAL SESSIONS (INCLUDING AUDIOVISUAL AIDS)
- INDIVIDUAL COUNSELING
- SPECIAL INSTRUCTION
- PAMPHLETS

Figure 4

therapists. They will help the staff to gain insight into the complex psychosocial problems of cancer and assist the patients and relatives in accepting and adjusting to the problems of diagnosis, therapy, and rehabilitation process. It is unfortunate that there are very few institutions in the country where this type of integrated program is available.

It is not enough merely to discuss the problem; our concerns and ideas need to be translated into action. This will require an intensive effort to change prevailing biased attitudes and a vigorous and adequately financed commitment to the development and support of such programs.

MANAGEMENT OF THE TERMINAL PATIENT

Although we stated that cancer today is, in many instances, a highly curable disease, a significant proportion of patients go through an unrelenting downhill course with widespread disease, multiple organ involvement, and progressive deterioration of their general condition. Often these patients are in a severe state of depression and despair, submerged in hopelessness or self pity. If in the initial phase, at diagnosis, the cancer patient may react with denial or depression, in the terminal stages many patients develop a more realistic view of their disease and ultimately accept the perspective of unavoidable death. Often the physicians and associated health professionals react negatively to this hopeless situation and tend to abandon the patient, who then feels rejected. Hinton (1974) interviewed 60 patients receiving treatment for terminal cancer; 40 of them had some awareness of impending death and none disapproved of an open discussion of death. However, 21 patients reported little or no meaningful conversation with the medical staff concerning their illness or their prognosis.

Moreover, the patient should be given the necessary psychological support to cope with the anxiety and depression that usually appears. The relationship with relatives and associates must be strengthened, and at the same time a measured free flow of information should give all parties involved a realistic picture of what is happening. Kubler-Ross (1969) has stressed the need to assist rather than judge the patients in this trying period. She feels the patient should be told the diagnosis and prognosis by the physician, although she advocates not telling the patients that they are dying or are terminally ill. The patients need to know that they may have to "get things in order," but usually they will bring up the subject. On the other hand, the family should be told of the actual prognosis.

It must be stressed that these patients will have many uncomfortable symptoms and that palliation is one of the main goals of our therapy. As much comfort as possible should be afforded to relieve the patient of pain, distressing symptoms, and uncomfortable feelings. It is imperative to avoid the unconscious tendency to abandon the terminal patient, and physicians, assistant staff, and nurses should spare no efforts not only in delivering the best supportive medical care but also in showing a solicitous and understanding attitude.

In the presence of recurrent or metastatic cancer, and particularly if the patient follows a downhill course, the physician and associated staff can do several things to reassure the patient that their interest and concern is not diminishing. Narcotics for pain can be changed or increased and electrolyte balance corrected, efforts can be made to improve nutrition, physical therapy can be instituted if tolerated, an ulcerated lesion can be kept meticulously clean and tranquilizers may be used to reinforce the outlook of the patient (Clark, 1976). If the patient suggests it, a psychiatrist or a religious individual may provide spiritual assistance, although the physician must avoid the temptation to relegate the entire responsibility of the patient to them. The creation of hospices for the terminally ill may foster the appropriate environment and specialized and devoted teams that may contribute to the comfort and understanding of patients and their families. Finally, a great judgment and sensitivity should be exercised in not employing heroic measures that will prolong the life of a distressed and physically battered terminal cancer patient.

REFERENCES

Achte, K. and M. Vauhkonen. 1970. "Cancer and the Psyche." Monographs from the Psychiatric Clinic of the Helsinki University Central Hospital, 1.

Bard, M. 1966. "Clues to the Psychological Management of Patients with Cancer in Psychophysiological Aspects of Cancer." *Annals of the New York Academy of Sciences*, 125:995-999.

Blumberg, E.M., P.M. West and F.W. Ellis. 1954. "A Possible Relationship Between Psychological Factors and Human Cancer." *Psychosomatic Medicine*, 6:277-286.

Brown, F. 1966. "The Relationship Between Cancer and Personality in Psychophysiological Aspects of Cancer." *Annals of the New York Academy of Sciences*, 125:865-873.

Butler, M. and W. Paisley. 1976. "The Potential of Mass Communication and Interpersonal Communication for Cancer Control." In J.W. Cullen et al. (eds.), *Cancer: The Behavioral Dimensions*, New York: Raven Press, 205-229.

Clark, R.L. 1976. "Psychologic Reactions of Patients and Health Professionals to Cancer." In J.W. Cullen et al. (eds.), *Cancer: The Behavioral Dimensions*, New York: Raven Press, 1-10.

Fedor, S.L. 1966. "Psychological Considerations in the Care of Patients with Cancer in Psychophysiological Aspects of Cancer." *Annals of the New York Academy of Sciences*, 125:1020-1027.

Goldfarb, C., J. Driesen, and D. Cole. 1967. "The Psychophysical Logical Aspects of Malignancy." *American Journal of Psychiatry*, 123:1545-1552.

Hayes, D.M. 1976. "Impact of the Health Care System on Physician Attitudes and Behaviors." In J.W. Cullen et al. (eds.), *Cancer: The Behavioral Dimensions*, New York: Raven Press, 145-157.

Hinton, J. 1974. "Talking with People About to Die." *British Medical Journal*, ii:25-27.

Kubler-Ross, E. 1969. *On Death and Dying*. New York: Macmillan Company.

LeShan, L.L. and R.E. Worthington. 1956. "Personality As a Factor in the Pathogenesis of Cancer." *British Journal of Medical Psychology*, 29:40-56.

Parkes, C.M. 1974. "Comment: Communication and Cancer—A Social Psychiatrist's View." *Social Sciences in Medicine*, 8:189-190.

Peck, A. 1972. "Emotional Reactions to Having Cancer." *American Journal of Roentgenology, Radium, Therapeutic, and Nuclear Medicine*, 114:591-599.

Stehlin, J.S. and K.H. Beach. 1966. "Psychological Aspects of Cancer Therapy: A Surgeon's Viewpoint." *Journal of the American Medical Association*, 197:100-104.

THE RADIOTHERAPIST'S PSYCHOLOGICAL APPROACH TO CANCER

Sucha O. Asbell

As an x-ray therapist, one must deal daily with the dying patient. Frequently referring doctors ask, "How do you stand facing so much death and dying? Don't you get depressed?" The reply is not simple and usually is initiated by another question: "In general practice what diseases do you cure? Diabetes? Atherosclerosis? Emphysema?" These chronic relapsing illnesses are in many ways similar to cancer. In radiation therapy the number cured provides sufficient gratification and stimulus to continue to handle the large numbers of terminally ill. One can find gratification through prolonging comfortable life. The palliation of bleeding and pain or the reversal of neurological symptoms with radiation therapy is rewarding for many physicians.

Patients assist the physician in developing a philosophy toward death. They give their insight into the problem, thus enabling the physician to offer a solution for other patients. How much easier it is to explain a fatal illness to someone by asking, "Is not death another phase of life?"

It has become standard policy in many departments of x-ray therapy to interview the patient while some other family member is present. When family and patient have been made aware of the patient's diagnosis previously, relating the prognosis as a consequence of the therapy advised is an easier task. The family member tends to give emotional support and frequently diminishes misinterpretation and misunderstanding. If the patient has been made aware of the diagnosis prior to the interview with the radiation therapist, he or she can pay full attention to the consequences of therapy and its results rather than handling the distraction of the initial shock of learning the diagnosis. Prescribing weeks of therapy and describing its side-effects and late complications can only be accomplished successfully when the patient is aware of the serious nature of the illness. It is important when relating the diagnosis to provide the patient with some hope, no matter how slim the chances. Sometimes it is necessary to use terms other than "cancer." Euphemisms such as tumor, growth, or malignancy do not portend such a horrible demise. They are generally accepted with the idea that cure is conceivable, while cancer is assumed to be synonymous with death. It must be explained to patients that their malignancy may be a chronic illness with which they can live for many years. It is important to provide examples and anecdotes. Comparing the survival of the severe cardiac patient whose life style is curtailed because of diminished ambulatory capacity with the general life style of a cancer patient reduces the fear of this dreaded illness.

If the therapist maintains an honest approach, the patient feels secure and has confidence in the physician's knowledge. The sincerity between patient and physician is usually sufficient to sustain the patient through the trying periods of the treatment.

Telling the prognosis to a cancer patient whose status is terminal in several weeks to months is quite difficult. If left without hope, the patient tends to spend the rest of his or her days dying a little each day. That is, the quality of survival is disturbed by emotional depression. Stressing a slim chance for longer survival based on any attributes such as youth, good respiratory or circulatory system, or a limited tumor size balances fear and assists in achieving more cooperation with treatment. Those terminally ill patients who have lived with cancer for years suspect when death is imminent. It is easy for the physician to hide from them and avoid facing their death. After years of association it seems cruel and unkind to abandon the patient in these hours of need. Patients expect continued honesty and deserve it. Many have been heroic, having survived experimental cancer regimens. They are frequently emotionally stable and handle the honest relationship far better than anticipated.

It is easier to work with the patient whose near-term prognosis is fair but, nevertheless, will be terminal in many months or years. One can offer the philosophy that during the interim newer drugs and techniques of radiation treatments may be found. Life can be kept comfortable when an acceptable expectation of survival is assured. Frequently, the requirement for medication and treatment for maintenance is far less than for chronic benign diseases. One patient anticipating death since 1969 has coped with her illness with the following philosophy: "It is not just cancer that is terminal but rather life itself. I enjoy each day to the utmost, for that is what we should all do even when in the best of health."

The perspective is more clearly understood if the physician assures the patient that an anticipated survival is beyond one year. Although the prognosis is terminal, the anticipated survival is sufficiently long to postpone the anticipation of death. Knowing this, the patient can come to deal with death in a more leisurely way and in a way similar to that we all must accept.

PSYCHOLOGICAL PROBLEMS OF PATIENTS RECEIVING RADIOTHERAPY

Tapan A. Hazra, Carol Rose Martin, and Vincent Rose

Patients who are referred for radiation therapy must face not only fears common to all cancer patients but also some special fears of their own. In addition to accepting the fact that they have a potentially fatal disease, patients for radiation therapy must also deal with a new and somewhat awesome situation. Some psychological problems result from their trying to accept and cope with the reality of the situation.

The diagnosis of malignant disease may be very recent, and the patient may not possess the coping skills necessary to accept the situation. The uncertainty brought about by the threat to the individual's survival may be difficult to accept. Moreover, the referral to radiation therapy may follow a major surgical procedure, and the resulting mutilation often produces a deep psychological impact and depression. The individual may have lost body parts during the surgery, causing both physical and psychological adjustment problems. For example, surgery to the head and neck area may destroy sensory organs vital to the individual's interpretation of his environment. Mutilation in the area usually has a greater psychological impact than extensive surgery in other parts of the body.

In addition to the problems brought into the radiotherapy department, there are many difficulties associated directly with the radiation therapy. There appear to be three definite time periods when different psychological problems are encountered. These time periods are pretreatment (when the patient is being evaluated for possible radiotherapy), during treatment, and posttreatment (when the patient has completed a course of therapy and returns for follow-up examination).

PRE-TREATMENT PERIOD

All patients referred for radiation therapy have fears of one kind or another. Initially, the patient comes to an unfamiliar place and meets and is examined by nurses and doctors he has never seen before. Often patients have many misconceptions about radiation therapy, perhaps becuase of information acquired from well-meaning friends or relatives. The most frequent fears patients have involve fears of pain, radiation sickness, becoming radioactive, and the false belief that radiation therapy is only used as a last resort. How well fears will be dealt with depends largely on the relationship that develops between the patient, the radiotherapist, and other members of the treatment team, such as the nurses and technicians. The better understanding the patient has of what is to occur during treatment, the better he will be able to handle the situation.

For many patients the period of treatment may be prolonged and costly. This may threaten their economic security, which may be further complicated by loss of employment. Transportation can present difficulties, since many patients live a good distance away from the hospital. Few patients have friends or relatives who are able to accompany them for a long trip five days a week for four to six weeks. Instead of waiting for the patient to exhibit or verbalize his fears, it is better to explain things on the first visit to allay his anxiety. One should attempt to establish a relationship in which the patient is able to trust the staff. It is also important to be aware of the patient's philosophy of life and his plans for the future. Questions should be encouraged by the staff, and truthful answers given to the patient.

It is imperative that the relatives have a good understanding of the patient's treatment and prognosis. Often they will request the physician not to tell the patient that he or she has cancer because the patient may be unable to accept the diagnosis. It is extremely difficult to understand how an intelligent person can be expected to receive a course of radiation therapy in a center where mainly cancer patients are being treated without being aware that he has cancer. When the physician attempts to withhold the truth and gives evasive answers, the patient quickly loses confidence in the physician and often will seek unorthodox treatment methods. The successful management of a patient with cancer always requires teamwork and close cooperation among the professional staff. The pretreatment problems that can arise when the patient is referred for radiation therapy will be minimized if the patient and family are kept well informed and dealt with honestly.

TREATMENT PERIOD

Many patients do not comprehend or remember everything the physician tells them on the first visit. In view of this, it is a good practice to reiterate some of the important aspects of the treatment. In very frightened patients as well as young children, a dummy session of treatment will allay some anxieties. It must be a very frightening experience to be placed in a large room with a big machine and be left alone during the course of treatment. Great care must be taken to explain why various gadgets are being used in the treatment.

During the course of radiotherapy, the patient's fears about some of the acute adverse reactions of the treatments are a reality. The reactions that occur depend on the anatomical area being treated—for example, abdominal or pelvic radiation may cause vomitting, diarrhea, and weakness. Total cranial irradiation will cause loss of hair. The patient needs to know the possible side effects before they occur, since some patients will attribute these symptoms to the spread of the cancer and not to the radiation therapy. Much anxiety can be prevented by telling the patient what reactions to expect and what will be done to control these. For example, a patient receiving pelvic irradiation should be told that diarrhea may occur and if it does the staff should be informed. The physician will then be able to advise the patient concerning medication and diet to control the diarrhea. Encouraging the patient to report side effects and letting the patient know that the staff is concerned about his progress and problems will promote and strengthen a good patient-staff relationship.

Psychological problems such as depression often are precipitated by physical problems (especially pain) and/or the patient's inability to cope with them. An example of this would be Mrs. S., a 70-year-old female who was irradiated for colon cancer post-operatively. Mrs. S. had difficulty accepting her colostomy, and was embarrassed to discuss her problems with anyone. She began to experience weakness, lack of appetite, and diarrhea. The only food she would eat was fresh fruit, which only increased her diarrhea. Mrs. S. finally developed severe irritation around her stoma from the diarrhea, which brought her problems to the attention of the staff. In her anxiety concerning the diarrhea, which she attributed to recurrence of her cancer, Mrs. S. was unable to care properly for her own colostomy, and refused to allow her husband to help her. Despite diet counseling, medication, further instructions concerning colostomy care, and emotional support from the staff, Mrs. S. discontinued her radiation therapy, since she was "going to die soon anyway." With this patient the staff needed to develop an earlier supportive relationship before the patient began experiencing problems. With modern megavoltage therapy, skin reactions are not a major problem. However, skin problems can be minimized by advising skin care.

POSTTREATMENT PERIOD

After the completion of a course of radiation therapy, a definite follow-up program is established with the patient. This is essential to prevent feelings of rejection by the patient and also to observe for long-term effects of therapy and to check for recurrence or progression of disease. Often a close relationship is developed between the patients and staff, and it is difficult for both when this is ended abruptly at the completion of treatment. During this period, the needs of the family should continue to be of concern to the treatment team. If the patient is doing well and has responded well to radiation therapy, both the patient and the relatives should be kept informed about the good prognosis. The patient, with the help of the family, should be encouraged to maintain a sense of independence. It is very important to determine how well a patient is coping with the problems associated with cancer and radiation therapy, and to meet his expressed and covert needs.

HUMANIZING THE RADIATION THERAPIST

Leonard M. Liegner

> It is a rare blending of learning and humanity, incisiveness of intellect and sensitiveness of the spirit which occasionally come together in an individual who chooses the calling of medicine; and then we have the great physician.
>
> Hans Zinsser

THE INITIAL INTERRELATIONSHIP

The radiation therapist develops feelings of omnipotence as he ministers to the needs of the cancer patient. Initially, his response is one of optimism and confidence in his own technical and oncological capabilities. However, the radiation therapist as physician may react defensively to questions put to him by patient and family regarding his modality of treatment, its efficacy, and his ability to cure. These questions may annoy the therapist since it appears that his experience, training, judgment, and modality are being challenged.

Much depends on the attitude of the patient and/or the family toward the therapist. Likewise, much depends on the counterfeelings induced in the therapist by the patient's and family's attitudes. From these interactions, either a meaningful relationship and plan of treatment can emerge or, contrariwise, an unrewarding, untenable interaction can result.

This initial setting can determine the extent of the radiation therapist's involvement. Assuming that the radiation therapist has any positive feelings for his patient, the first meeting will be optimal. One can observe that even the most isolated, withdrawn person can, during the initial meetings, mobilize himself sufficiently to appear to make human contact with the patient. It is in this initial interchange—in which the physician is willing to handle questions and to respond honestly within the limits set by the patient's understanding and desire to know—that the patient constructs his idealization of the radiation therapist as a potent force in the curative process. The extent to which the therapist can do this is many times predetermined positively or negatively by limitations imposed by the primary referring physician as well as the family.

On the other hand, unrealistic expectations are aroused in the patient during these initial interviews. This occurs despite realistic statements by the therapist regarding prognosis, ultimate cancer control, or cure, as well as possible adverse effects of the treatment.

What are the possible factors determining the initial patient-physician relationship?

The radiation therapist as the physician in control of a radiation modality represents to the patient a powerful force. Since the ill patient is in a regressed dependency state, he usually reacts to the therapist much as he would in a psychotherapeutic relationship, as though the physician were the parent or person of significance in his early life (transference). Since all relationships, especially earlier ones, have ambivalent—positive and negative aspects—a clue may be given as to the expected cooperativeness of the patient in following recommendations, or in arousing negative feelings in the therapist, especially feelings of rejection. To complicate matters, the physician also reacts to the patient based on his own early life experiences with significant persons in his life. This can result in a receptive or negative stance toward the patient.

Fortunately, in most instances the initial reactions of the physician and patient are modified as each cautiously judges the other. Depending on motivation and ability to understand each other, progress is made in accepting their respective deficiencies. It is during these initial contacts that human involvement, measured neutrality, or even outright rejection takes place between patient and physician.

I would like to suggest additional factors that may be important in shaping the feelings of physicians toward their patients, especially toward the cancer patient although the factors that I will discuss seem to be counterproductive to the sensitiveness of spirit that Hans Zinsser refers to in the making of the physician.

The medical student in his preclinical years (modified in more recent programs by earlier clinical exposure) has as his first model of scientific detachment the preclinical scientist who, by choice or chance, does not have contact with patients, nor is he involved in their direct care. The medical student views the human body through its microscopic, biochemical, and molecular components. This places an almost insurmountable barrier to the psychic process of reintegration of the patient as human. Dissecting the cadaver contributes further to the future physician's ability to depersonalize the patient. This depersonalization occurs despite the physician's ethical beliefs in the sanctity of the human being.

This experience, whereby the medical student, ill equipped to understand his own emotional makeup, delves into and dissects every structure and fiber of the cadaver, must impose an everlasting imprint on the psychology of each and every medical student. It leads to repression of what under normal circumstances would lead to emotions of caring, bereavement, and identification with the cadaver and later, as physicians, with their patients.

I am not suggesting that we eliminate basic science and dissection of the cadaver from the medical curriculum. What I am suggesting is that medical students be entered into group psychotherapy seminars during their entire education. The purpose is obvious: to facilitate the recognition by medical students of their feelings, offering them the opportunity to verbalize both positive and negative feelings and yet, despite the pleasantness or unpleasantness of these emotions, to carry on and function. The ultimate goal would be to graduate doctors of medicine who are fully human, who can experience a complete range of feelings in their relationship with patients without acting improperly.

The alternative is to leave things as they are and continue to train physicians who must stand aloof from the patient and suppress or block their feelings in order to survive. We know what price physicians have paid and are paying in the stress involved in caring for patients. The high rate among physicians of alcohol and drug abuse, divorce, mental breakdown, and suicide attests to this fact. Yet the scientific stance and the emotional detachment of the physician form the basis of the public outcry that physicians are not concerned about their patients.

The ultimate cure of those deficits, it appears to me, rests primarily on the positive influences exerted by the physicians' early family constellation as well as subsequent life experiences. Ultimately, the emotional reeducation suggested above may produce physicians who are sensitive to others, aware of their own feelings, and capable of a full range of human responses.

How can we bring about the humanization of the present generation of practitioners, including those of us who identify ourselves as radiation therapists?

"Know thyself" is the first recommendation. But to do so in dealing with the cancer patient requires us to be aware of our own feelings about our own death and mortality, and of feelings of failure, of hopelessness, of depression, of anger, of frustration, of omnipotence, of disgust, of revulsion, of indifference, of impatience, of empathy, of pity, of identification, of need for closeness, of need for affection, of need for love, of need for isolation, of our own dependency needs, of feelings of hatred, destructiveness, and aggression. I mean the full range of positive and negative feelings, pleasurable as well as painful.

In this era of specialization and distinction of roles, the need for diffusion and blurring of roles in medicine is vital to the process of full humanization.

I have an admission to make! I am a member of all the most prestigious societies an oncologist can strive to join, which marks me as a man of the physical and biological sciences. In addition, however, broadening my perspective, I am a member of the American Psychosomatic Society, a multidisciplinary organization, open to all those interested in the mind-body-body-mind complex. I have also run groups of cancer patients under the auspices of the New York Division of the American Cancer Society. I have co-led groups of cancer patients at St. Luke's Hospital (New York City). Furthermore, I have participated in national symposia in the psychophysiological aspects of cancer held at the New York Academy of Sciences.

I was invited to act as a consultant for a hospital-based, multidiscipline medical oncology group, headed by a medical oncologist and including psychiatrists, social workers, nurses, and technicians, who were all interested in possibly learning from me how to organize and run therapy groups for cancer patients. The medical oncologist was becoming more and more frustrated by my not giving him specific information on how to form and maintain such groups. Instead, I used these interactions as a paradigm of a group and directed investigative questions to the members of the group. My goal was to create a climate conducive for a cooperative experiential learning experience. I did not wish the group members to be passive recipients of a didactic lecture. The medical oncologist questioned me in an angry tone. I continued to frustrate him by questioning him as to the value of giving him the answers. He retorted sharply, "That's what you are here for." I indicated that he was being very cooperative in being able to express his anger toward me. I told him that although I might feel angry in reaction to him, I was aware of how I felt and its cause, and I did not have to counterattack. I told him this was much the feeling his patients had toward him at times yet were afraid to express since their fate was in his hands. He had confirmed his attitude previously by saying proudly that he was completely in charge of his clinic and no doctor or patient dared challenge him. He then, after the interchange of anger with me, asked how was it that he and I, both doctors involved in cancer, were so different. How could he become like me? I said I normally would not reveal myself, but since he had been so cooperative in verbally expressing his anger toward me and since I really believed he wanted to know as a means of improving himself, I was willing to tell him.

I thereupon told him that we as physicians were both molded as scientists but one element was missing in our training. I told him my wife, as a psychoanalyst, had humanized me, made me aware of human emotions. Furthermore, if he desired to pattern himself after me he could attend meetings of the American and Eastern Group Psychotherapy Association, attend their seminars, and finally gain personal understanding by entering group and individual psychotherapy. This was thoughtfully received. As a result of this demonstration that verbally expressed anger between the director and myself did not lead to a destructive scene, the psychiatrists were able to point out to the director things that he did that angered them.

What I am saying is that before dealing with the cancer and dying patient at the psychological level, insight must be gained into what makes each one of us tick. Do we allow all feeling to permeate our being? Do we put out our antennas and allow ourselves to be aware of patients' moods and feelings (including fears)? Are we willing to interact with the dying patient in a human, meaningful, rewarding way? Does fear of our own emotions and fear of our own resultant behavior cast us in the role of the cold, calculating minister of magic emanations, rather than the physician who understands and has compassion?

The following case is offered as an example of the range of attitudes and emotions that a patient is willing to express to the physician who is interested in listening and who is willing to develop confidence in his role as a facilitator.

Case of M.R.: Mrs. M.R. was a 43-year-old, Italian female, with unresectable Stage III cancer of the ovary; married, with children 16 and 19 years of age. Her mother was alive, although she had suffered a mild stroke.

Mrs. R. was in a responsible supervisory position in an insurance comapny and managed the affairs of the entire family. Her husband would give her his entire paycheck and say, "Don't bother me; you'll manage and you'll worry about it."

The medical situation was somewhat tragic in that despite excellent gynecological care over the years, the pelvic tumor was discovered belatedly. The patient stated to me that she had lost complete faith in any kind of medical work-up and would in the future refuse further investigation.

The first meeting with the patient was the day following surgery. She was lying in bed in no unusual distress. She responded pleasantly to my being there. She stated she knew why I was there—to discuss the radiation program for her treatment. Her mother was in the room. With annoyance, she asked her mother to leave stating, that she had no right to be involved or ought not to know what was going on. The mother left. The patient then said, "If I have cancer, Dr. Liegner, I want you to inject something and make sure that I don't survive." I responded, "I will let you know when that time comes, and we'll tell you when you can do away with yourself." She did not react with shock, but merely stated, "I depend on you to do it."

I realized that the patient assumed she had cancer, although the attending physician requested she not be told. I had not violated the physician's orders, yet had communicated by my response that she and I were operating on the same wave length.

Following this interview I met with the mother, who knew that her daughter had cancer and expressed her wishes that "if this were so, God willing," she would die. I did nothing to reassure the mother but permitted her to express the wish that her daughter die rather than suffer. The mother further wanted me to be kind to her daughter and do everything I could to make her existence easy. She wished I would not allow her daughter to come home because she herself could not manage it and she did not want the family to suffer either.

At the first visit to the radiation therapy department in the treatment planning room, the patient sat up and cried, "Dr. Liegner, I don't want to have cancer. I have too many responsibilities to take care of at home, and they need me." She continued, "I cannot afford to have cancer." Four days later I revisited the patient in her room. She was up and about, smiling, very active, wearing a nice robe. She stated she had decided that she would make it. She had called for the hairdresser, and her hair was done beautifully. She had put on lipstick and seemed quite adjusted.

We sat face to face and started to speak quite frankly. She said, "Dr. Liegner, if I have cancer, you know what to do." I responded, "Well, suppose you did have cancer, what would your reaction be to this?" She did not answer. I continued, "Well, let us assume that we could not guarantee that your cancer had been completely removed and it would take one, two, or three years to prove that there is no cancer. So why don't you work on the thesis that you do have cancer at this time?" She responded that she could tolerate the knowledge of early cancer and live with it. However, advanced cancer means being an invalid, having to ask the family to give her water, even to cope with her bowel movements. This thought was intolerable to her and she would rather be dead.

There was a difference in her mind between dying of an acute disease like coronary occlusion or other acute accidents, because it was over quickly. Although your family did mourn you, there was no undue prolonged suffering of the family.

She pointedly asked, "Dr. Liegner, if you knew you had advanced cancer, would you want to live?" I responded, "I might and I might not." The discussion continued, but at no time did she say she would commit suicide. She only wanted me to perform a mercy killing.

She had gas pains the next night and was in great discomfort. However, she was able to tolerate this pain with the belief this was not due to advanced cancer but due to surgery and radiation. She stated that if the pain had been caused by advanced cancer she would have found the pain intolerable and she would have wanted heavy sedation. She did not ask for sedation.

We wanted her to go home for Christmas. She thought that this meant we believed it would be her last Christmas. She did not want to go home because she also thought it would be a tremendous burden to her family.

I responded to this by asking her, "Why can't you be a dependent when you are ill and enjoy the care that your family gives you?" Her 16-year-old daughter was present and said, "Please come home; we love you, and we want to do everything for you."

The patient asked about going back to work. I said, "Look, enjoy your illness; be dependent. Why can't you be a burden to them? They have been a burden to you long enough."

The model offered by the radiation therapist, as a person sensitive to the needs of his patients, sets the mood of his department and assures the active involvement of his entire staff. This includes secretarial, technical, and professional, including the physicist.

The needs of the departmental staff for psychological counseling must also be considered. In our department group sessions are held, which include the patients as well as staff. The unusual talents of the staff members become evident in these groups. They demonstrate great insight and emotional understanding of themselves and the patients. The key to both individual and group sessions is to permit people to talk and to facilitate discussion, especially about feelings. Little or no intellectual interpretation of behavior is offered. The group leader and co-leader must be aware of the mood and emotions of all members and by indirection assure that the group permit all members to participate and express negative or positive feelings. Most important, the right of participants to be quiet and not participate is respected. However, it is the group leader's role to understand the resistance to communicate and at appropriate times to work toward reducing the resistance to verbalization. Many obstacles exist that prevent patients from expressing feelings, especially negative attitudes. Some of these are:

1. Fear of punishment by the staff if the patient should express anger or annoyance toward them.
2. Denial of their disease.
3. Feeling that they as cancer victims are among the living dead. Feelings reinforced by family withdrawal and the avoidance by them of open discussion with the patient.

Behavioral patterns of family members attempting to diminish the patient's fears and depression, when expressed by them through excessive joviality, sadness, depression, withdrawal and diminishing human interaction and contact.

4. The attitudes of the primary physician and family that mitigate against honest response: their desire that the patient not suffer, have bad feelings, have cancer, or know he is dying. The physician, family, nurses, technicians, and so forth want the cancer and dying patient to be happy and feel good at all times.

The expressed feelings of cancer patients are contrary to the unrealistic goals of the physician and family. The cancer patients have a myriad of feelings and thoughts—guilt, disgust with themselves, fear, hopelessness, thoughts of suicide, hatred for loved ones, anger at the physician or other staff members, depression, sadness, abandonment, loneliness. These feelings and attitudes are normal, and patients feel better by expressing them rather than suppressing them. The physician and family cannot deny them their human reactions even though by their demeanor and behavior they force the patient to play the game of making *us* feel better, their physician or family.

As a final thought: Envision the patient—or in fact envision yourself—alone in the radiation therapy room; the door closes; no human contact; the treatment commences. Are we so foolish as to believe our patients do not feel? They do not know? Would you?

STRATEGIES OF PSYCHOLOGICAL INTERVENTION

L.D. Hankoff and Joseph A. Braun

While there may be some disagreement among professionals on issues involved in the psychological care of the cancer patient, we feel that the family and friends of the patient are able to plan and followup a rational course of psychological help just as the direct medical treatment is pursued in a rational framework. In order to provide rational and effective psychological and emotional care, consideration must be given to the *total* array of participants in the cancer patient's current life situation. Involved with the patient in the course of his illness will be a social network of friends and relatives as well as a wide variety of caregivers. While the patient progresses over time, members of the caregiver group may pass on and off the scene as the patient's condition and the setting of his care change. The issue of psychological management, that is, a concern for the emotional aspects of the illness, may never be raised by the caregivers, who may even reject it as unimportant in the middle of the highly complicated medical treatment. It is important to note, however, that although the caregivers may change, the network of family and friends remains relatively unchanged.

The psychological management of the cancer patient, as opposed to the more clearly defined medical management, is made difficult by potential problems in setting direction and in assuming authority. There are many decisions to be made in the course of the illness which are very personal in nature and are not just medical questions. The whole interrelated circle of friends, relatives, and caregivers may provide a confusing and conflicting set of directions and opinions about the patient's life course and life situation, at times even becoming involved in decisions that can be made only by the patient. Such divisions among the individuals in the social network will possibly cause tensions and barriers to communication throughout the network.

Moreover, as more than one physician is usually involved in the care of the cancer patient, the line of authority even within the medical portion of the network may be unclear to the family. The medical specialists may well agree on the plan of medical treatment, but these same specialists may have differing attitudes and values toward helping a patient with emotional aspects of the illness. The specialists will have different personality styles in relating to the cancer patient, and they are not likely to achieve any spontaneous coordination of psychological assistance for the patient. Further complications almost inevitably arise on the introduction of a new specialist who is to take over the medical treatment; for example, the patient who has had cancer surgery may move on to receive chemotherapy or radiotherapy from a new specialist who takes over the prime authority with regard to the course of the illness and any other questions of a medical nature. These questions of medical authority are highly relevant to the matter of psychological management.

The changing or expanding array of physicians caring for the patient may create obstacles for relatives and friends who offer to help the patient cope with his or her illness but who feel that the final authority over communications with the patient rests with the physicians. For example, a close relative may develop an intense working relationship with a cancer patient but feel inhibited in imparting "medical" information to him when questions of diagnosis or prognosis arise during conversations. Similarly, a friend with day-to-day contacts with a cancer patient is often in a natural role to assist him in airing feelings on the subject of his illness. In many cases, however, frank discussion along with an easy sense of freedom to communicate is seldom achieved by family and friends.

The attention given to the cancer patient, particularly when he enters a chronic or terminal phase, is not derived solely from medical and paramedical caregivers and from family and friends. The clergy play a key role in the lives of many patients and may have important times also with patients' relatives and friends. In his role as comforter and counselor, a clergyman may greatly facilitate the psychological management of terminal illness; a well-intentioned cleric may, however, intensify the problems of coordinative responsibility if he is not *integrally involved* in the planning network.

> Mrs. E.R. had a recurrence of cancer of the colon and following a second operation discovered herself with a colostomy plus a scheduled series of radiotherapy treatments. Her family had never shared the original diagnosis with her, but after a discussion with a psychiatrist friend decided along with the family physician to respond openly to her questions and tell her the status of her illness, namely, that she had recurrent carcinoma that had spread locally, was inoperable, and was likely to advance in the next few months. In particular, she needed an explanation of the colostomy and radiotherapy. The family was preparing for free discussion when the patient was visited by her local rabbi. He spontaneously launched into a lengthy reassurance to the patient, told her that new cures for illnesses are being discovered daily, and that, if the present hospital and doctors were not satisfactory, she could transfer to a much finer nearby hospital. The rabbi's uncalled for "support" raised many doubts in the patient's mind and for the time being postponed the clarification toward which the rest of the network was working.

THE NEED FOR COORDINATION OF EFFORT

The conclusion seems clear that, although sound medical care for the cancer patient may be abundant, there is, nevertheless, a great need for coordination of effort among all persons in order to give the cancer patient organized and sustained assistance in resolving emotional problems. There must be a resolution within the patient and within the caregivers, relatives, and friends of any attitudinal conflicts that may hinder the patient's psychological mastery of the situation. The patient's *total* well-being must be promoted in a restorative and rehabilitative manner while medical treatment efforts specific for the cancerous process are carried out.

The above generalizations are of little practical value to the persons involved with the individual patient and we certainly are not suggesting that every terminally ill or cancer patient requires the direct attention of a behavioral scientist or psychotherapist. We do note, however, that in the same way that human strengths and cultural patterns have supported individuals in resolving nonmedical personal crises or a mental illness there does exist a common pool of wisdom and of coping mechanisms for dealing with the challenge of a serious or fatal illness. The question as we see it is *how* to initiate and mobilize these mechanisms within the complexities of modern medical treatment and, more specifically, *who* the initiating source of the organized effort will be.

The initiating of a plan for emotional care of the patient would be greatly simplified if we could say with confidence that each patient had a primary physician who occupied the team leader position. However, since the care of the patient is often divided among several physicians who view one another as co-equal participants, no single individual is clearly designated as the leader of psychological management. Accordingly, those persons who understand the particular patient's needs and personality and who have at least some awareness of the emotional aspects of terminal illness must act as the initiators of psychological care regardless of how they view themselves in the line of authority of caregivers. Indeed, one must take the view that the person most sensitive to issues of psychological care must at that time be the leader in seeking such care. He or she has the task of uniting the persons involved with the patient in consideration of the patient's unique psychological make-up in order to plan and carry out their cooperative strategy of participation in relation to the patient and his familial and social network.

INTERVENTION TECHNIQUE

A total strategy for the emotional care of the cancer patient begins with an understanding of the patient and of the social and caregiving network within which he lives. From this evaluation key persons are located and developed in their roles as helpers in the psychological management of the patient. The completed task involves the ongoing application of coordinated psychological management effort for the individual patient.

Understanding of the Patient. An understanding of the patient is basic to any strategy of psychological management. We believe that most persons involved are able to reach such an understanding independently of a behavioral specialist if the assessment is conducted in a systematic and comprehensive fashion.

A full understanding of the patient should include a review of facts and observations pertaining to: (a) the patient's general personality quality or type; (b) particular strengths, abilities, and ways of dealing with stress; (c) known difficulties of adjustment, past and present; (d) past crises and the manner in which the patient handled them; (e) financial status; and (f) medical status and prognosis of the cancerous illness.

Finally, an assessment of the patient's knowledge of and his attitude toward his illness should be made. How open is the patient to discuss the illness? To what degree does the patient appear to be accepting or denying his illness? Is the patient depressed? What is the patient's attitude toward the future? What is he or she actually doing in relation to the future apart from talking about it? What is the patient's daily routine now in comparison with his routine before the illness?

The Interpersonal Network. The growth of a strategy of intervention depends next on an assessment of the patient's immediate social network and the team of caregivers involved. Again we believe that such an assessment can be made systematically by the person actually caring for cancer patients. The assessment calls for identifying: (a) friends or relatives living with the patient; (b) other friends or relatives of significance in the patient's life; (c) interpersonal relationships that are a source of support to the patient; (d) interpersonal relationships that are emotionally harmful to the patient; and (e) caregivers of all types and levels who may have formal or informal relationships with the patient. An important aspect of this assessment lies in examining the total medical care extended to the patient and locating areas where it is not well coordinated.

The Key Person or Persons. A major goal in the leader's understanding of the patient's interpersonal network is the locating of a key person (or persons), whom we define as that person in the patient's immediate social network who exerts the most powerful and far-reaching emotional influence on the patient. The key person may already be the same sensitive person who is trying to take a leadership role in providing emotional care. The influence by the key person may be through a direct relationship with the patient or an indirect one exerted via family members close to the patient.

The key person already favorably influences the patient and the psychological climate around him. We presume that the key person is potentially more powerful in his influence if given more initiative and direction.

The Non-issue: To Tell or Not To Tell. The debate continues unresolved among professionals over the pros and cons of revealing to a patient that he has a life-threatening illness or that he has entered a terminal phase. We feel, however, that the issue must be carefully faced by those concerned with the emotional care of each cancer patient. It is more important to achieve agreement on a strategy of psychological management in each *individual* case than to resolve varying philosophies related to the general issue of revealing a bad prognosis.

When disagreement persists among relatives, friends, and caregivers over the issue of informing the patient, there is little purpose served in forcing the issue; any agreement is not likely to be achieved through persistence. On the other hand, caregivers and relatives *are* always in basic agreement that the patient should receive the best care possible. The next step—obtaining agreement that this care should include psychological management—is an easy one. Attention can now be focused on positive efforts to assist the patient in his adjustment. Assistance to the patient can now progress and the area of controversy regarding informing the patient can be circumvented as not essential, at least at this phase of initiating emotional care.

Initiating Psychological Management. Theoretically, the psychological management of the patient might take the form of the resolution of psychological problems by the patient himself. In this simplest and ideal form the patient is his own initiator of the process of psychological solutions. A second-level alternative consists in a key person who initiates and maintains a strategy of psychological intervention, possibly in conjunction with one of the existing caregivers. A third-level lies in the initiation coming from an outsider (usually a caregiver or clergyman) who in turn relates to a key person in the social network of relatives and friends.

In terms of these three alternatives for the initiation of psychological management, our main focus in this paper is on the second alternative in which the initiative comes from someone within the circle of friends and relatives, who wishes to develop a plan for emotional care where none exists. We propose, in this instance, that this interested person initiate the development of a program of psychological management through outreach efforts in relation to whoever is perceived as the key person or through a realization by the initiator that he or she *is* the key person. The beginnings of this task may be difficult owing to the initiator's own emotional reaction to the patient's illness. If the initiator is also the key person, he or she may well seek a friend, clergyman, professional counselor, or one of the physicians in order to come to grips with the feelings and conflicts related to the loved one's illness. If the relative or friend who sees the need for emotional care is not the key person, he or she can begin by helping the key person in an informal, appropriate, and flexible way adjust to and cope with the reality of the illness and by developing a working relationship with the key person that focuses on issues around the crises at hand.

The next step is for the key person to explore and to utilize his relationships to the rest of the network. The key person must be helped in his ties to the other individuals so that his impact on the network of persons and on the patient will be maximized.

An overall goal of any program of emotional care is the opening up of channels of communication. The key person will by definition have better channels of communication than anyone else in the situation. On some issues, however, even his or her channels of communication may be insufficient for a given issue and the key person must ask for assistance or some assistance must be arranged. For example, the various individuals—relatives, friends and professionals—may experience great difficulty in communicating the facts of the cancerous illness to each other or to the patient. There may even be agreement that the patient should be told, but no one in the network appears able to assume this responsibility. An outsider such as a clergyman may be sought to act as an intermediary. The providing of such a volunteer or alternate informant in the social network is, however, not without its disadvantages. The outsider may simply provide more information but may not really change the lines of communication. His efforts are likely to be quickly negated. It is common experience for patients or family members who have been informed of a serious illness to fall back on the defense of denial as soon as they are informed. Thus, a single heroic effort by the outsider is by itself not likely to change the situation. On the other hand, such a demonstration of openness or improved communication by the outsider may start a new chain of events or may change people's *attitudes*.

The limitations of an outsider underscore the need for *continued responsible effort* by the key person, who alone can really provide the foundation and the continued support and monitoring necessary for progressive and substantial change in the quality of interrelations within the social network. The ultimate benefactor of these efforts is, of course, the patient, who as a result will not exist in an atmosphere of emotional isolation deprived of the support and full presence of his or her most meaningful people at that point in life when they are most needed.

GROUP WORK WITH CANCER PATIENTS IN RADIATION THERAPY

Patricia Fobair, Abby Wolfson, Norman L. Mages,
Joan Hall, Irene Harrison and Julia Vose

Working with cancer patients in "groups" is one of the most satisfying, touching, and patient enabling processes a clinical staff might consider in reaching out to meet the psychosocial needs of the cancer patient in radiation therapy. While nothing will replace the one-to-one relationship in providing clinical services, the group process offers a unique way of enabling cancer patients to mourn, to grieve, to express anger and doubt, to recognize themselves in others, and to experience themselves as "not alone." Although all patients will not want a group experience, those who *do* will find a new source of emotional support to help them tolerate the uncertainty of their illness. Cancer patient groups, like other group therapies, tend to attract the verbally able, yet these patients also suffer from feelings of being isolated from others and from themselves.

This chapter describes the group work with cancer patients at Mount Zion Hospital and Medical Center in San Francisco. We will discuss some of the needs of cancer patients and how these needs are met in group therapy. We will also mention the goals established by the group leadership, and how these goals are determined.

Originally, group therapy was introduced by physicians on behalf of the chronically ill patient at the turn of the century (Buchanan, 1978; Yalom, 1975, p. 479). Yet the popularity of working with physically ill patients in groups seems to be a recent development. Since the early 1970s, reports have been published in medical journals about the benefits of group treatment for epileptics, diabetics, cardiac, and dialysis patients. The authors derived positive information about having patients meet together from additional sources:

1) The encounter group movement (very strong in California) which enables unhappy but otherwise well-integrated people to use a group process to improve their lives (Yalom, 1975, p. 486).

2) The observation of a need: some patients undergoing radiation therapy had found their lives dramatically changed and seemed depressed, immobilized, in a state of limbo.
3) The positive group experiences with breast cancer patients and with head-and-neck cancer patients reported by various institutions.

Our group history began in February, 1972, when ten patients and two apprehensive social workers met to explore whether this kind of weekly event might be useful. For several months, I (P.F.) thought each session would be the last, fearing that no one would come, worried that the patients were talking about subjects that might hurt rather than help them. Gradually, it became clear, from the number of patients, family members, and hospital staff who wanted to attend our weekly two-hour sessions, that we really had something of value.

In January of 1973, several younger patients joined the group. After a few sessions, they asked for a group of their own. They had trouble identifying with the problems of the older patients, and wanted a place to discuss more intimate topics, pertinent to the difficulties of their own age. Recognizing a new need, I sought the help of staff from the Department of Psychiatry at Mount Zion. Under the leadership of psychologist Abby Wolfson, a pilot group was organized for the young patients for a nine-week period, June through July, 1973. We were reluctant to see this brief series end, as the young people had been able to reveal among themselves troubling issues they could not have shared so easily with older patients.

Later that summer, a young master poet from San Francisco State University was employed by Mount Zion Hospital to bring the "Writer-in-Residence" program to a hospital setting. At first, I felt she could enrich our group by providing the less verbal patients with a regular means of expression. Later, however, it turned out that we all found writing twice a month to be a most creative way of expressing thoughts and feelings. Because of this collaborative effort, the reader will be able to enjoy the patient's words, phrasing, and expressed ideas.

In April, 1975, a planning grant from the National Cancer Institute made it possible to extend our group services as part of a larger project to study the rehabilitation course of cancer patient survivors. This additional staff funding enabled us to organize three separate groups, and we devised a system for evaluation. Group I continued to serve most of the middle-aged and older patients, while family members were offered a support group for themselves. The third division offered an ongoing group to young cancer patients, aged 18 to 35 years. The success of our program is affirmed by the many moving entreaties from members that the groups be continued, as well as by the increasing flow of referrals from physicians, social workers, agencies, and patients throughout the Bay Area.

PATIENT NEEDS MET IN GROUP THERAPY

A summary of cancer patient experiences along the disease continuum reveals the many problems that can be shared in a group. For example, the trauma of the new diagnosis and acute illness produces feelings of shock, anger, grief, and uncertainty for many patients. Newly diagnosed patients will fear recurrence and progression of disease (Mages, 1976). Having to tolerate the thought of damage to one's body either from the illness or from its treatment is another bitter concern, not easily managed by patients. They need to maintain a sense of self-sufficiency and control over themselves, and to continue with their lives, yet they must absorb all the changes that have occurred. This "see-saw" requirement is yet another area of trouble. Patients facing chronic illness must deal with the dilemma of regression versus mobilization. Terminal illness forces a patient to come to terms with the prospect of death, so that the remainder of life can be lived in as satisfying a manner as possible.

These are universal problems occurring with most patients, but to the individual experiencing them with the full intensity of feeling, each segment seems unique. In a patient group, these experiences are shared, with the effect of reducing the vulnerability and sense of aloneness of those involved. The patients have expressed these ideas poignantly in their creative writing over the months of our working together.

TRAUMA OF THE ACUTE ILLNESS

Several patients have written about the feelings of shock, anger, fear, and grieving which they felt during the first few months of illness. After entering the group, they tell us why they are there.

Sarah, a 50-year-old educator, acknowledged vividly: "My anger is what I'm coping with. I feel ashamed of my body, and I'm angry with the doctors for not finding it earlier."

Nelson, a 50-year-old businessman, said: "I have a sense of outrage! I've made the shocking discovery that I, a middle-aged athlete, have cancer of the lung. I thought it was fraud until the doctor came back with the biopsy."

Maria, a 35-year-old mother, wrote this poem to her husband:

> I'm scared. I'm scared
> This thing is going to kill me!
> What about Jimmy? What about Bobby and Lisa?
> They don't need what I've taught them;
> They need *me*—my presence. . . .

Tom, a 60-year-old insurance broker told us: "I couldn't stop crying for two days straight when I found out I had myeloma. My son said, 'Did you cry?' I said, 'Sure, I've been pouring all over the bed. I've had a two-day shakedown.'"

Forms of fear and anger appear in the conversations and related experiences of many patients. In the early days of the group, anger towards physicians was *the* initial topic and source of group cohesion. I had not realized that this was such a common feeling. At first I worried that it would mobilize destructive behavior, but later it became clear that initial anger toward doctors is universal. With group support, patients are able to sort out the "rational" from the "irrational" aspects. Here is a partial conversation between several patients who knew the same doctor:

"I think Dr. G. is the coldest guy I've every seen."
"Well, I liked the way he gave me the cold facts."
"*You* want the straight facts; *I* want a little empathy and straight feeling."
"I thought he was a warm, out-going person."
"Doctors! I really needed him to be able to say what I was feeling."

Part of a patient's anger is often reasonable, but patients also reveal an irrational demand that the doctor be all-knowing. Some patients wish that the diagnosis could have been made before the evidence was in hand. This magical thinking suggests a basic anger with the illness *per se,* and with the self for not being healthier. "My body let me down," said a patient, "and it's profoundly distressing."

Yalom has written:

There is a shattering of the narcissistic position that we are the center of the universe, that takes place when a person faces his illness. That the world can exist without us is a horrible thought; it destroys our delusion of vulnerability and immortality and causes the patient to search for control, perhaps finding in the doctor, the ultimate rescuer (Yalom, 1976).

Some anger must occur when the doctor cannot satisfy the magical thinking of the patient. Helping patients to sort out their reasonable and unreasonable feelings is an important task of our group.

FEAR OF RECURRENCE

Someone in the group is speaking: "It's such an insidious thing. I can't see it; I feel it. It's eating away inside my bone. . . my bone marrow; not like a cut or black eye or broken nose; you can't stitch it or patch it or set it."

During an interview, Martha, a 44-year-old teacher and mother who was a prospective patient for the group, said, "My early experiences with diagnosis and surgery weren't hard; I had a lot of help from my friends; but when I had to have chemotherapy, my fear of recurrence drove me to look into your group." Later, she realized that she had the most trouble accepting her cancer in regard to the fear of recurrence and its implication that death was a possibility. Her family's support was no longer sufficient to meet her needs. "My daughter feels that I am looking for sympathy, and I see myself as a victim. I need to be with others who are going through what I am." She was thinking about quitting her job and was fighting with internal urges to withdraw.

Don, a 39-year-old psychologist, had not only resigned from his job, but also had withdrawn from almost all relationships and was living in a state of limbo, marking time and awaiting the next event in his unknown medical course. The possibility of recurrence and progression of disease evoked an intense and immobilizing anxiety in this man. For many patients, the fear is paralyzing, or at least affects major life decisions. The following poem by Don reflects his feelings of helplessness and uncertainty:

> What the hell's happening?
> Think I know... then know I don't.
> How to find out?
> Check it out! Check it out! Check it out!
>
> Now I've checked.
> Back where I started.
> That man is right,
> Never know what the hell's happening.
>
> What's going on?
> Can't be there and here at the same time.
>
> Might as well relax
> Get a few laughs
> Take care of the human as best I can
> Let the sun fall on me
> Make sure Doc's the center of it
> Take a trip
> Enjoy the stereo
> What's changed? A little? A lot?
> Maybe nothing.

Tolerating the uncertainty of not knowing what is going to happen is one of the greatest sources of anxiety for some patients. The leaders help the patients to tolerate this uncertainty by providing in the group a safe and stable atmosphere where they can expose their vulnerabilities and regain their equilibrium. The task of the group is to recognize and accept the uncertainty of the future and the inability to change this ambiguity.

Peter, a 45-year-old poet laureate in our group, really puts his finger on this issue when he wrote:

> Control, Control, know what it's all about,
> Where it came from, where it goes,
> What will happen, when it will happen,
> How it will turn out.
> B — — s——, there is no certainty
> All the above is a waste of time
> An energy drain,
> A mind f——, a circle of nothingness.
> This is it here and now,
> The future doesn't add meaning
> To the present, just gives it more significance.
> Just flow with it

> Make choices even though you don't know the point
> Like all searches,
> You come back to where you are.

If fear of recurrence brings patients into the here-and-now, and helps them focus on their current values and philosophy of life, the issue of "damage to one's body" has the effect of forcing them to focus on how they feel and how they see themselves internally and externally.

DAMAGE TO ONE'S BODY

Much of our sense of self-esteem is based on how well we look to ourselves and in each other's eyes. Cancer cells intrude upon healthy cells and displace tissue on the face, in the throat, in the breast, in the groin, and in the lungs. If the tumors themselves don't destroy appearance, the surgery or radiation surely will. Is it any wonder that many patients need to tell us their sadness over the changes in the body? A group of patients is a wonderful setting for mourning lost parts and lost energy; to grieve over losses is a human need that is seldom met in the current practice of medical centers.

Listen now to dialogue from several months of group sessions, as Martha and Sarah describe some of their feelings about their bodies and themselves. Martha said, during her first few months in the group:

> Depression is to be immobilized
> These drugs take it out of you
> I've always been athletic, jogged and skied...
> I don't know if I can this year.

> You know, it's tough to accept losses.
> I feel like I'm sitting on a rock, but I don't feel secure.
> I'm afraid of being afraid; of being dependent.

> Somehow I need to feel 'special.'
> I hate to say this, but I feel a loss of sexual eagerness;
> A loss of femaleness; of what makes me feel like a woman.
> It's vanity, but my body let me down.

Later she said:

> I'm angry over the loss of my breast; pissed off that I have only one breast. I'm not good enough. I'm angry with the doctors for not knowing.

Then, towards the end of her ten months in the group; these thoughts:

> I need to move on. I've seen myself as 'less than' rather than 'more than.' It's time to stop using cancer as an excuse.

> "Want to go jogging with me around Lake Merrit?" she asks another patient.

Sarah had similar things about herself; in her own words:

> I feel maimed, not whole anymore since my breast is gone. I gagged when I looked at myself in the mirror; had trouble using bath oils. *They* did it to me on purpose! Nobody really cares. . . I'm invisible; nobody pays attention. I don't look okay; I'm hiding my body; it's a piece of garbage. It's a fight not to give up. I used to love hot tub parties; now I can't go.

In Martha's dialogue, you can hear the slow move toward expressing her feelings more vividly, then letting them go and moving back into her more active life stance. With Sarah, the depressed words come through with more projection. Both women function in their outside lives as completely adequate, professional women, but, as Sarah says:

> I'm trying to live in the here-and-now; when I come here I can talk crazy; I don't have to play a role like on the outside. It helps me get my head straight for the rest of the time.

Talking about losses helps many patients drain off the excess feelings of sadness and regret, helps them tolerate what has happened and cannot be changed.

MAINTAINING SELF-SUFFICIENCY AND CONTROL

How does a patient maintain the thread of his life? How does he deal with the sense of loss of control, the relative inability to affect the course of the disease? We see the adaptive task here as "exercising choice" when possible, and "accepting one's helplessness and dependency" when necessary, without excessive regression or turning to a magical solution. This is another ongoing issue that presents tremendous difficulty to many patients. The group becomes a place for patients to describe the daily events of life, the intrapersonal and interpersonal struggles to maintain a sense of equilibrium.

Tom and Nelson were two men who used the group during chronic and terminal illness periods. Their words express some of the problems in maintaining a sense of continuity. During February, 1975, Tom told the group that:

> "Your whole life structure stops. . ."
> "I threw the whole burden on my wife."
> "It's a complete change, you see."
> "We're closer, seeing things together; much happier."
> "But for a while I couldn't dust or dress myself."
> "Today, I feel very calm about myself."

> Two months later, he said:
> "I'm 60 and, gosh, I'm not doing anything."
> "I wake up in the middle of the night and pace the floor and my wife paces with me; and then she puts me back to bed and I feel like a baby."

Tom and his wife were willing to change the formula of their life together to include the new events that cancer brought, but it was difficult for *him* to give up part of his masculine role. He fought against regression and loss of face, and used the group to mourn the changes he had to endure.

Nelson was a proud, bright man, who had built a small empire in the shipping industry in San Francisco. He came to the group only a few months before he died and said:

"I'm bored out of my mind; confined to the home."

"Normally I'm athletic. I'm developing theories of disc jockeys on the pop stations; they really are of limited character, but they don't realize it. Each one has an identity which he projects. After a few minutes listening to them, I can figure out what they're after."

"Feel like I'm in jail. I'm in a holding pattern. I'm breaking the monotony like any prisoner would."

"Ah, Nelson, now you're a spineless jellyfish. Resistant to change."

"Wasn't interested in yoga and meditation before I got sick, so why should I be now?"

"What's good for my cancer is what I'm getting here at the hospital."

Giving Nelson a place to share his wit and observation on disc jockeys and jails, a chance to tell us how he wanted to handle the last threads of his life, was all we could offer him, but it was enough to help sustain him for those weeks before his illness made him too sick to join us.

Some patients, whose illness stabilizes or goes into remission, can use the group to regain a sense of control over themselves and their own destiny. Martha used the group for a ten-month period to regain a positive view of herself. She joined us when her chemotherapy sessions were making her feel like a victim and she worked through a lot of issues about body image; how she was similar or different from others, her need to feel "special." By the time her chemotherapy was terminated, she had gained control over her view of herself, felt less guilty about having "caused" her illness, and was able to move on to her other concerns about her husband and children and to resume her normal life.

Peter summarized many of these issues and quandaries when he wrote:

Why is being powerless so scary? But, of course, I have no control over my cancer. It's in the hands of God. But don't you dare tell me what to do and give me no choices. Set the clocks each morning as if I were in control of the day.

I take my pills to control my disease, but of course, it's all in the hands of God. Of course I'm not responsible for my illness; I'm only responsible for how I live with it. God help us all.

CHRONIC AND TERMINAL ILLNESS

Many patients join the group long after their diagnosis and initial treatment period. Perhaps groups like ours meet the needs of the chronically ill best of all. Having to tolerate the continued losses, the need for further treatment, the recognition that the disease is progressing and may not be controlled, can be overwhelming to experience alone.

Louise wrote the following poem about a monthly incident in her chronic illness:

> Once a month there comes that day.
> Admission for an overnight stay
> For chemotherapy
> How I dread it!
> Why?
>
> First of all the tests:
> Cardiogram, blood analysis, chest x-ray;
> Next, what kind of roommate?
> Cheerful, sick, obnoxious?
> No sleep!
>
> Every thought brings back the same fears
> I've experienced for six years
> Why?
> Because it all started *here*
> In this atmosphere
> Where is your patience, Louise?
> You've always had it.

Writing and talking about an experience difficult to tolerate, that goes on and on, are helpful to many patients. For some, the group acts as a focused reminder that they have cancer. This allows them to forget about it with greater comfort between sessions—a kind of planned forgetting. One patient said, "I deal with it here so that I can forget it when I leave."

It occurs to most cancer patients that they are "victims" of their situation, but the chronically ill patient needs to take a look at this position. Forming an identity around being a cancer patient and developing interactions based on other people's feeling sorrow for you may be tough to avoid altogether, but it is worthwhile examining. Cancer patients, like patients with other disease, are vulnerable to regressions. They are in a position to use their illness to manipulate others to get their own way.

Patients tell stories of the "Look what so and so did to me" variety, sometimes with a great deal of anger; then we hear more and realize what the patient has done to provoke the incident. Sometimes they reveal their story reluctantly and with chagrin. The punch line is inevitable "But, I'm a cancer patient, you can't do that to me"; or, "Now look what you've done! I'm a cancer patient and

I may not live long." To help them avoid indulging in such secondary gains, we encourage group content around such issues as "self-pity," "envy," "being a victim," and "feeling exploited." Here is a partial dialogue from one session:

"How long does it last—that you feel sorry for yourself?"
"Oh, don't indulge yourself in pity; it's a waste of time."
"Self-pity is a cancer."
"Perhaps you have to go through the self-pity before you can know it's useless."
"I came here to express feelings I couldn't express any other way."

Along with "getting it off their chests," group members share the personal situations of self-pity that they have experienced and the ways they have found to extricate themselves from the regressive pulls of dwelling on their misfortunes, envying their healthier friends. Finding real choices, learning to say "no," sorting out the feelings from the facts, figuring out the reality in the situation, all help people to find ways to move ahead in their lives.

Some dying patients seek entrance to our group close to the point of their terminal illness, while others, chronically ill and long-term members of the group, will sometimes find themselves suddenly in a terminal phase. The new patient who comes in near death is often terribly lonely. Terminally ill patients may be "cut off" from their families and friends as a result of earlier problems, but sometimes, too, they increase their isolation by a reluctance to discuss their most central concerns with others.

Such a patient was Ted, a man in his thirties, confronted with terminal illness resulting from a mesothelioma. He and his wife had used the group for a while but dropped out when he grew better. The day this dialogue was recorded, he had returned to the group, very sick:

"If I hadn't gotten married, things would be a little easier. You're always on the fence. As good as Peg is, you still can't get to the point of saying, 'Well, I'm gonna die and you have to be strong.' Seems like you can never face the truth together; you can't finalize it; you're not sure. We got burial plots back East, but it's not going to happen. Didn't want to tell her; I want to hide it. I want to look around in myself and find the superman who knows exactly how to handle the problem."

Ted and Peg were finally able to talk about dying and his plans for himself and for her. His description of his sense of isolation and the difficulty in accepting what was happening was adeptly and poignantly phrased. The cancer patient who is dying goes through the emotional phases of denial, anger, bargaining, and depression, all over again. One young man in his twenties came to our group after a recurrence, following a long remission, shortly before death. He said: "There's got to be a way out; seems like I'm getting rushed into something. I was just learning more about this cancer and my body. Now, I feel like I just got gypped. I just got out of school and everything. I've been zapped by God. Well, I'm just going to have fun. I told my parents that it's a good feeling to be free. All that I know right now is these drugs are keeping me alive. I know that I'm sick and since I'm alive, I'm going to have fun. I got life in one fat package; sickness, aging, all that in one."

Hinton has said: "Our own death is not unimaginable, but can be imagined only with a considerable degree of distance, blurring and denial."

Gullo, Cherico and Shadick wrote in 1974: "In working with dying patients, one realizes that there are a variety of responses to the prospect of death; there are people who are "death accepters,' and there are people who are 'death deniers.' "

An older journalist joined our group during his last year of life, because he knew it was to be his last, and he wanted to celebrate the last days with new friends who would understand him as well as with old friends whom he saw at home. During one of his first creative writing sessions with us he wrote:

> The poet in me is still
> I'm ready to laugh at death
> But, life is absurd too
> And being alive — still
> I prefer to laugh at life
> But the poet in me is still
> Wake up, Poet, and tell me a funny story.

Bill celebrated life until the end, while accepting death with as much humor as ever I have seen.

Was Betty denying or accepting of her death when she wrote:

> I, of course, am not as others
> I, alone, am immortal
> Forever young
> The obituaries will be great
> But none, I think, do there embrace

This well-known, local educator used the group only briefly in our setting. Her purpose in coming was to learn how we did it, so she could help another hospital set up a group of its own.

After an active group member has died, there is recognition, discussion, and mourning of the lost person for one or perhaps several sessions. Mary wrote this to Bill after he died:

> Bill, I miss seeing you today
> When you walked into the room
> The whole place seemed to light up
> I loved the way you hugged me one day
> It made me feel so good

Reminiscing and sharping regrets for the person who died, having our own memorial service, has become an important folkway in our group. Those who remain know that they too will be mourned should they die. It is reassuring to look around the room into the eyes of one another and remember that *we are* still here, alive, and feel "let's go on."

GROUP GOALS

What goals might leaders consider for cancer groups? Our groups evolved over time, through a natural growth and development process. However, we have sharpened our focus and sense of direction since April, 1975, when funding allowed for expansion of staff. As group leaders, we have found it helpful to have weekly discussions about the issues that develop within the group. Although each of our three groups is concerned with particular tasks and group problems, we have identified a number of goals that may be pertinent to all ongoing groups of cancer patients and their families. Here is a short description of group goals as we see them currently:

1) *Provision of a support system:* Whether for a short or long period of time, we are providing a place where patients can come and talk about problems and develop an ongoing relationship that sustains or mobilizes them in relation to the rest of their lives. It is a place where they can reveal themselves in a regressed fashion and find that they are accepted. For example, listen to Larry's complaint:

> Don't like being such a fool.
> Don't feel my problems are as important as others.
> Much ado about nothing.
> Joseph Heller knew what he wanted to be...
> A little boy
> The group is a part of health
> Creates mirrors that otherwise might not exist

In the adult patient's group, creative writing is an important part of the support system too. Patients and leaders find ways of saying things through writing that might have been only hinted at during the verbal exchange. We share the writing orally with one another immediately after it is completed, then Julia Vose, our poet leader, brings it back to us the following week, typed and copied for distribution. Bill made this written observation about the value to him of the writing:

> I love this group
>
> Even reading our history in the group is exciting
> Samuel Johnson said, 'The knowledge that he is to
> be hanged doth wonderfully focus a man's mind.' I
> want a new poem, "Intimations of Mortality," maybe

that's what the group is writing week by week. I
see the group as a flower garden, beautiful doubts,
healthy fears to smell and savor.

We see the cancer group bridging the medical and nonmedical lives of patients during the tough times in their medical course. We also see ourselves helping some patients to refocus needs so as not to use the group when another means might do as well.

2) *Catharsis:* We are providing a place for the release of pent-up feelings of anger, grief, and fear in an ongoing structure. Patients can count on seeing us and each other on a regular basis. The sharing of feelings with others who have experienced them, and the merging of experience, reduce a patient's sense of isolation. Sometimes we see patients relax from a previously constricted or stereotyped reaction that existed when they entered the group. It is beneficial for them to have a place to repeat stories of trauma until they have mastered the feelings that have gone along with the experience. Peter described a blow-up with his son that came at a time when he was worried about further recurrence of his disease:

Generally bothered, I blew up at my son last night. My head hot in trouble thinking I had more cancer. Have to see the doc next week. Moody. . . emotional. . . I can't control when I get a recurrence. I cook dinner and he's supposed to put the dishes away. *SMOKING!!!* I *hate* smoke; I screamed and ranted like an ass at things I can't stand in myself. "Get out of the house," I said. "There's a lot of things about me you don't like." Can't control my cancer, can't control my son. Said a lot of things I wish I hadn't. When I see myself in him, Oh! I think, it's heredity when you see those bad things.

The initial traumas of the early diagnosis and treatment period are surprising and often catch people unaware of a new role they must respond to, but the ongoing worries that chronic illness brings create a periodic stress for many patients, reawakening feelings of anger, grief, and fear.

3) *Help in Overcoming Regressive Pulls to Passivity:* Group members offer help to each other in a number of ways. They are first tolerant of the new or sicker members' regressive behavior. By sharing information on medical treatment programs, they offer each other *hope* that treatments are beneficial in extending life and reducing pain. The altruism of offering help to one another assists the cancer patient to move from the passive position of victim to an active stance. We encourage patients who are physically able to become volunteers in our hospital or in another beneficial health organization, such as the American Cancer Society. Those who do so feel less helpless about themselves. As the weeks go by, group members hear how they might behave differently, and they benefit from "imitating" one another's successful behavior in coping with familiar problems, such as asking questions of busy physicians.

4) *Reality Testing:* Patients use the group to sort out their feelings and ex-

periences that have been unfamiliar and frightening. Hearing from others how they dealt with a variety of issues helps all patients feel less crazy and less alone. Yalom (1975, p. 26) states that reality testing is part of all group process and has been experienced by some as part of the curative factor, for example, when the patient learns that some initial reactions were not suited to the situation. In follow-up interviews with long-term cancer-patient group members, we found this to be true too. For example, one angry patient realized that she was expecting too much of her doctor.

5) *Facilitating Adaptive Communication:* Patients often avoid discussion of feelings or practical issues with their families. Sometimes they have difficulty saying "no" to family members' requests of them. For example, some relatives wish the sick member to continue in all family activities as before, denying to themselves the seriousness of the patient's illness. Many benefit from rehearsing how they might get points across to important others. Group cohesiveness is often most evident as members help one another find ways to be more direct in their communication of facts and feelings that have been difficult for them to get across in the past. "I used to have your problem, and here is how I dealt with it," one often hears in group. Group members borrow self-esteem from one another as needed, which is particularly helpful when they are feeling so battered and diminished by their immediate circumstances.

6) *Relief from a Sense of Omnipotence and Guilt:* Though it is one of the "regressive pulls," this issue is so important that it deserves individual mention. We have noticed that both cancer patients and family members often share the irrational and magical belief that they themselves have caused the illness. They believe that if they only had the proper attitude or strategy, they could cure it. Currently, patients talk about using medication as a way of controlling their disease. Some patients enter the group verbalizing concern about having caused their illness: "My cancer is my punishment for all my evil thoughts," a group member confided.

Sarah entered the group feeling guilty about having caused her cancer: "I'm responsible for causing my cancer. It has to do with my game of being dependent. I delayed seeing a doctor. It's their fault, I couldn't trust them."

Anthropologists have found that under stressful circumstances, the need to find *cause* increases in proportion to the immediacy of danger. Abrams and Finesinger (1953), in interviewing patients on their attitudes toward cancer, found that 56 out of 60 patients made statements indicating that they considered their illness to be their fault or the fault of others. Guilt seems to be a universal part of the life experience in illness.

In our own experience, both with cancer-patient survivors and currently diagnosed patients, we have found, anecdotally, that most of the patients interviewed recognized a moment or two of feeling personally guilty for their illness but dismissed the notion or refused to dwell on it when they saw themselves getting better.

Patients most troubled with guilt feelings seem to be those who do not have satisfying support systems currently, or those for whom the present illness is a reminder of sadness and loss in the past. Two case examples come to mind.

Sarah felt that her bitterness toward her husband led to her later development of breast cancer. Martha felt that her cancer was connected to the loss of her parents during her teenage years. Both women felt relief in exposing these irrational connections and in sorting out, verbally, the various parts of the unfinished business from the past. Connecting old guilts with new problems is a common human predicament that can be a great source of unhappiness for patients. Talking about childhood problems that have persisted within us down through the years and seeing the connections with our feelings about ourselves today can be a gradually liberating experience. We find that patients who enter the group with a heightened sense of personal guilt tend, as time passes, to relax the feelings of omnipotence and guilt. As Peter wrote:

> What causes cancer? Not living right?
> Not feeling right? Pollution?
> Anger? Loss? Grief?
>
> But those things are *LIFE*
> Life causes cancer
> The dreams point to the Bull of Lascau
> The DNA way back from the big bang
>
> So cancer makes you religious
> In the sense of *MYSTERY*
> That the real sources are unknowable
> And so remains the future
> Another religious mystery

We have shared with you some of the history of the cancer groups at Mount Zion Hospital, some of the patient needs that are met by the groups, and some of the goals that we as leaders set for ourselves in providing such groups. It is a fascinating growth and development experience for us as leaders, as well as a potentially helpful process for patients. It is, as described by our poet-patient, "a part of health," creating "mirrors that otherwise might not exist."

REFERENCES

Abrams, R. and J. Finesinger. 1953. "Guilt Reactions in Patients with Cancer." *Cancer*, 6(3):474-482.

Buchanan, D.C. 1975. "Group Therapy for Kidney Transplant Patients." *International Journal of Psychiatry in Medicine,* 6(47).

Gullo, S.V., D.J. Cherico, and R. Shadick. 1974. "Suggested Stages and Response Styles in Life-Threatening Illness." In B. Schoenberg et al. (eds.), *Anticipatory Grief,* New York: Columbia University Press.

Mages, N.L. 1976. *Psychosocial Change and Adaptation in Cancer Patients.* National Cancer Institute Grant Application.

Yalom, I.D. 1975. *The Theory and Practice of Group Psychotherapy.* New York: Basic Books, Inc.

———. 1976. *Cancer and the Group Experience.* Keynote address, Social Work Subcommittee, American Cancer Society, Los Angeles, California.

PATIENT GROUP THERAPY SESSIONS

Joan M. Liaschenko

The utilization of group therapy began in 1904, when Dr. J.H. Pratt of Boston treated groups of tubercular patients in private homes because they could not afford care in a sanatarium. Dr. Pratt observed that in addition to learning to care for themselves, the group created an environment that fostered emotional support. For the following 50 years, Dr. Pratt continued to experiment with the use of groups in helping his patients and eventually in 1956 coined the term "group psychotherapy." Definitions of group psychotherapy have varied from the extremes of rigid, clearly delineated purposes aimed at patient defenses to the concept that anything happening between more than two people in a therapeutic situation is group therapy. Generally speaking, group therapy may be defined as "that form of therapy which is practiced by clinicians in groups formed for the specific purpose of helping individuals with their psychological and emotional difficulties, the depth of such therapy depending largely on the individual technique of the therapist."

Since the initial work of Dr. Pratt, group therapy has become an accepted psychiatric treatment modality. Recently, however, there has been a renewed interest in using group techniques as a method of helping medical patients cope with the emotional aspects of their illness. This paper briefly describes, from the author's viewpoint, the experience of group therapy sessions conducted under the auspices of a department of radiation therapy.

Hodgkin's disease, frequently a disease of adolescents and young adults, places great stress on these persons who must cope with their disease at a time when major developmental problems occur. For this reason, we elected to work with this group. With the exception of this homogeneous classification, no other criterion was determined by design. All physiological stages of the disease were represented except Stage IV, and all cell types, with one exception, were mixed cellularity. Seven patients, five females and two males, constituted the group. The group lasted 15 sessions, with one female and one male terminating prior to that time. The ages ranged from 16 to 34 years.

Perhaps the most interesting variation was the time intervals in relation to completion of radiation therapy, which ranged from those currently in treatment to five years post-treatment. Patient selection was made by the attending radiation therapist, with the explanation to the patient that this group would serve two purposes: first, it would provide a supportive environment where they could share their concerns with people facing similar difficulties, and secondly, they would be helping the staff to learn more about people with Hodgkin's disease so that we could provide optimal care. The patients responded very positively, especially to the second reason. Group sessions were videotaped with the patients' permission and proved to be a helpful adjunct to the group process itself. Two women—a psychiatric resident and the author, a psychiatric nurse—were the group leaders. Weekly one-hour sessions were held for 15 weeks. This paper is descriptive rather than analytic and interpretive, and the group process will not be readily discernible. However, it is hoped that the reader will gain an understanding of both the salient themes elicited and how patients were helped with them by the group.

Because physical difficulties were a common experience, this subject became the logical focal point of the group. Initially, much attention was given to procedures such as biopsies and x-rays, which were recounted in vivid detail. However, few emotions were expressed in relation to them. As the focus continued, a sense of group cohesiveness began to develop. As a result, patients felt less isolated and more comfortable in participating. In addition to this development, the therapists made a gradual attempt to help patients relate feelings to descriptions of physical distress and changes.

With this discussion came the realization that the group members had received variations in the standard treatment regimen. Knowledge of this disparity produced anxiety and was initially dealt with in a manner of intellectual acceptance and a denial of affect. Members continually made the group aware of information they had received through others and from various publications. As the group progressed, the awareness of the anxiety increased and culminated in the group's request to have a radiation therapist present to answer their questions. A few weeks prior to the termination of the group, a physician spent a session with us, which was very therapeutic. The majority of patients were able to ask very direct questions such as the meaning of staging and why treatment regimens varied. The serenity, humor, and sincerity displayed by the physician had an extraordinary effect in relieving the patients' anxiety.

It should be noted that the author, unlike the patients, was quite anxious because of the expectation that they would become acutely distressed. That this did not happen demonstrates the fact that, most often, staff's expectations of patients' behavior are a projection of their own feelings. Because anxiety had been alleviated and concrete information provided, the patients felt comfortable in asking about the possibilities of producing defective children as a result of exposure to radiation, a topic that had not been previously mentioned. They asked the physician for his advice on having children, which he answered in a sincere, humane, and ethical manner. For some patients this was a resolution to many months of anxiety.

The diagnosis of a potentially fatal disease seemed to precipitate in many members feelings about the loss of relationships and persons and concerns about their families. Members began to reflect on the losses they had experienced, which ranged from the death of close relatives to neighbors moving, and their subsequent reactions. It was striking to realize the amount of psychological isolation they felt, which interfered with their expression of affection, grief, and anger. It should be kept in mind that this sense of isolation existed prior to the diagnosis of Hodgkin's disease. Patients often reported the fear of crying and/or inability to cry in front of family members for fear of upsetting them. This method of coping frequently resulted in their being the main support to their families, often at the expense of loss of emotional support to themselves.

Inability of family members to communicate their needs and anxieties to one another resulted in several forms of tension. For example, there were the feelings of guilt if a mother could not completely care for her husband and children, resentment because everything was being done for them, which left them with the feeling that they were no longer part of their families, and guilt because they were placing emotional, physical, and financial burdens on their families. Not only did these patients have difficulty in verbalizing their needs, but they also felt guilty about needing support at all. As one young woman phrased it, "My husband is too good."

Because the purpose of the group was not to provide intensive therapy, the etiology of these difficulties was not an issue. It was stressed, however, that similar feelings and experiences were shared by the members and their families, with the result that in the group patients learned to express emotions that they had been unable to convey at home. Members began to move beyond their isolation to some degree, and they were able to take this new-found strength back to their families and friends.

"What causes cancer?" became a very important issue that was repeatedly introduced into the group. Punishment from God, pollution, emotional difficulties resulting from childbearing and the death of loved ones, and the need to suffer were reasons given. Much literature exists on the personality characteristics of cancer patients and the psychosomatic aspects of neoplastic disease. Much of the material elicited in this group lends support to those hypotheses. Intensive research needs to be done in this area, and groups may prove to be a useful clinical methodology in addition to providing therapeutic assistance to the patients. In this group, these issues were not directly worked through in any depth or detail, but the mere verbalization of them was helpful.

Regardless of the prognosis, people who receive a diagnosis of cancer live with the threat of death. This theme—although it varied in intensity and form—was present throughout the duration of the group. All patients except one reported that upon diagnosis they immediately "looked it up," in everything from dictionaries to technical medical journals. From their reading all believed that

Hodgkin's disease is fatal. The shock and horror felt at this time was assuaged by the positive yet serious attitude conveyed by the physicians and the support given by the technicians who actually treated them. With this initial help they were able to mobilize some of their resources. However, the importance of time cannot be overestimated. The amount of acute anxiety experienced seemed proportional to the length of time from completion of treatment. Perhaps the belief in an absolute cure after five years of survival contributed to this. It may be necessary for a given amount of time, which understandably would vary between patients, to elapse before someone can deal creatively with the possibility of death.

In summary, this group was formed to provide a supportive environment for patients with Hodgkin's disease to share their experiences and concerns and as a method of education for the staff in how these patients perceive their illness and function with it. Five major themes were consistent throughout the group; namely, physical difficulties, the disparity in treatment methods, loss and difficulties communicating with family, the etiology of cancer, and the threat of death. The group attempted to provide support, decrease feelings of isolation, and help one another reflect on some of their problems. Intervention on the part of the therapists was minimal, being primarily limited to helping them relate feelings to experiences and encouraging them to support one another, and to be more accepting of themselves and their needs.

Many more questions were raised than answered, but this uncertainty is a positive step. Perhaps more research will be directed toward this area, with the result that group therapy will become an effective, accepted modality in helping patients deal creatively with serious illness and death.

CONCEPTS OF ADAPTATION AND LIFE CHANGE IN CANCER PATIENTS*

Norman L. Mages, Gerald Mendelsohn, and Joseph Castro

As part of a cancer rehabilitation project, the authors studied the longterm effects of cancer on patients who have survived their illness for up to six years. Perhaps, because we were primarily studying survivors, rather than acutely ill or dying patients, we found that existing conceptual approaches did not do justice to the material that emerged. Many older psychodynamic concepts, derived from the study of neurotic patients, were relevant but were not precise or specific enough when applied to the reality-based problems of cancer patients. We discovered that 1) we required more carefully drawn concepts of adaptation in order to understand the normal range and course of patient responses, and 2) we needed an appropriate way to formulate and account for the profound life changes observed in these long-term cancer survivors. To meet the first requirement, we extended and applied accepted psychodynamic principles to the realities faced by cancer patients; for the second, we drew on some promising newer perspectives in adult development that have not yet been systematically employed in studying reactions to cancer, but that provide illuminating ways of viewing long-term life changes. The following is a presentation of the basic conceptual approach which we adopted, along with the considerations that led to its development, and some results of our investigation which illustrate its use.

Our study is based on interviews with about 60 adult cancer patients drawn primarily from a population treated with radiation therapy, and their families, and on group discussions with an additional 40 other patients and their family members. The interviewed subjects were selected consecutively from lists of patients admitted for cancer treatment. They included three- and six-year survivors as

---

*This investigation was supported in part by U.S.P.H. Grant CA 16873 from the NIH National Cancer Institute.

well as newly diagnosed patients, in order to provide cross-sections at different points in the course of the illness. Our contacts with them were both intensive and extended in time. Multiple individual interviews with each patient, and sometimes an additional family member, generally totalled four to eight hours. Two patient discussion groups and a group of family members met weekly for over a year, providing ample opportunity to explore common problems in considerable depth.

These efforts produced an enormous amount of clinical material. Our attempts to organize the data in a meaningful fashion took us through phases of assembling individual case histories, examining psychological responses and defenses, gathering overall impressions, quantifying some types of observations, and striving to define the existential realities of such an illness. It soon became evident that our spontaneous efforts were an abbreviated recapitulation of the historical development of cancer studies.

Thus, in the 1950's and early 1960's many psychoanalytic and psychodynamic studies appeared that described the meaning of cancer for an individual and the psychological reactions and defense mechanisms of patients in adjusting to living with the acute stages of cancer. Examples are studies of series of patients by Shands and Finesinger (1951), Abrams and Finesinger (1953), and a group of papers from Memorial Hospital in New York (Sutherland et al., 1952; Orbach and Sutherland, 1953; Bard and Sutherland, 1955; Drellich et al., 1956). There were also individual case studies, such as those by Norton (1963) and Renneker et al. (1963). As such studies accumulated, some authors attempted a general overview, e.g., Senescu (1963); Bronner-Huszar (1971); Peck (1972); Holland (1973). More recently, the trend has been toward quantitative study, as exemplified by the work of Worden and Weisman (1975) and Weisman (1976). Other clinicians have emphasized the existential aspects of the patient's situation (Krant, 1974) and the individual physician's relationship with his patients (Rosenbaum, 1974). Psychoanalytic case studies have tended to be replaced by first person accounts of the cancer experience, such as those by Harker (1972) and Harrell (1972).

While a great deal has obviously been learned about how people react to cancer, we found that some of the questions in which we were most interested were still unanswered. In two areas especially, there were gaps in the literature relevant to our own work, which required new ways of thinking about the issues:

1) Most studies in the literature report work with troubled patients who are seen at one particular phase of their illness; relatively little has been established regarding the normal range of patient reactions to cancer, and the progression of these responses over time. In our own work we are following a sample of "normal" patients who do not present because of psychological difficulties. We needed a conceptual approach that would allow us to depict the entire psychosocial course of these patients, along with its typical variations. Central to such an approach is the identification of the major issues that confront cancer patients at different stages of their illness, and of the methods patients use to deal with

these issues. Identifying such issues and coping methods makes it much easier to determine the manner and effectiveness with which a given patient deals with his illness and provides a basis for delineating and comparing different types of patients.

2) Most investigators have focused either on the patient receiving acute treatment or on the dying patient. The large group of cancer patients who have no recurrence, or those who are likely to live for a considerable period of time with their illness, receive much less attention. A few follow-up studies have begun to appear: Schottenfeld and Robbins (1970), Izsak and Medalie (1971), Schoenfeld (1972), Izsak et al. (1973), Craig et al. (1974). Though useful, these have mainly been surveys that provide little clinical material, are based on an assessment at a single point, and consequently do not yield much information about what processes lead to different outcomes. Our own retrospective interviews with three- and six-year cancer survivors impressed us with how profoundly many of their lives had been changed by their experience with cancer, even when there was a good medical result. We needed conceptual models which could do justice to such long lasting changes and the processes producing them and that could place these changes within the developmental context of patients' lives.

In pursuing these objectives we have begun to make use of three overlapping models, each of which will be discussed in turn. Though each model has immediate and long-term aspects, we found it helpful to view immediate responses in terms of adaptational concepts, mid-range effects in terms of psychosocial transitions, and long-term changes in the context of adult developmental life stages.

ADAPTIVE MODEL

As increasing attention has been paid to responses to major illnesses and other types of life crisis, a psychological point of view that emphasizes stress, adaptation, and coping has become more prominent. (Janis, 1958; Hamburg and Adams, 1967; Katz et al., 1970; Lazarus, 1966; Coelho et al., 1974; Horowitz, 1976). In applying this approach to cancer patients, we used our individual interviews and group discussions to identify and sort out the various themes expressed by patients. We found that their concerns tended to cluster around certain basic issues. For each issue one could conceptualize an adaptive task that needed to be accomplished successfully to enable the issue to be resolved and the patient to proceed with the business of living. While these issues must be faced by every cancer patient, the intensity and significance of each will vary with the individual, the stage of the illness, and his other external circumstances.

For the cancer patient in the earlier stages of illness, these issues and tasks may be grouped as follows:

1) *Issue: Trauma of the acute illness; symptoms, diagnosis, treatment.* For many patients, this has the characteristics of a traumatic experience; a sudden catastrophic event, assault on one's body, disruption of normal

life—all of which lead to a sense of being overwhelmed with shock, numbness, flight, outbursts of feeling, or repetitive reliving in fantasy or dream. *Adaptive task:* To be able to recognize and deal with the realities of the situation, regulate the emotional reactions, and integrate the experience of illness with the rest of one's life.

2) *Issue: Possibility of recurrence and progression of disease.* Usually this intense fear gradually eases over the years, especially with the successful passage of the five-year point, but it seldom disappears entirely. The fear may be paralyzing or may profoundly influence life decisions. *Adaptive task:* In order to live with this fear, it is necessary to be able to put it out of mind most of the time, yet at the same time be sufficiently aware of it to continue appropriate medical follow-up and to take it into consideration in making long-range plans.

3) *Issue: Damage to one's body from the illness and/or treatment.* (compare Adsett, 1963; Schoenberg and Carr, 1970; Blacker, 1970). This includes loss of energy, body parts, important functions, and disfigurement. The damage varies greatly with cancer site and with the stage of the illness and the type of treatment, but it is often permanent. *Adaptive task:* To mourn the loss, replace or compensate for lost parts or functions, where possible, and maximize other potentials so as to maintain a sense of self-esteem and intactness.

4) *Issue: Maintaining continuity; finding a way to return to the fabric of one's life after the dislocation of illness and treatment.* Patients frequently report that they are changed by the experience of cancer and develop new attitudes toward time, mortality, work, relationships, and their priorities in life. In addition, they frequently find that they, in turn, are treated differently by family, friends, and employers. *Adaptive task:* To understand and communicate one's changed attitudes, needs, and limitations in a way that permits formation of a new balance with the environment. Ideally, this should proceed with a minimum of constriction of one's life and activities and without becoming socially excluded or assuming an identity based solely on being a "cancer patient."

5) *Issue: Maintaining a sense of self-sufficiency and control.* The sudden realization of life-threatening illness, inability to personally affect the course of the disease, and damage to one's body, relationships, and career, often lead to a profoundly disturbing sense of powerlessness and lack of control over one's life. *Adaptive task:* To become able to exercise choice, where possible, and to accept one's helplessness and dependency, where necessary, without excessive regression or seeking a "magical solution" in lieu of appropriate treatment.

If recurrent, disseminated disease is discovered, the issues a patient faces are changed radically. In most cases he is no longer a cancer "survivor" and so must be prepared for new physical symptoms and the likelihood of disabling treatment, pain, progressive infirmity, and death. Though there may be extended remissions and periods of comfortable and productive life remaining, such a patient lives in a different experiential world from the disease-free survivor. The tasks that must be faced include maintaining emotional equilibrium so as not to succumb to fear and despair, preparing to leave family and friends, providing for loved ones, and using medical assistance and one's own resources to minimize pain and disability. In brief, it is essential to come to terms with the prospect of death so that the remainder of life can be lived in as full and satisfying a manner as possible.

The issues and adaptive tasks faced by patients at different stages of illness have their counterpart in those faced by the family. Each issue places certain stresses on family and other close relationships, and each adaptation is influenced by the support (or lack of it) from family and intimate friends. Our interviews with patients and families have revealed a fairly high incidence of problems in communication, difficulties because of role shifts, and interference with family tasks and activities. Family disruption occasionally occurs, and children are affected in many ways, such as increased difficulty in separating from parents and a tendency to identify with the ill parent.

We may organize the methods by which patients cope with their illness into three main groups:

1) Use of some of the many varieties of avoidance and denial is very common, perhaps universal (Weisman, 1972; Weisman and Hackett, 1967). Most patients find these techniques helpful in managing their anxiety and in keeping themselves from dwelling unnecessarily on their illness. We have been impressed that patients are careful to maintain appropriate medical follow-up treatment and use avoidance and denial in very specific and selective ways that typically do not endanger their survival. These latter techniques would include remaining unaware of facts, not perceiving the implications of known facts, and not registering that knowledge on an emotional level. Avoidance is often reinforced by keeping too busy to think and by restricting one's life so as not to be confronted by painful realities.

2) Efforts at active mastery may co-exist or alternate with the need to avoid (Hamburg and Adams, 1967). A patient may adapt by actively seeking information about his illness, the problems it imposes, and the ways in which other cancer patients have handled these problems. He may take an active role in his own medical care and in other ways control the course of his life as much as possible. A mechanism that we have observed in a number of patients is the turning of the passive patient role into one of actively caring for and helping others.

3) Because a patient is realistically limited in his own ability to meet all of his needs and to influence the course of his illness, he must turn to others for help. This may take the form of appropriate and realistic dependence

upon medical caregivers, family, and friends. It may become an exaggerated and childish dependence in which the illness is used to extort excessive care, or, on the other hand, the patient may avoid even an appropriate degree of dependency. In their helplessness and desperation, we have sometimes seen patients turn for rescue to "higher powers," in the form of an excessively idealized physician, through religious faith, or in a belief in miracle cures and magical thoughts. While a few of our patients made their physicians into gods and an occasional patient could not develop a trusting relationship with any doctor, most patients looked to their physicians for facts, understanding, and skillful treatment of their cancer. With an occasional exception, they did not discuss much of their personal lives with their physician but still derived tremendous support from knowing that he was interested, competent, and available.

Most of our observations support the view that cancer patients handle their illness more easily if they are securely imbedded in a social matrix. Patients tended to turn to family or friends to talk things over. In our study it was rare for a patient to seek professional psychological counseling. Although religion was important to some, they seldom talked to clergymen about their personal difficulties. These data are similar to Krant's (1976) findings and emphasize the importance of various kinds of informal support systems (Caplan and Killelea, 1976). We have seen some patients who always lived relatively isolated but stable lives and did not find it comfortable or useful suddenly to seek out close supportive relationships with others. These patients often rely heavily on another type of support that is frequently overlooked—the important stabilizing influence of the routines of work and daily living. We have been impressed with the degree to which each patient develops and structures an individualized support system, based on his interacting with others. Unfortunately, some patients with the greatest needs have the least skill in enlisting the aid of others.

A patient's choice of coping methods depends partly on his own personality and partly on the realities of his illness. Sutherland (1967) has emphasized that each patient's reactions can be understood fully only if one investigates the individual meaning of the illness. In our own material we have seen how unresolved conflicts around dependency, sexuality, and aggression, along with their attendant guilts, become intensified or rekindled. In some of these cases, past experience with cancer in a close relative or friend had a profound bearing on the personal meaning of the disease. Our impression is that, in dealing with both the realities of illness and the psychological conflicts which are reactivated, a patient will first rely on the methods which have worked most successfully in the past, resulting in a characteristic coping style. Along with Katz et al. (1970), we found that, aside from certain primitive defenses such as massive denial or projection, effective coping may occur by means of a variety of different strategies. We have seen patients handle their illness well by avoiding thinking about cancer, by actively seeking information and control, by gathering a supportive coterie around them, or by going it relatively alone. The specifics of the medical situation also play an important role in determining the availability of certain coping methods. For example, we have found, not surprisingly, that the greater the symptoms, functional impairment, and degree of bodily damage, the harder it is for a patient to avoid being reminded continually of the illness with all its associated fears. We were impressed with how patients use denial much more readily when warding off feelings associated with hidden internal damage than when they must constantly face a visible deformity such as a facial disfigurement or absence of a breast. Somewhat similar observations have been made by Plumb and Holland (1974) and by Krant (1976).

PSYCHOSOCIAL TRANSITIONS

Recently, there have been attempts to develop the concept of psychosocial transitions to apply to those human circumstances in which resolution of a crisis leads to an altered state of mind, lasting life changes occur, and the person experiences himself and his world in a new way. This approach, as used by Parkes (1972) to understand bereavement and loss and by Weiss (1975) to conceptualize changes around divorce, seems to us to offer considerable promise as a way of viewing the course of many cancer patients.

In the crisis model often employed in conceptualizing reactions to stress, it is assumed that the stress upsets an initial equilibrium and that the task of the individual is to resolve the crisis situation so that he can return to the original state. However, our observations and the observations of others (Abrams, 1966; Gullo et al., 1974; Quint, 1963), indicate that adaptation to cancer proceeds through a sequence of phases that evolve over time. Thus, one can speak of periods of: 1) initial turmoil, 2) trials of various modes of coping, and 3) formation of a relatively stable adaptive pattern that often differs considerably from the pre-illness state. Although one must take into account individual differences between patients, it is our strong impression that absence, distortion, or arrest of this sequence may well herald a serious difficulty in rehabilitation. We also found, in discussions with radiology technicians, nurses, and physicians, that experienced medical personnel frequently use an intuitive knowledge of this sequence to predict that the patients who deviate from it are likely to encounter future difficulties. Nevertheless, it can be extremely difficult to predict long-term outcome from antecedent factors or from observations made early in the course of illness. New events occur which can change a patient's medical and personal situation. Probably the most important single factor affecting the patient's future emotional state is whether the cancer recurs. Non-cancer related events such as the death of a spouse or a new crippling illness may also have a profound impact.

One reason for selecting the particular six-year retrospective sample of patients used in our study was that a number of observations about their emotional responses had been recorded by social workers and residents at the time of initial treatment. When we looked at the interviews with the survivors, there was little correlation between the initial judgments of distress, understanding of illness, or appropriateness of response, and their emotional state and daily functioning six years later. Although it is possible that more refined initial observations might make a difference, we are inclined to attribute the lack of correlation to the influence of inter-current events and to the difficulties inherent in making long-term predictions about someone who is seen in a state of acute turmoil. A more valid hypothesis may be that a patient's state at six or twelve months after diagnosis correlates better with long-term outcome than does his initial state.

In our studies we found that most patients experience a marked change in themselves as a result of having cancer, and only a few reported that they returned to their previous mode of living, unchanged by the encounter with illness. The great majority described changes in self-image, values, capacities, and sometimes, in the direction of their lives. The changes in self-image were highlighted in our retrospective study by use of the Gough-Heilbrun (1965) Adjective Check List, on which patients were asked to describe themselves as they were before becoming ill and as they saw themselves at the current time, three years later. A rather consistent picture emerged. Although patients reported little alteration in the level of dysphoric affect, nervousness, and the like, an increase in distractibility, absent-mindedness, and loss of concentration was frequent. Ambition, drive, aggressiveness, the striving for achievement and recognition were seen as having declined, while tolerance, humane concern, and understanding were reported to have increased. Overall, the impression is of lowered intensity and engagement in the external world, coupled with a more mellow focus on the smaller world of home, family, and friends. An unexpected finding was a significant difference between men and women in the way they perceived themselves. For the women, positive and negative changes tended to balance out, and they were able to preserve their self-esteem relatively well over the three years. Among the men, the perceived decline in activity, assertiveness, and striving for achievement led to a much less positive self image.

By the use of family interviews, it was often possible to confirm the patient's own impressions of how their work, family, social, and sexual lives had changed. Frequently, these changes took the form of a withdrawal or constriction of activities. Situations that evoked unpleasant memories or feelings of being less attractive or desirable were avoided. Patients who felt overwhelmed by the multiple physical, emotional, and practical burdens of illness often narrowed their interests to create a smaller and more manageable world. Such outcomes appeared to be the result of a process beginning early in the course of illness. We found a number of instances in which unsuccessful early adaptive efforts resulted in chronic psychological symptoms, diminished self-esteem, reduced functioning, or use of illness to obtain gratification from or power over others.

LIFE STAGES

The importance of viewing psychosocial processes in the context of the human life cycle has become generally accepted (Erikson, 1950; Lidz, 1968) but, historically, the emphasis has been placed on unraveling the complexities of childhood development. Only in recent years has more adequate attention been paid to adult development and aging (as reviewed, for example, by Neugarten, 1968a, and by Schaie, 1975). In similar fashion, we find that while the developmental stage in which cancer occurs has been recognized as a crucial variable in children and adolescents (Easson, 1968; Binger et al., 1969; Moore, 1969; Schowalter, 1970), a life-stage perspective has seldom been used to understand how adults deal with cancer or other life-threatening illnesses. A notable exception is the study by Rosen and Bibring (1966) which demonstrated that the manner in which men react to myocardial infarction is markedly different for different age groups.

Adult development is not tied as closely to biological maturation as is childhood development, and therefore adult life stages are not as neatly demarcated, but there is wide agreement that adult life may be usefully grouped into stages that differ with respect to biological changes of aging, level of experience, social norms and expectations, time perspective, economic status, and position in the family life cycle (Neugarten, 1968b). These differences result in particular concerns and conflicts becoming uppermost at each stage of life (Erikson, 1959), concerns that sometimes are congruent and sometimes quite different for men and women (Lowenthal, 1976). Lowenthal examined the normative transitions that mark the entrance and exit of each life stage and found that idiosyncratic transitions, such as serious illness or impairments, may have a profound bearing on growth or regression. Many of her subjects reported considerable change in themselves, their values, and their behavioral patterns accompanying or following such events.

We use life stage concepts in two ways: 1) as an independent variable that partly determines the mode of experiencing cancer and the personal and social resources available for coping with it and 2) as a framework to help evaluate long-term outcome. Changes in life patterns can be viewed in terms of shifts in the developmental course of an individual's life and can also be compared with the norms for that person's age group.

In our studies we found it most feasible to arrange patients into the three broad categories of young, mid-life, and older adults. While somewhat arbitrary, the grouping by age alone represents a first approximation of a meaningful classification, especially if one also uses other developmental landmarks, such as marriage, the presence of children at home, or retirement.

Young Adults (18-35): In keeping with the findings of many observers, we noted that the young adults in our study were concerned primarily with separation from their parents and with establishing stable, intimate relationships, marriages, families, and careers. The experience of cancer at this stage tended to impede the development of self-sufficiency, and, for some young people, it resulted in delay and disruption of their efforts to establish themselves in adult roles. Their uncertain future made it difficult to embark on a commitment in any direction. The sense of soberness and altered priorities that came with facing possible death left some of the younger people feeling out of touch with their more carefree, "childish" contemporaries. Resolution of "intimacy vs. isolation," the conflict that Erikson found most characteristic of this age group, is greatly complicated by the patient's increased needs for comfort and support, which place great stresses on intimate relationships and young marriages. Some couples are able to grow closer in the process of dealing with these pressures, but in other relationships we have seen the demands of illness lead to excessive clinging or to avoidance of communication and intimacy.

Mid-Life Adults (36-55): In middle life (Butler, 1975a; Neugarten, 1968a), there is a gradual change in time perspective. The passage of time is clocked by career and family milestones, and life comes to be viewed in terms of time left to live. For some, this period may be experienced as the prime of life, with a maximum sense of mastery and control. A trend towards introspection usually begins, which includes taking stock of one's accomplishments, failures, and unfinished business. Adult roles and position in life have become firmly established, for better or worse. Erikson emphasizes the need to contribute to and care for others, to be "generative" rather than "stagnant."

In adults of this age whom we studied, the occurrence of cancer threatened disruption of the roles that they had built through so much effort, and of the important tasks that they had yet to carry out. They experienced a foreshortening of the future and increased concern about their remaining time. Working men and women worried about being able to maintain their occupations, financial security, and self-sufficiency. Parents feared that they would not be able to care for their children and help them grow to maturity. Husbands and wives were afraid that they would no longer be adequate partners and might become unable to meet their spouse's economic, emotional and sexual needs.

In our study this age group showed the greatest variation in response; it included some patients who were the most able to take their illness in stride and some who were the closest to open panic. The men seemed to have an especially difficult time dealing with their illness and appeared most vulnerable to adverse emotional reactions. These impressions are in keeping with the differential age responses that Rosen and Bibring (1966) observed among men with myocardial infarctions and with the sex differences that we observed on the Adjective Check Lists. For a possible explanation, we look to the fact that men in their forties and fifties ordinarily have considerable time in which to adapt to the gradual decrease in vigor, strength, and potency that occurs with aging and to accept, and even enjoy, the passive and nurturing qualities that they commonly develop. For some of these men, cancer, with its accompanying bodily damage and threat to life, may undermine their sense of masculinity and self regard in too abrupt and traumatic a fashion. We have seen some catastrophic reactions precipitated in this manner.

Older Adults (56-75): A voluminous literature has started to appear on problems of aging (Busse, 1969; Butler, 1975b) in recognition of the previous neglect of these issues and their increasing social importance. Many sources document the accumulation of losses faced by the older person—losses in regard to health, vigor, friends, job, and economic status. For many older persons the world becomes increasingly difficult to deal with, and there is a tendency to withdraw into oneself and to disengage from external investments and struggles. Sometimes this disengagement is a welcome choice, a simplification of life and relief from burdens; in other situations it may be imposed by social restrictions and personal limitations (Cumming and Henry, 1961; Havinghurst et al., 1968). At the same time the older person may be forced to become more dependent on others because he cannot do as much for himself as before. There appears to be a need for the aging person to review his or her past in order to come to terms with life as it now is. If it is possible to take pride in one's accomplishments, forgive oneself for sins and limitations, and find meaning in past experiences, then one can deal with the future with integrity and dignity rather than despair (Butler, 1963; Erikson, 1976).

In older adults, we have observed that cancer commonly leads to an acceleration of these aging processes, imposing new losses, and resulting in more rapid disengagement from work, social, and leisure activities and in greater dependence on others. For example, we have found that as a result of their cancer, adults in their late fifties and early sixties frequently decide to retire earlier than they had planned, even when their medical condition would permit them to continue working. Many factors appear to be involved, such as having less energy, feeling that future ambition is pointless, feeling embarrassed at facing others because of deformity, or wanting to enjoy what life remains as fully as possible.

Another impression is that many of the older, already retired adults seem to face cancer with less anger than younger people. Patients at each life stage express specific kinds of anger when their hopes and wishes are thwarted; the young are angry because they may not ever have a chance to develop their lives; the midlife adults are angry because their lives may be cut short before they can finish their tasks; the pre-retirement and retirement age group are angry because they may not be able to enjoy the leisure earned by a lifetime of work. Nevertheless, at least some of the older people, who have reviewed their past and feel that they have lived their lives fully, are able to deal with their illness with a greater degree of equanimity than the younger patients.

While we have emphasized how cancer may interfere with optimal adult development, it would be misleading to leave the impression that cancer affects adult development only in negative ways. We have seen dramatic instances in which patients who were floundering in managing their personal affairs were able to use their experience with cancer to reorganize their lives, taking advantage of new opportunities and new sources of help that became available. Less dramatic, but more frequent, is the quiet reassessment that many patients go through, which may lead to a keener appraisal of what is important in life and to more satisfying choices regarding the style and direction of their lives. The impact of illness leads some patients to become more constructively self-centered and more assertive in pursuing their personal goals. Moreover, for those couples and families who are able to cope with the stresses of cancer, the experience of surmounting crises together—and perhaps communicating in ways in which they never have before—may lead to a satisfying growth and deepening of relationships.

SUMMARY

This paper arose, in a sense, from our dissatisfaction with the concepts available for ordering and explaining the thoughts, actions, and emotional responses of people with cancer. Our attempts to understand our individual interviews and group discussions with cancer patients brought out the need to integrate psychodynamic and environmental approaches in a way that can do justice to both inner emotional life and the realities of illness and life circumstances. Many psychodynamic concepts, derived from experience with neurotic people in relatively stable external circumstances, are not immediately applicable to mostly non-neurotic patients who are faced with a severe and sometimes overwhelming threat to health and well-being. In fitting these concepts to cancer patients, we have chosen to use an adaptational approach in which we construct, from our clinical material, a schema of issues and tasks faced by cancer patients, and categorize the types of coping methods used by these patients.

The other major area that we have addressed, that of long-term life change, comes out of our observations on cancer survivors. These indicate that such people often undergo profound and long-lasting changes in attitudes, values, and self-image, even when their cancer has been treated successfully. Here, we have drawn on some promising new perspectives on adult change and development that have not yet been used much in work with cancer patients. We see the idea of psychosocial transition as a way to conceptualize the phases that patients go through in struggling with their illness which often lead to a new outlook and equilibrium. We employ an adult developmental framework to illuminate how, at each life stage, there are differences in the way cancer is perceived, in which concerns are most relevant, and in the resources available to cope with the illness. Within this framework, the psychosocial outcome of cancer is conceptualized in terms of how it affects future development. Some effects may be detrimental, as by interfering with maturation, threatening stability, or accelerating decline, but they often are positive, with the experience with cancer leading to opportunities for constructively reorganizing one's life, understanding oneself and others better, and deepening close relationships.

ACKNOWLEDGMENT

We wish to acknowledge the important contributions of our co-investigators, Patricia Fobair, M.S.W., Joan Hall, M.S.W., Irene Harrison, M.S.W., and Abby Wolfson, Ph.D.

REFERENCES

Abrams, R.D. and J.E. Finesinger. 1953. "Guilt Reactions in Patients with Cancer." *Cancer*, 6(3):474-482.

Abrams, R.D. 1966. "The Patient with Cancer—His Changing Patterns of Communication." *New England Journal of Medicine*, 274:317-322.

Adsett, C.A. 1963. "Emotional Reactions to Disfigurement from Cancer Therapy." *Canadian Medical Association Journal*, 89:385.

Bard, M. and A.M. Sutherland. 1955. "Psychological Impact of Cancer and its Treatment. IV. Adaptation to Radical Mastectomy." *Cancer*, 8:656-672.

Binger, C.M., A.R. Arlin, R.C. Reuerstein, J.H. Kushner, S. Zoger, and C. Mikkelsen. 1969. "Childhood Leukemia." *New England Journal of Medicine*, 280:414-418.

Blacher, R.S. 1970. "Losses of Internal Organs." in B. Schoenberg et al., eds., *Loss and Grief: Psychological Management in Medical Practice*, New York: Columbia University Press.

Bronner-Huszar, J. 1971. "The Psychological Aspects of Cancer in Man." *Psychosomatics*, 12(2):133-138.

Busse, E.W. and E. Pfeiffer (eds.). 1969. *Behavior and Adaptation in Late Life*. Boston: Little, Brown.

Butler, R.N. 1963. "The Life Review: An Interpretation of Reminiscence in the Aged." *Psychiatry*, 26(1):65-76.

Butler, R.N. 1975. "Psychiatry and Psychology of the Middle Aged." In A. Freedman et al. (eds.), *Comprehensive Textbook of Psychiatry II*, 2nd edition, Vol. 2, Baltimore: Williams & Wilkins.

Butler, R.N. 1975. *Why Survive? Being Old in America*. New York: Harper and Row.

Caplan, G. and M. Killilea. (eds.). 1976. *Support Systems and Mutual Help*. New York: Grune and Stratton.

Coelho, G.V., D.A. Hamburg, and J.E. Adams. 1974. *Coping and Adaptation*. New York: Basic Books.

Craig, T.J., G.W. Comstock, and P.B. Geiser. 1974. "The Quality of Survival in Breast Cancer: A Case-control Comparison." *Cancer*, 33(5):1451-1457.

Cumming, E. and W.H. Henry. 1961. *Growing Old: The Process of Disengagement*. New York: Basic Books.

Drellich, M.E. et al. 1956. "The Psychological Impact of Cancer and Cancer Surgery. VI. Adaptation to Hysterectomy." *Cancer*, 9:1120-1126.

Easson, W.M. 1968. "Care of the Young Patient Who Is Dying." *Journal of the American Medical Association*, 205:203-207.

Erikson, E.H. 1950. *Childhood and Society*. New York: W.W. Norton.

————. 1959. "Identity and the Life Cycle." *Psychological Issues*, Monograph I. New York: International Universities Press.

————. 1976. "Reflections on Dr. Borg's Life Cycle." *Daedalus*, 105(2):1-28.

Gough, H.G. and A.B. Heilbrun. 1965. *The Adjective Check List Manual*, Palo Alto, California: Consulting Psychologist Press.

Gullo, S.V., D.J. Cherico, and R. Shadick. 1974. "Suggested Stages and Response Styles in Life-Threatening Illness: A Focus on the Cancer Patient." In Schoenberg et al. (eds.). *Anticipatory Grief*, New York: Columbia University Press.

Hamburg, D.A. and J.E. Adams. 1967. "A Perspective on Coping: Seeking and Utilizing Information in Major Transitions." *Archives of General Psychiatry*, 17:277-284.

Harker, B.L. 1972. "Cancer and Communication Problems: A Personal Experience." *Psychiatric Medicine*, 3(2):163-171.

Harrel, H.C. 1972. "To Lose a Breast." *American Journal of Nursing*, 72:676-677.

Havinghurst, R.J., B. Neugarten, and S.S. Tobin. 1968. "Disengagement and Patterns of Aging." In *Middle Age and Aging*, ed. (1968a), Chicago University Press.

Holland, J. 1973. "Psychologic Aspects of Cancer." In J.F. Holland and E. Frei (eds.), *Cancer Medicine*, Philadelphia: Lea & Febiger.

Horowitz, M. 1976. *Stress Response Syndromes*. New York: Jason Aronson.

Izsak, F.C. et al. 1973. "Comprehensive Rehabilitation of the Patient with Cancer—Five Years Home Care." *Journal of Chronic Diseases*, 26:363-374.

Izsak, F.C. and J.H. Medalie. 1971. "Comprehensive Follow-Up of Carcinoma Patients." *Journal of Chronic Diseases*, 24:179-191.

Janis, I.L. 1958. *Psychological Stress: Psychoanalytic and Behavioral Studies of Surgical Patients.* New York: John Wiley and Sons.

Katz, J.L., H. Weiner, T.E. Gallagher, and L. Hellman. 1970. "Stress, Distress and Ego Defenses." *Archives of General Psychiatry,* 23:131-142.

Krant, M. 1974. *Dying and Dignity.* Springfield, Illinois: Charles C. Thomas, Publisher.

Krant, M. 1976. Personal Communication.

Lazarus, R.S. 1966. *Psychological Stress and the Coping Process.* New York: McGraw-Hill.

Lidz, T. 1968. *The Person: His Development Throughout the Life Cycle.* New York: Basic Books.

Lowenthal, M.F., M. Thurner, D. Chiriboga, et al. 1976. *Four Stages of Life.* San Francisco: Jossey-Bass.

Moore, D.C., C.P. Holton, and G.W. Marten. 1969. "Psychological Problems in the Management of Adolescents with Malignancy." *Clinical Pediatrics,* 8:464-473.

Neugarten, B.L. (ed.). 1968a. *Middle Age and Aging.* Chicago: University of Chicago Press.

Neugarten, B.L. 1968b. "Adult Personality: Toward a Psychology of the Life Cycle." In *Middle Age and Aging,* Chicago: University of Chicago Press, 137-147.

Neugarten, B.L. 1968c. "The Awareness of Middle Age." In *Middle Age and Aging,* Chicago: The University of Chicago Press, 93-98.

Norton, J.E. 1963. "Treatment of a Dying Patient." *Psychoanalytical Study of the Child,* 18:541-560.

Orbach, G.E. and A.M. Sutherland. 1953. "Psychological Impact of Cancer and Cancer Surgery. II. Depressive Reactions to Surgical Treatment for Cancer." *Cancer,* 6:958-962.

Parkes, C.M. 1972. *Bereavement: Studies of Grief in Adult Life.* New York: International Universities Press.

Peck, A. 1972. "Emotional Reactions to Having Cancer." *American Journal of Roentgenology, Radium Therapy and Nuclear Medicine,* 114:591-599.

Plumb, M.M. and J. Holland. 1974. "Cancer in Adolescents: The Symptom Is the Thing." In B. Schoenberg et al. (eds.), *Anticipatory Grief.* New York: Columbia University Press.

Quint, J. 1963. "The Impact of Mastectomy." *American Journal of Nursing,* 63:88-92, (November).

Renneker, R.E., R. Cutler, and J. Hora. 1963. "Psychoanalytic Explorations of Emotional Correlates of Cancer of the Breast." *Psychosomatic Medicine,* 25:106-123.

Rosen, J.L. and G.L. Bibring. 1966. "Psychological Reactions of Hospitalized Male Patients to a Heart Attack." *Psychosomatic Medicine,* 28:808-821.

Rosenbaum, E.H. 1975. *Living with Cancer.* New York: Praeger.

Schaie, K. et al. 1975. "Adult Development and Aging." *Annual Review of Psychology,* 26:65-96.

Schoenberg, B. and A. Carr. 1970. "Loss of External Organs: Limb Amputation, Mastectomy and Disfiguration." In B. Schoenberg et al. (eds.), *Loss and Grief: Psychological Management in Medical Practice,* New York: Columbia University Press.

Schoenfield, J. 1972. "Psychological Factors Related to Delay Return to an Earlier Life-Style in Successfully Treated Cancer Patients." *Journal of Psychosomatic Research,* 16:41-46.

Schottenfeld, D. and E.F. Robbins. 1970. "Quality of Survival Among Patients Who Have Had Radical Mastectomy." *Cancer,* 26:650-654.

Schowalter, J.E. 1970. "The Child's Reaction to His Own Terminal Illness. In B. Schoenberg et al. (eds.), *Loss and Grief: Psychological Management in Medical Practice.* New York: Columbia University Press.

Senescu, R.A. 1963. "The Development of Emotional Complications in the Patient with Cancer." *Journal of Chronic Disease,* 16:813-832.

Shands, H. and J.J. Finesinger. 1951. "Psychological Mechanisms in Patients with Cancer." *Cancer*, 4:1159.

Sutherland, A.M. 1967. "Psychological Observations in Cancer Patients." *International Psychiatric Clinics*, 4:75-92.

Sutherland, A., C.E. Orbach, R.B. Dyk, et al. 1951. "The Psychological Impact of Cancer and Cancer Surgery. I. Adaptation to Dry Colostromy." *Cancer*, 5:857-872.

Weisman, A.D. 1972. *On Dying and Denying: A Psychiatric Study of Terminality*. New York: Behavioral Publications.

Weisman, A.D. 1976. "Early Diagnosis of Vulnerability in Cancer Patients." *American Journal of Medical Science*, 27(2):187-196.

Weisman, A.D. 1967. "Denial as a Social Act." In S. Levin and R.J. Kahana (eds.). *Psychodynamic Studies of Aging*, New York: International Universities Press.

Weiss, R.S. 1975. *Marital Separation*. New York: Basic Books.

Worden, J.W. and A.D. Weisman. 1975. "Psychological Components of Lagtime in Cancer Diagnosis." *Journal of Psychosomatic Research*, 19(1):69-79.

THE MALE PATIENT IN CANCER CRISIS

Richard O. Lowy

When the male cancer patient deals with the crisis of cancer, he relies on behavior patterns that have worked for him in the past and is thus usually locked into an established role. The specific ways he deals with the cancer problem are related to who he is as an individual, where he is in his growth as a male, and his socioeconomic situation. The crisis of having cancer may create such turmoil in his emotional behavior that a complete and clear resolution is almost impossible for him to achieve. The purpose of this report is to clarify certain problems the male cancer patient has in coping with his disease crisis and to propose solutions that will facilitate his adjustment to this difficult situation.

THE MALE

In our technologically oriented society there has arisen a well-defined profile of a man with clearly established and accepted characteristics. From early childhood the male is oriented toward specific career goals and is seen ideally as an achiever and provider. To reach these goals he relates on the intellectual plane in combat with his fellow man. From early adolescence to retirement he is oriented toward achievement and recognition in a highly competitive milieu. Very often the competition becomes the end rather than the means, and the "fantasized" goals are obscured in the heat of the battle. Usually when the much sought-after goals have been reached, a feeling of letdown and emptiness results and new goals and new battles may be created.

Accompanying the competitive spirit is the necessity for the boy and the man to maintain strong control over his internal emotional forces. To express honest emotions is identified as a weakness and therefore would place him at a disadvantage in the competitive forum. The basic emotions, such as fear, sadness, joy, and tenderness, are so buried within him that the only way they can surface is as expressions of depression or anger. During his lifetime, most of the energy is channeled into living up to his masculine image, so he rarely takes time to look within himself at his own emotional needs. A serious health crisis such as cancer may produce a breakthrough of feelings when a man's priorities have shifted from maintaining his external facade to examining his internal basic needs. Even with the greatest incidence of cancer either in early childhood or after middle age, males of all ages may be under treatment. In the average radiation therapy department one may find a cross-section of men, from the student to early career and family man to the man near or at his professional peak, to the elderly or retired.

A MAN AND HIS CRISIS

When confronting his cancer crisis, a man remains within his familiar intellectual and physical spheres of involvement. The male cancer patient instinctively avoids revealing feelings of deep emotion, as he would expect those feelings to impede him from working through the crisis. In his reactions to the crisis, various behavior patterns occur that are usually more typically "masculine." Many individuals react by attempting to dominate and overpower all aspects of the crisis. Intellectual domination by researching his diseases and treatment may be his first step, symbolic of a power struggle with those in the health profession involved with his treatment. He often attempts to strengthen his dominant role in his family to ensure and perpetuate his place of power. These expressions of increased power and dominance often occur unconsciously. He usually continues to maintain his "cool" with emotion remaining deeply obscured. Traumatic insults such as the confrontation of his diagnosis, surgery, radiation therapy, and courses of chemotherapy may allow suppressed emotions to surface. He may become unpredictable, obstinate, and irrational, lashing out at his spouse and children or at the physicians or other health personnel. Another possible reaction is his finding the need for withdrawal, separating himself from his distressing external environment and sliding into deep depression and isolation. He may revert to a passive childlike role in his family, seeking protection and comfort, relinquishing the control of and responsibilities for his life. He becomes incapable of making decisions and handling direct confrontation with authority figures. The above reactions may be a temporary stage of his life-threatening crisis. At the point he recognizes the futility of continuing these destructive processes, true growth and communication can occur.

THE MALE AND RADIATION THERAPY

In order to understand better the dynamics of a male cancer patient during therapy, it may be helpful to observe the interaction with the personnel in a radiation therapy department. The radiation therapist is usually a male (and a physician) and therefore represents a dominant authority figure, one with tremendous power and control. The male patient will probably react to the therapist as he has to other authority figures. The spectrum of his responses may range from one of submission in a dependent manner to attempted forceful domination of the therapist, expressing the patient's show of power and control. In this relationship, one of the most overlooked personalities is that of the radiation therapist; where he is in his career, how he deals with his emotional life, and how he interacts with other males. Often the therapist is not well equipped to deal with the emotional aspects of his male patient, as he himself has spent considerable time and effort controlling and burying his own emotions in pursuit of his own career. In most physician-patient interactions, usually the therapist feels most comfortable in dominant-intellectual roles, to achieve his goal of providing the most effective treatment and maintaining his own omniscient position.

The radiation-therapy technician and nurse may be seen symbolically by the patient as the nurturing partners to the physician. This professional male-female relationship may have many characteristics of the typical dominant-passive or parental relationship. In this situation, the male patient may envision the technician and nurse as caring, mothering individuals to whom he can communicate much of his concerns and feelings and from whom he may receive security and warmth.

Radiation-therapy treatments are given as a continuing course, lasting from four to eight weeks. Repeated treatments administered on a daily basis may often produce a great deal of fear and anxiety. The continual exposure of the patient to radiation treatment reaffirms the diagnosis and prognosis. This process can have a tremendous impact during treatment, painfully reexposing many of the deeply buried emotional forces. An important aspect of the trauma is that irradiation is feared by many as an invisible force producing severe damage or death. Presently there is an additional anxiety concerning radiation-induced malignancies produced by diagnostic x-ray tests or atmospheric testing of nuclear weapons. During radiation destruction of a tumor there are side effects produced by damaging of normal tissues. The side effects may be felt necessary by the patient in order to achieve the goal of cure or palliation.

With the awareness of having cancer and experiencing radiation side effects, the patient may be more conscious of various body functions and of a variety of minor discomforts, previously ignored. These signs and symptoms, though usually minor, produce considerable anxiety, and each must be evaluated by the therapist. In contrast, a patient may experience a counter-reaction to the disease and may feel divorced from his body because he interprets the cancer as a failure of his body.

Precise measures of progress and success are difficult, if not impossible, for the majority of radiation-therapy patients. Though there may be measurable or palpable tumor mass, the ultimate goal of total elimination can only be measured by time, sufficient to determine total control or recurrence of the disease. With completion of the treatment course, the patient may be left in a state of limbo and be faced with the reality of having to live with the uncertainty of his future, a waiting game that may continue for years.

DEALING WITH THE CRISIS

With a life-threatening disease, the patient usually relinquishes a great degree of responsibility for managing his medical care. His fears associated with having cancer accelerate the acquiescence of the control of a portion of his life to those in the medical profession who have the expected knowledge and ability to save his life. The cancer patient may feel quite powerless and may not desire to share responsibility with the medical profession, but may wish to instead place himself totally in the therapist's hands. In such an agreement the subtleties and deeper implications of the relationship are not always fully appreciated by either the patient or the physician. The patient gives up a significant portion of control of his life in following the directions and treatments of the physician. In essence, there is a loss of status and stature and dominance. This is exemplified by the hospitalized patient who loses his individuality upon entering the hospital in the anonymity of admitting number, floor numbers, room numbers, etc. The physician accepts this acquiescence of responsibility but often is not aware of the tremendous power he holds. Gestures or single words, communicated from health personnel, can have a significant impact on a cancer patient looking for any sign of hope in his critical situation. If both the physician and the patient were aware of the process of control, they might be willing to share more equally the responsibility of care and treatment.

In a radiation-therapy department the implications of the responsibilities assumed by the physician and the technical-nursing staff in treating cancer patients should be thoroughly recognized. In the well-organized radiation therapy department the patient is expected to follow specific rules, regulations, and orders that are "in his best interest," so that the treatment is delivered most effectively. Some of the most upsetting situations that occur in a radiation therapy department are with those patients who resist this type of control, becoming angry, irritable, questioning, or belligerent. Awareness by the department personnel of the processes within the patient may permit satisfactory resolution of these problems.

When a man is labeled as having cancer, his status and relationships in his profession may alter significantly. Often, he may continue to work regularly, though often his productivity will diminish and his general attitude will change as he perceives a shift in his own priorities. These changes may be accepted by his employer and coworkers, though he often is treated quite differently. He is no longer the same person to others, and significant communication becomes more difficult. The sensitive male has probably begun to shift his priorities, and this may alter internally his own definition of his manhood, his profession, and his career.

Interpersonal relationships with his family and friends may change abruptly. Often friends "politely" pull away, not knowing how to relate to someone with cancer. Finding it more and more uncomfortable to be close to him, they begin to withdraw. This is met with sadness and confusion by the man and implies to him a further loss of control of his life. His changing relationship with his family is often the most critical one. When his physician assumes the dominant position, the patient may experience a radical change in his own family role. He might totally acquiesce dominance to his wife, becoming childlike, demanding protection and caring. He may become more assertive, becoming angry and less rational in his behavior toward his wife and children. This may be a destructive attempt to demonstrate that he still is dominant and that he can at least hold power over some individual, even though he may have lost power in his relationship with his physician. Within his family, the result of increased power or acquiescence of power may lead to verbal and physical isolation. True communication may become impossible as long as the man is preoccupied with his loss of status and with never-ending thoughts of his disease and the threat to his life.

With such radical life changes appearing beyond his control, an individual often visualizes himself as a victim of the disease. The victim role is commonly assumed during stressful situations, and it is more comforting not to take responsibility. It is remarkable how often people are unaware how they thrive in the victim role and are never aware how it interferes with honest communication. Victimization is often accepted and nurtured by the medical and health professionals and by patient, family, friends, and fellow workers. This acceptance of his victim role strengthens his own image of one who has lost control and responsibility.

A man with cancer may therefore undergo changes in behavior toward himself and others, from that of the morosely depressed (sad and unable to communicate his feelings) to the angry and hostile (keeping people at a distance and constantly on the defensive). In all these reactive states, the man is forced into an old familiar role, the only one he knows how to play, burying powerful emotions of fear and guilt, yet aware of overwhelming sadness and aloneness. It is a very sad situation and most difficult to deal with.

HELPING THE MAN TO COPE

As previously stated, the objective of this paper is to clarify a man's dilemma in coping with cancer and its treatment. Ideally, many facets of a man's personality might need some modification in order for him to deal with such a serious crisis. Yet, this very individual usually has significant physical disabilities or a significantly shortening lifetime, which may interfere with in-depth communication and counseling. The major step in communication is awareness—awareness of his interpersonal relationships and emotional reaction with his family, his friends, and health personnel. Within a radiation therapy department there exists the opportunity to take an active role in identifying his needs and developing a program toward support and modification. Often, a trained counselor or social worker, sensitive to a man's needs, can deal most effectively with the problem. The counselor may be viewed by the patient as his own advocate, with their relationship separate from that between himself and the physicians, technicians, and nurse. The counselor may be in a good position to evaluate his previous experiences, his family interrelationships, and his career, and to integrate this information into active counseling activities.

The patient may become aware of the repeated intellectual-physical struggles he is utilizing and the need for recognition and acceptance of deeply buried emotions. Many standard techniques for communication in one-to-one and group sessions may be utilized, and structured but flexible programs, including individual patient counseling, family communications, and cancer groups, can be used to form such a foundation. With the problems of the male, consideration should be given to group sessions with men with cancer and to male counselors to whom the male patient may better interrelate. These may facilitate communication in more empathetic surroundings and allow for growth beyond the cancer crisis.

The course of radiation therapy may provide an ideal entrance into counseling, with treatment usually occurring shortly after diagnosis and being continuous with daily visits over a number of weeks. It is imperative that counseling begun during treatment be continued after completion of radiation therapy whether the patient goes on to further forms of therapy or not. It is important that all those individuals concerned with the patient's care, health professionals and family, be educated as to the interpersonal and communicative problems the male patient may be struggling with through similar awareness processes such as group or individual sessions.

SUMMARY

The specific problems of the male cancer patient coping with the emotional turmoil of his disease need greater attention from the health professional. The crisis of having cancer may be a period of growth for the man. Prior to cancer, his recognition and expression of emotion had probably been sacrificed in the pursuit of career-oriented goals that gave him definition as a man. A reorientation of his priorities and a greater awareness of his emotional needs occur during diagnosis and initiation of treatment and throughout the course of his therapy. All people involved need to be aware of his needs in order to be able to provide positive assistance.

THE IMPACT OF PEDIATRIC RADIATION THERAPY

Giulio J. D'Angio, Nancy Ann Osman and Judith W. Ross

Cancer diagnosed in childhood identifies not only a sick patient, but a sick family as well. The mother and father often are young, and just developing financial resources and a place in the community. The blow is, therefore, doubly cruel, affecting the family not only emotionally, but also threatening its fiscal integrity. The "ripple" effect on other members of the family is appreciable, too (Evans, 1968; Fellner, 1973; Lansky and Lowman, 1974; van Eys, 1976). Siblings share the anxiety and emotional and financial deprivation that inevitably ensue. The decision to give radiation therapy often results in additional stress for the already distraught family. It is therefore important for medical personnel and supporting staff to be aware of the psycho-socio-economic impact of the disease and of the special problems inherent in radiation therapy. They then can take steps to provide the requisite total support, which includes a willingness not only to discuss problems in depth, but also to mobilize the resources provided by the community to help meet the needs of the family (Evans, 1968; van Eys, 1976). At the same time, the patient must not be neglected. Staff members must be attuned to the special needs of the pediatric patient which will vary with the child's age and illness.

Fear is the predominant emotion to be overcome; and it is a different kind of fear for each member of the family. The young patient is afraid of pain and of the unknown. For the siblings, as shifts of parental attention inevitably take place, the seeming loss of affection causes concern. The siblings and the patient are frightened by the distress, uncertainty, and disequilibrium they observe in their parents and by the loss of security and stability this represents to them. The parents, in turn, have fears of the effects of irradiation added to those engendered by the disease and the threats to the solidity and continuity of the family unit.

THE PATIENT

The infant usually requires only comfortable surroundings and minimal, if any, sedation. The latter can be provided by such simple means as a brandy nipple; that is, sugar syrup with brandy that is often sufficient to take off the "edge," and allow therapy to proceed with relative ease. Immobilization of the child by strapping and other means often heightens fear and resistance and can be counterproductive. On the other hand, some restraint is necessary for safety purposes. This often can be provided by means of elastic bandages and sand bags or specially constructed immobilization devices (D'Angio and Pearson, 1975). When extraordinary precision is required, anesthesia can be avoided by the use of ketamine and similar agents proven to be of value in these patients.

For older children—that is, those who can reason—"confidence" is the key word. A preliminary discussion with the child in his new "home" environment on the ward is beneficial. The physician introduces himself, and reassures the child that no "needles" will be used and that the procedure has no pain or sensation of any kind. Thus, when the child is brought to the radiation therapy area, a now familiar figure greets him. Once again, reassurance regarding the lack of pain is given repeatedly, and the procedure of marking the skin to outline the treatment portals can be made a game by suitable jocular comments during the procedure. It is advantageous to schedule treatment early in the day when the child is fresh and has not had any "needle sticks" for laboratory studies and the like.

It is the treatment room itself that makes the greatest impact, however. Curiously, children are less frightened of the huge machines than are adults. They fear more the isolation necessary during treatment. Therefore, it can be useful to sham the irradiation procedure at the first session. That is, the child is placed in the treatment room, all the set-up procedures are followed, and the staff leaves the room. The machine is not actually turned on, however, and the staff re-enters the room promptly. The turn-around time is thus abbreviated; the child is reassured that there has been no pain and that someone is waiting to take him back to the ward or back home. This becomes particularly important if the patient has been in the hospital and treatment is either being continued or initiated on an out-patient basis.

It is advisable, whenever possible, to separate pediatric from adult patients. The disfigured adult after surgery for head and neck cancer is a shocking sight for the sensitive child, as is the debilitated, cachetic adult with late stage disease. On the other hand, the presence of children often gives support to the adults. They empathize and consider their own problems less severe than those of the afflicted child.

Staff discussion of the technical details of the treatment should be kept at a minimum in the presence of the child because jargon and medical terms can easily be misinterpreted. "Cut the edge here," meaning, "Reduce the size of the field," while pointing to a spot on the leg is heard as, "Amputate the leg here." On the other hand, both the parents and child should be reassured that all questions will be answered truthfully. It sometimes is difficult for parents to accept this; nonetheless, it is by far the better policy (Karon, 1973). The physician once detected in an evasion or a lie is not trusted again. On the other hand, details regarding diagnosis, treatment, complications, and outcome can be explained in terms that are understandable for the child of a given age. This is comforting for the child who feels he can manage such information and is reassured that the illness is not so bad as to be "unmentionable." Analogies are appropriate. Dandelion seeds in a lawn is an image the average child can understand; indeed, the analogy will often help clarify matters for the parents. Application of "weed killers" and the dangers they pose to ornamental borders (normal tissues) are easily understood, and the need to hold still during treatment so that the weed killer will not get into the flower bed makes the point clear.

The older child, who has a better awareness regarding cancer, sometimes poses a more difficult problem. Again, it is best to be frank and straightforward, answering questions by asking others so that the levels of understanding can be tested even as communication proceeds. "Do I have cancer?" can be countered with, "What does that word mean to you?" Usually, it connotes an invariably lethal, horrifying illness. Appropriate reassurances can be given point by point depending on the diagnosis and stage of the disease. On the other hand, evasions of direct questions should be avoided, and the gravity of the situation imparted directly and in simple language. It sometimes results in a more cooperative and trustful patient (Karon, 1973). Reassurance should also be given that the fears and concerns expressed are completely understandable; that it is normal to be apprehensive when confronted by such a major medical problem, and that questions no matter how "crazy" should be asked.

It is wise to be sensitive to the unasked question. "Will I be able to play football in the Fall?" really is, "Will I be here in the Fall?" "What is heaven like?" is really "Am I going to die?" Superficial or off-putting answers are not appropriate because they can be misunderstood. "We'll see," or "Let's not worry about that now," is heard as, "We don't have to worry about football in the Fall; you won't be here."

It is essential that both the immediate and late complications of treatment be explained fully to the parents and patient in terms appropriate to the latter's age and level of comprehension. Failure to do so, and to provide medications to alleviate the discomfort of radiation reactions, leads to loss of confidence and resentment (Harper, 1973; Peck and Boland, 1980).

Deformity, disfigurement, loss of hair, and other stigmata of treatment are felt acutely by the teenager so conscious of peer acceptance and approval. Preparatory counseling with the social worker as to what to expect and how to meet the situation should be given. Additional support should be offered during periods when the patient cannot be competitive or attractive, or just feels "low." Relatively simple expedients may make all the difference in tiding the patient over temporary but difficult periods—a wig or a home tutor for the epilated, for example. Talking with the social worker about feelings of low self-esteem, of difference from peers, of anger or despair may be quite helpful at this time.

It is not surprising that older children and teenagers sometimes retain unhappy memories of the irradiation experience because of the complications encountered. Added to this is the resentment at being kept "in jail" (hospital) solely because a long course of radiation therapy was necessary. Treatment on an out-patient basis, whenever possible, is therefore to be encouraged.

SIBLINGS

Siblings should be made welcome in the department and should be recognized as individuals. The focus of attention on the sick child inevitably makes the sibling feel left out and unwanted. It will be easier for the whole family if this is explained to the parents, that this reaction can be expected and is entirely natural. It can be mitigated to some degree if the parents adopt an even-handed policy regarding the sick child and do not shower attention on the patient. Such a policy is best for the whole family, the patient included (Lansky and Lowman, 1974).

The staff can help by deliberately taking notice of brothers and sisters who accompany the child. Siblings can be brought back to the treatment area with the patient once confidence has been attained and treatment is proceeding smoothly on a day-to-day basis. The younger sibling can be allowed to twist inoperative dials and push inactive buttons, watch the television monitor, share in any "treats" that are made available to the patient, and otherwise be made to feel a participant (van Eys, 1976).

It is also helpful if siblings are prepared for the side effects of treatment so that they are not overly distressed when these occur. They can be helped by being told they did nothing to cause the illness, that it is not "catching," and that they need not worry about becoming sick themselves. During follow-up visits, the sibling should be present, acknowledged, and engaged in conversation, however briefly.

PARENTS

The parents will already have made a partial adjustment at least to the sudden and crushing blow to their young hopes and plans. Added to these concerns are those engendered by radiation therapy. Many have heard or read of the hazards of irradiation and may have a more or less clear idea regarding radiation oncogenesis, disturbance of normal bone growth, and possible genetic effects. The interview with the radiation therapist may serve only to confirm these fears. Therefore, the discussion must be conducted with great care so that the facts can be presented in proper perspective. It is advisable for the therapist to attempt to learn what the parents know about radiation. He thus can respond to possible misinformation and alleviate unnecessary apprehension. At the same time, full information must be given, as to both the reasons for treatment and the possible early and late complications that might be encountered. It is best to provide written information regarding the side effects, so that these can be reviewed by the parents later (Harper, 1973). The physician must empathize with the dilemma offered: treatment is necessary to save life, but deformity and disability may result. During the initial stages of the disease, at least, the parents hope for a perfectly normal child at the end of a nightmare experience. It is at this stage that acceptance of radiation therapy may be particularly difficult. Indeed, as the disease progresses, the compromises with this idea are among the sadder moments in a therapist's life. Expectations change, and at the end, the plea may be only for relief of discomfort and an early, merciful death.

Radiation therapy on an out-patient basis makes necessary exceptional demands in that daily visits are required, often over a long period. The practical arrangements that must be made sometimes tax the parents' physical and emotional resources to the utmost. Someone must be found to look after children left at home, time must be taken from work, a driver is needed because public transport is impossible, and so on. The parents find themselves dependent on relatives, friends, neighbors, or total strangers. For those of independent bent, the experience can be shattering and humiliating.

The financial burden of prolonged treatment has anxieties of its own. Outside agencies may be able to help as the family resources become depleted and the patrimony remaining for the other children lessens.

THE FAMILY UNIT

It is very difficult not to "spoil" the involved child. Nonetheless, it is important to stress to parents that they should make every attempt to treat the youngster as he was managed in the past as much as his medical circumstances permit. Even-handed treatment supports not only the patient, who will sense unwonted attention and fear the reason, but also reassures other children of the family. Otherwise, they may demand attention by extraordinary behavior; for example, truancy in a previously well-behaved youngster (Lansky and Lowman, 1974; van Eys, 1976). When parents view the illness as a "family problem"—that is, affecting all members of the family—successful adaptation is more likely.

It may well be that the least severely affected member of the family is the young patient. A study by Ferguson (1976) showed that patients surviving childhood cancer did not develop psychological disturbances. Since radiation therapy was a part of the process for many of these children, it can be assumed that the procedure does not leave scars of this type.

The extra stress placed on family relationships may trigger latent hostilities among its members. It is the impression of some who deal with childhood cancer that the divorce rate in parents of cancer patients is high (Lansky and Lowman, 1974). In some cases this appears to be the result of one partner's wishing to proceed aggressively in the face of widely metastatic disease, and the other wishing to spare the child rigorous treatment perceived as having only a small likelihood of success. Generally, however, divorce appears to result from the marital stress produced by discrepant means of coping with the problem. Profound disturbances may develop in the husband-wife, father-mother roles that had become established prior to the illness. Father must work, and the burden of the daily visits is carried by the mother, who often has little time left for herself and the other members of the family. A period of initial understanding and solidarity gives way to mutual disaffection and recriminations (Fellner, 1973; Lansky and Lowman, 1974).

Anticipatory counseling and guidance is to be encouraged for vulnerable families. It is helpful if a social worker skilled in counseling such families forms a relationship with the parents soon after the diagnosis is made. An assessment of the kind and intensity of support needed can thus be made before the family becomes dysfunctional. Discussion groups for parents are another means of providing support through open sharing of problems and anxieties, and the means some have found to surmount them (van Eys, 1976).

STAFF

The child undergoing radiation therapy has a considerable impact on hospital staff members. Trained and experienced paramedical personnel—technologists, physicists, nurses, and others—who are accustomed to dealing with the adult cancer patient find the management of the child with malignant disease especially trying. Because of an inability to face the problem, staff personnel sometimes become short in tone and mechanical in approach. This often is a defense mechanism and not a reflection of a dislike for children. Nonetheless, it is best to have on hand a team of trained individuals who are willing and able to work in pediatric radiation therapy. The extra patience and understanding required can be acquired in some degree, but attitude and motivation are by far the most important, if not the essential, ingredients. The same applies to other members of the supporting staff, such as social workers, who should be familiar with the special problems of the families of children with chronic diseases, and know the resources available to support the "sick family." Social workers can also assist other members of the team by helping them to understand a particular family's psychosocial needs or behavior, or to understand and cope with the staff member's own reactions to a specific patient or family (Lansky and Lowman, 1974; van Eys, 1976).

It is important in choosing staff to select individuals who can relate to the patient and be gentle but not become too deeply involved emotionally. An unfavorable turn in the course of the child's illness can have shattering repercussions on the too deeply attached staff member. Deep attachments cannot always be avoided, however. Supervisory senior staff can be helpful by detecting deepening relationships at an early stage, and by providing guidance and support as needed.

Staff members should have similar goals, based on an understanding of the strengths and the limitations of treatment, and of their own roles as members of the team. No one should be permitted to feel he or she carries the burden alone.

Personnel elsewhere in the hospital often regard radiation therapy as a mysterious and frightening procedure. They often react sharply and with dismay to the mucositis, epilation, and other acute responses that, at times, are the expected results of irradiation, especially when radiation-enhancing chemotherapeutic agents are used concomitantly. Every attempt should be made to educate these individuals regarding radiation therapy. This can be done by regularly scheduled lectures and tours of the radiation therapy facility, and by meeting with the staff members concerned when an unusually brisk reaction is encountered or anticipated.

Hospital chaplains should be accessible to patients, and all members of the staff should be familiar with their names (Evans, 1968). Availability of this service should be brought up in a matter-of-fact way so that parents can feel free to use it if they so desire. They should not be made to feel it is expected or that it has been suggested because the patient's demise is anticipated momentarily.

COMMUNITY RESOURCES

The stresses felt by the patient and the family can often be relieved by agencies in the community; thus, a knowledge of available resources becomes extremely important. Tutors, for example, may be needed while a child is in the hospital so he can return to school without undue scholastic strain (Lansky and Lowman, 1974). Financial help or volunteer drivers may be available to assist the patient and the family in coming to the hospital for daily treatment. Comfortable, safe, low-cost living accommodations may be crucial if the family must come from out of town for radiation therapy. Governmental benefits such as public assistance funds will be important to the working parent obliged to remain at home with a sick child. Putting parents in contact with people and organizations that can help often keeps a difficult situation from becoming an overwhelming one.

LATER YEARS

Radiation therapy may continue to have psychosocial consequences years after the treatment has been completed. At best, the patient is alive without appreciable residua, and gratitude and satisfaction because of the result achieved are the predominant emotions. Memory of the therapy itself fades, and there remains only a dim recollection of the treatment process. The parents of the patient who did not survive may retain only a sense of gratitude for the alleviation of pain or disfigurement that may have been achieved by irradiation. It is not unusual for the parents of surviving patients on their way to or from the clinic to stop by for a social visit with a fondly remembered radiation technologist, nurse, or physician. Sometimes, bereaved parents do the same once or twice, and may continue for years to write a few words of appreciation at Christmas.

There may be unpleasant memories. Radiation therapy may become intermixed with recollections of the difficult declining days, or there may have been an unusually brisk reaction, so that the radiation experience itself was painful and is remembered that way.

The psychosocial sequence becomes complex for the patient who survives with pronounced post-radiation sequelae. At first there is a difficult period when the problems of the radiation therapy course must be surmounted. After that, there is the interval, measured usually in years, when the disease remains under control, there are no appreciable sequelae, and life goes on normally. Then, the late radiation complications begin to become manifest insidiously. These may take any of several forms—for example, bone growth shortening, asymmetry of the face, or disruption of function of a vital organ. At first, the concerns may be largely medical. There soon are added the psychological stresses, often precipitated in the younger child by the gibes and taunts of unthinking playmates. They become severe particularly for the teenager, when deformity becomes an intolerable burden. It is at this point that the patient may well berate the parent, "How could you let them do this to me! I would rather be dead!" The reaction of the parent can be imagined. Sorrow, remorse, and guilt develop all too easily. Hostility of all family members against the therapy team is another logical consequence. Forgetting the explanations given before treatment began, parents may blame staff for failure to explain the long-term complications.

The really difficult social problems may also become manifest at this time. The handicapped patient must choose a suitable career, sometimes entailing a compromise with earlier aspirations (van Eys, 1976). The severely deformed patient, although functionally capable, may require considerable counseling and psychiatric support when leaving the home to face the wider world. Material assistance may be needed in order to provide special facilities or training, depending on the complication encountered.

Medical, emotional, and social counseling helps mitigate these difficulties and should be offered in all cases in which severe residua can be predicted.

THE BRIGHTER SIDE OF THE COIN

Not all the circumstances surrounding radiation therapy are unpleasant or unhappy. There is the relief and gratitude of the parent and of the patient when pain is assuaged rapidly and easily by a few treatments. Sometimes, the fact that the child is ready for radiation therapy marks a favorable way-stop in a complex series of planned treatments. The parents, knowing that irradiation was to be given only if preliminary remission was achieved with chemotherapy, arrive in the department elated, aware that a major hurdle has been cleared.

After the radiation therapy course is completed, both the patient and the family may derive considerable satisfaction from the fact they were able to surmount the many difficulties inherent in the procedure. The patient has tested his courage and has not been found wanting. The family has been able to manage daily visits to the institution despite the severe disruption of family life that might have been necessary. Patients or parents may find that they were able to tap unknown inner resources and to provide support and encouragement to other patients or members of other families. Many volunteer the information that the experience has given them new self-confidence and maturity; that they have "grown" in the process.

It is, perhaps, surprising to learn that the parents of dead children often share at least one happy memory among the many unhappy ones. Because of the problems associated with radiation therapy, they were obliged to seek the help of family members, neighbors, and strangers. Commonly, they state that this was one of the most heartwarming episodes of their lives because of the ready and willing assistance provided by others.

Finally, there often is the satisfaction of learning from the physician in charge that the treatment has been successful and that the perhaps unpleasant or unsettling experience was worthwhile after all.

REFERENCES

D'Angio, G.J. and D. Pearson. 1975. "Radiation Therapy." In H.G.J. Bloom et al. (eds.), *UICC Cancer in Children*, Berlin: Springer-Verlag, pp. 29-47.

Evans, A.E. 1968. "If a Child Must Die." *New England Journal of Medicine*, 278:138-142.

Fellner, C.H. 1973. "Family Disruption After Cancer Cure." *American Family Physician*, 8:169-172.

Ferguson, J.H. 1976. "Late Psychologic Effects of a Serious Illness in Childhood." *Nursing Clinics of North America*, 11:83-93.

Harper, P.M. 1973. "Radiotherapy and the Patient." *Radiography*, 39:257-261.

Karon, M. 1973. "The Physician and the Adolescent with Cancer." *Pediatric Clinics of North America*, 20:965-973.

Lansky, S.B. and J.T. Lowman. 1974. "Childhood Malignancy: A Comprehensive Approach." *Journal of the Kansas Medical Society* (March), pp. 91-94.

Peck, A. and J. Boland. "Emotional Reactions to Radiation Treatment." Personal communication.

van Eys, J. 1976. "Supportive Care for the Child with Cancer." *Pediatric Clinics of North America*, 23:215-224.

APPROACHES TO MALIGNANT DISEASE

(including Chemotherapy): Disease Entities, Alternative Modalities, and Patient's Responses

CO^{60} RADIATION: LIFE OR DEATH?

Isamettin M. Aral

> *A useless life is an early death.*
> Goethe

Written from the perspective of the radiotherapist, the purpose of this paper is to demonstrate his daily struggle in trying to educate physicians and laypersons concerning the exact place of radiation therapy in general, and Cobalt^{60} therapy in particular; to observe the radiotherapist's daily efforts in trying to describe that tool called "Radiation Therapy," with its merits and dangers, its indications and contraindications.

Case Report

A 47-year-old male patient was admitted to the hospital with an enlarged right testicle of three weeks duration. His father died of heart disease at a young age. His aunt had succumbed to metastatic breast disease after suffering for five years. Intelligent and very ambitious, the patient had gained wealth and prominence on his own. His family life was very happy. Now this successful man is confronted with a serious medical problem for the first time in his life. He must have surgery. He must lose a testicle. This is a trauma—to lose an organ of his body so closely related psychologically to his virility. How can he survive this? What will it do to his marriage? His wife is still young. These are only some of the questions that haunt him. If he survives, will he ever be the same again?

At this time, he is in desperate need of reassurance from his doctors. He has the surgery and the pronouncement is made: "You have cancer." Now he is confronted with, for the first time, the thought of an early death. He thinks of his aunt, her pain and her suffering. The thought of dying is frightening, but the fear of living racked with pain, as she did, is devastating. He thinks to himself, "I have only had surgery. She must have been worse, she had to have cobalt treatments." He tries to allay his fears.

One week after the surgery, his urologist comes to him with the final pathology report—good news—pure seminoma. This is very frequently curable. Through his apprehension, he tries to derive confidence from his surgeon's encouraging words. His surgeon mentions that he would suggest a source of prophylactic radiation. This does not seem to unnerve Mr. M. He is not equating radiation with cobalt. In his mind, there cannot be a relation. His aunt had cobalt treatments; he is only going to get radiation. This radiation is only going to be a prophylaxis.

(We, as physicians, know there is no prophylactic radiation. Why, then, are patients told this? Is it ignorance on the part of the physicians and organizations at local and federal levels, or is it an ill-advised "passepatient" to hide the shortcomings of surgery in curing solid cancer in 100 percent of the cases? Let one's conscience decide.)

When I met Mr. M. for the first time, I met a very nervous and frightened man. Following my review of the chart, x-rays, and referring physician's consultations, and my own examination, I decided the type of radiation to be used, the parts of the body to be treated, the frequency of treatments, the daily increments, and the total dose in rads to the site of the potentially involved lymph nodes. I presented the problem to the patient and his wife in the following manner:

"Mr. M., you had a tumor of your testicle that has been successfully removed. There was no gross evidence of spread of cancer to the rest of your body; these are the findings of your surgeon. They are confirmed by various tests, all of which are normal except for moderate calcification and widening of your aorta, which is suggestive of arteriosclerosis. Although the studies are normal, there is a 35 percent chance that the lymph nodes surrounding your aorta may be microscopically involved. For this reason, a preventive course of radiation is highly recommended. My radiation therapy in combination with your surgery will give you a chance of cure that is over 95 percent.

"You would do well to cut down on your food intake, as your weight may kill you first, if you are not careful. You will be coming for treatments five days a week, for a period of four weeks. It is possible that you have not been told about the secondary effects of your radiation therapy. The only things to expect will be a mild case of loose bowels and/or burning on urination. If either of these should develop, please advise me and I will give you medication. There will be no anemia or hair loss as a result of these treatments.

"One final point: During your treatment the door of the treatment room will be locked for protection purposes, and you will be lying on a treatment table. The equipment is rather large and ominous, but don't let it frighten you. It will never touch your body. There will be no sensation, as radiation is not seen, felt, or heard. Good luck to both of us!"

When I had finished my explanation, I asked if there were any questions. "What is your machine called?" asked Mr. M. "You will be treated on our cobalt unit," I replied.

That was it! A sob from him and a scream from his wife. What was wrong?

What had happened? I tried to calm them, but to no avail. Finally, I quieted Mr. M. enough so that his words were intelligible. "If I am getting cobalt, I'm going to die. There is no hope! My aunt had surgery, chemotherapy and radiation, but she only got radiation when all hope was gone! Why didn't they tell me it was hopeless? Why weren't they honest? Cobalt is the last step before the box!"

After much explanation, I was able to convince him to take the treatments I was never able to convince him that this was not the last step before the box. This he found out for himself as, after the treatments were over, he began to feel better and stronger. After a few weeks he returned to work. It was my pleasure to have him come to me at his six-week follow-up and say, "Gee, Doc, I'm so grateful on the one hand and so embarrassed on the other. If only someone had explained the situation before I got here, I would have been prepared."

A sad commentary indeed. With whom does the fault lie? Is it with the surgeons, who explain in detail what they are going to do surgically, and then when they are in doubt as to residual tumor, mention radiation to the patient without explaining why and how it is to be given? Is it with the oncologist, who explains how his chemotherapy is to be administered and for what gains it is to be given, and then when it fails, says, "Maybe we'll try cobalt." Or is it with federal agencies, who are continually warning of the hazards of radiation?

It is said that responsible official and voluntary health agencies are propagating fears of radiation harm. Sometimes surgery and, more often, chemotherapy have their own morbidities. Radiation, in a clinical sense, is not a killer when employed by a qualified radiotherapist. It is time *now* to educate the public and perhaps health personnel that radiation is not to be equated with death. Let us place our medical tools against cancer in their proper perspective.

It is unfortunate to report that Mr. M. died four months after his surgery and radiation therapy—not from cancer but from rupture of his aortic aneurysm.

REFERENCES

Kubler-Ross, E. 1969. *On Death and Dying.* New York: Macmillan Co.
Norton, C.E. 1969. "Attitudes Toward Living and Dying in Patients on Chronic Hemodialysis." *Annals of the New York Academy of Sciences,* 164:720.
Pritchard, R. 1969. "Dying—Some Issues and Problems." *Annals of the New York Academy of Sciences,* 164:707.
Rhudick, P.J. and A.S. Dibner. 1966. "Age, Personality, and Health Correlates of Death Concerns in Normal Aged Individuals." *Annals of the New York Academy of Sciences,* 16:44.
Weisman, A. 1972. "Psychosocial Death." *Psychology Today,* 6:77.

THE PSYCHOLOGICAL IMPACT OF RADIATION THERAPY INSTEAD OF MASTECTOMY FOR EARLY CARCINOMA OF THE BREAST: A PRELIMINARY REPORT

Phyllis J. Ager, Jack Terry, Seymour Alpert, and Nemetalliah Ghossein

The profound emotional distress associated with the discovery of a breast mass has been well documented in the literature (Lee and Maguire, 1975). The common delay of women in reporting the mass is thought to be due as much to the fear of losing a breast as to the fear of the diagnosis of cancer itself (Hackett et al., 1973).

Twenty patients with breast cancer were interviewed and given an opportunity to discuss anything they wished. Most were seen for more than one interview and some for as many as ten. Eight had mastectomy and twelve had tumorectomy with postoperative radiation. All received radiation therapy. None were charged a fee for the psychiatric service, and most were comfortable and appreciated the opportunity to express and share their feelings.

In the group studied the choice of procedure was primarily determined by the attitude of the surgeon. If the surgeon informs the patient and her family that there is no difference in the survival rate between mastectomy and tumorectomy with radiotherapy, and the procedure is explained, the patient chooses tumorectomy rather than mastectomy. Some patients seek out a surgeon who will perform a tumorectomy because they have made up their minds, even before diagnosis, that they would not have a mastectomy.

Some patients who choose tumorectomy admit that they would have agreed to almost any radical procedure if they had been directed to have surgery immediately upon diagnosis. The interval between the diagnosis and surgery offers the patient the opportunity to participate in the decision.

Another factor is the patient's personal experience with cancer in her family or among friends. For example, a patient whose mother died one year after her mastectomy refused mastectomy for herself.

A patient, 26 years old at the age of diagnosis of a 2 cm tumor in her right breast, was unmarried and attractive, and took pride in her appearance. She was told by her surgeon that she had no chance to live without having a mastectomy, but she refused. Although her surgeon told her that she was vain and insisted on a mastectomy, the patient sought a surgeon who approved of tumorectomy and subsequent radiation therapy.

This patient's situation illustrates the difficulty in evaluating the quality of survival of patients who had mastectomies as compared with those for whom a local excision was performed. Although much has been written in an attempt to show that the majority of patients who have had a mastectomy returned to work and were able to live a "normal" life, the patient's feelings of self-esteem are not usually evaluated.

The breast is a highly cathected part of every woman's body. The significance of the breasts to the woman, and indeed to every person, changes throughout her lifetime, but it is never viewed as an insignificant organ. When it becomes the locus of pathology, especially cancer, it becomes reinvested with conflict.

Some women with depressive personality makeups see the disease and its treatment as punishment for their self-perceived sexual transgressions, such as masturbation, premarital or extramarital sex, or promiscuity, whether real or fantasized. In others, it revives early castration conflicts by stimulating memories of the mutilation fantasies of childhood. They speak of missing some part of their body, and of feelings of shame and disgust. "If only I didn't see this ugly scar." "Had they cut out something from the inside that I couldn't see it wouldn't bother me so much."

One woman complained of a disturbance of her sense of balance as a result of her mastectomy, feeling that she was leaning in the opposite direction. In another woman, the mastectomy revived her mourning for her son, who had died in an accident four years earlier. This is an indirect expression of mourning for the lost breast.

In contrast to those women with mastectomies, the tumorectomy patients were qualitatively less depressed. None of the women expressed the apprehension associated with retaining a diseased organ, although the general concern about having cancer remained.

These women gave direct and indirect expression of body-intactness and correspondingly a more stable self-esteem. They were acutely aware, however, of the scar, its size, degree of disfigurement, and skin changes during radiotherapy treatment. Younger women with tumorectomies retained their capacities for sexual fantasizing (a point that requires further investigation).

The diagnosis of cancer has a profound effect on any individual's outlook, no matter to what extent denial is used. It affects not only the patient but also those with whom the patient has contact. This fact is well documented. What has not been sufficiently emphasized, however, is that each individual has his or her own unique response to the life-threatening illness. This response is determined by the individual's capacity to tolerate anxiety, depression, and loss.

The type of denial varies from a very primitive, global, magical type to a more circumscribed and limited variety. Degree of maturity, level of object relations, and capacity to regulate self-esteem are of great significance in the patient's capacity to deal with the disease and with family members and to maintain a reasonable quality of life.

In most patients in our sample, very few significant changes were noted in the basic life patterns. For example, cases with a preexisting sexual pathology between husband and wife, such as frigidity or discontent with the partner's sexual performance, were characterized by a continuance of such traits after mastectomy or tumorectomy. Where there had been a well-adjusted sex life, it returned soon after immediate postoperative inhibitions were relieved. The most frequently reported inhibition among tumorectomy patients was fear on the male's part to touch the affected breast during foreplay.

The fear of radiation therapy that most patients have, because of the popular belief that radiotherapy is used as a last resort, was not found in our patients. Peck (1976) and his group found that cancer patients, in general, believed that their disease was far advanced and that they were to have a possibly damaging and carcinogenic treatment. However, our patients were optimistic about radiation therapy because of their original contact with a surgeon who explained that radiation therapy was a curative part of the treatment. These women felt that their cancer was not so advanced, rather than feeling that it was incurable.

SUMMARY

On the basis of interviews during treatment of patients referred to as for radiation therapy instead of mastectomy for *early* breast cancer, a preliminary impression of their attitude toward their more conservative treatment is that some will actively seek out a surgeon who will perform a lesser procedure. These women believe that their cancer is not too advanced *rather* than feeling that it is incurable.

The effect of a diagnosis of carcinoma of the breast on a woman's attitude toward her body image and sexuality is dependent on her preexisting character makeup.

Finally, if the *referring physician* believes that tumorectomy and radiation therapy are as good as mastectomy, the patient mirrors this hopeful attitude.

REFERENCES

Hackett, T.P., N.H. Cassem, and J.W. Raker. 1973. "Patient Delay in Cancer." *New England Journal of Medicine,* 289:14-20, July.

Lee, E.C.G. and G.P. Maguire. 1975. "Emotional Distress in Patients Attending a Breast Clinic." *British Journal of Surgery,* 62(2):162, February.

Peck, A. and J. Boland. 1976. "Emotional Reactions to Radiation Treatment." *International Journal of Radiation Oncology Biology, Physics Supplement,* 1:111, October.

PELVIC CANCER'S IMPACT ON A WOMAN AND HER FAMILY

William F. Finn

THE FIRST DISCLOSURE

The diagnosis of cancer of the pelvic organs has a profound effect on a female patient. After drying her eyes she asks in a tremulous tone, "What does this mean? What do I have to do now?" The physician sitting with her reflects, "What and how much shall I tell her now?" Knowing that this is not an abstract disease in a statistical person but a disease of widely different potentials in different individual human beings, he thinks of her age. If she is past a certain age, disease and death seem to be of importance. However, she may be in her middle years or may have been pregnant recently or, worst of all, she may be a young adolescent whose life has barely started and now is threatened with loss of menstrual function, loss of the childbearing function, and even death. What of her husband? Is the marriage a close intimate relationship of love or one of mere toleration? Or has her marriage ended in divorce? Is she a widow supporting a family? Are there young children at home or older ones at college or are they widely scattered with children of their own? What type of person has she been? Does she complain at the least little problem or is she stoical? Does she face problems head on? What of her more remote family? Have there been recent deaths of parents? Have there been frequent cancers and illness? Are one or more seriously ill or in nursing homes or in hospitals?

As these thoughts flash through the physician's mind, let us think of the symptoms that brought this patient to the doctor. She may have come for a routine, annual physical examination. At times, cervical smears have been diagnosed as positive, although there are no symptoms. Unusual bleeding, pain, vaginal discharge, swelling of the abdomen or the appearance of a mass may have led to the examination. Now her worse fears have been confirmed. At other times, pathological reports of curettages or operating table diagnoses are made.

What is the patient's reaction? There is an immediate fear of death, but this disappears as she comes to view it as less imminent. Loss of menstrual function, menopause, castration and loss of the capacity to bear children, even though she has not given birth in many years, cause deep concern. These are connected with the fear of aging. Loss of sexual function and coital difficulties loom large in her mind. In single women or in women with an insecure marriage, such fears may be unusually strong. Fear of mutilation occurs less frequently in this situation than it does in breast cancer where the results of surgery are obvious. Later, fear of pain that cannot be relieved occurs. The fear of death, and especially of separation from loved ones and familiar places, returns later.

How does the physician tell the patient that she has cancer? His appraisal of her as an individual guides him. Some patients are best told immediately and forthrightly. You must speak the patient's language. Forget long, esoteric medical words. Remember all questions have hidden meanings. "What is my outlook?" "Can I be cured?" Answer the covert as well as the overt questions. Some patients are best told in graduated doses that they are capable of absorbing at that time in the progress of their disease and at that stage of development of their personality. Some patients do not want to hear the word "cancer" spoken explicitly. Although they know their diagnosis and cooperate with all treatments, they prefer this method of veiled communication. Respect their defenses. Do not force knowledge upon patients. Many times it is desirable to inform patients in the presence of responsible family members. This helps the communication among members of the family and the physician since all know the stage of knowledge and degree of acceptance of each other. It is always the responsibility of the physician to inform the patient. Sometimes the physician may be the family doctor who has known the patient for years, or it may be the surgeon or radiotherapist or cancer specialist who has just begun to know the patient. The telling may occur at home or in the hospital near home or in a speciality hospital away from home. In any event, it then becomes the responsibility of the primary physician—as leader of the complex health team; nurses, hospital personnel, clergymen, social workers, and other medical specialists, to keep the patient, her family and all members of the team informed of her condition and of her knowlege of her state.

The initial interview also includes discussion of modes of treatment. Gynecological cancers are treated by combinations of surgical operations, irradiation and chemotherapy. A careful general outline of the plan of treatment allays many of the patient's fears of the unknown. When a new modality is introduced, she is reassured because the physician had already mentioned it. Otherwise, she might think that this new treatment means that she is getting worse. Careful explanation of the complications of treatment—the pain of surgery; the nausea and diarrhea caused by abdominal irradiation and the hair loss or mouth sores secondary to chemotherapy—does much to assuage the patient's genuine concern that these may not be normal. Preparation of the patient beforehand prevents unanticipated surprise that can shatter her emotional resources.

If not at the initial telling, almost immediately afterwards, the patient wants to know her prognosis. If the cancer has been detected in an early treatable stage, how comforting it is for the physician to impart this news to the patient. If, unfortunately, the diagnosis has been made in a far advanced or even metastatic stage, what can the physician say? He can tell the truth, but sometimes not all the truth! Always hold out hope. Occasionally, patients respond to treatment far better than the physician ever expected. Knowing the fallibility of human prophecy, the physician will not state the outcome in days or months. Patients are not interested in survival rate percentages; they want to know what is going to happen to them. Talking to the patient like an intelligent human being permits her some freedom in decision-making. It makes the treatment a cooperative venture between physician and patient. Unfortunately, many physicians find themselves uncomfortable in this role; hence, their patients have no opportunity to experience the advantage of such mutual cooperation. Physicians frequently find that they cannot communicate to the patient in a relevant fashion. Being dedicated to health and cure, they find it hard to give bad news or find it cruel to talk about certain diagnoses and their therapeutic and prognostic implications. Nurses, hospital workers, and clergymen have the same difficulty. Relatives, if not properly informed, cannot relate to the patient in a meaningful manner. Hence, the better the level of information, the more meaningful the communication and the more intimate the interpersonal relationships that can be created. Establishment of such relationships between patient, family, and physician as early as possible makes possible the highest degree of emotional support for the patient.

THE MIDDLE COURSE

Weeks and months have passed. The patient has been admitted to a hospital. Many diagnostic tests have been performed. She has met new doctors, new hospital personnel, nurses, residents, x-ray and laboratory technicians. All these encounters have aroused new emotions of anxiety, concern for others and fear extending even to stark terror. There has been at least one trip to the operating room and anesthesia and recovery in a surgical intensive care unit. The pain incidental to these events has occurred. Irradiation or chemotherapy may have been begun. Each new event in the unprepared patient leads to more fear. There must be a continued retelling of the original explanation by the physician who is sympathetic to the new emotional reactions of the patient. The physician must relate to the patient's position on the dying trajectory. This apt phrase was devised by Glaser and Strauss (1968) to depict the stages of dying. The trajectory includes the following phases: The first suggestion that the patient is dying; the preparation for death by the staff, the family and possibly the patient, leading to a final statement, "Nothing more can be done." The inevitable progression, gradual deterioration, lead to the last hours and the event of death, followed by the public and legal announcement of the death. We must concentrate on the process of dying, not on the isolated event of death. The physician must respond appropriately to the patient's state of knowledge and her emotional reactions.

Kubler-Ross (1969) has divided the emotional stages of the dying into five—denial, anger, bargaining, depression and finally acceptance. These phases are helpful, provided the physician realizes that they are not absolute and that the patient does not necessarily progress from stage to stage. The first four represent non-acceptance, in general, and also include guilt, anxiety, fear of pain, fear of separation from loved family members, fear of abandonment, regret, and infinite sadness. Not all patients go through all stages or in the same order or at the same rate. Many regressions occur before the ultimate stage of acceptance or acquiescence is reached. The physician should not expect the patient to be a good patient. Let her vent her disbelief, her anger, and her sense of incompleteness. Let her voice her concern about who will care for her children and her husband. Would you not have exactly the same concerns and worries if you had cancer and were dying? Sit down close to the patient. Hold her hand. Don't stand as an awesome, remote figure at the end of the bed. Even worse, don't stand poised at the door ready to dash on to the next patient. Do not see the patient less frequently and then say, "You were asleep when I was here yesterday."

There may be a favorable response to treatments. Then joy can be shown. When results cannot be appraised, uncertainties and anxieties will persist. Complications of therapy may appear. The incision may become infected. Urinary tract infection may appear. Fistulas may develop. The well-known complications of irradiation therapy—colitis, anorexia and skin irritation may occur. Worse still, the cancer may not respond to therapy or surgical removal may be incomplete. Such persistence or recurrence of cancer is disheartening to the patient who watches each little indicator of progress or regression. Readmission to the hospital with all its emotionally destructive events may be necessary. The patient says, "I was doing well and now this." Bad news may have to be given to the patient. She absorbs the meaning of "We could not completely remove the cancer" or digests the thinly veiled message, "We will see what chemotherapy will do." She immediately realizes that this is merely a promise of palliation and not definitive therapy. The pain and distortion of her troubled body adds to her emotional distress. Here kindness, frequent visits, administration of pain-relieving drugs, without fear of causing addiction, will help the patient.

THE END

As death draws near, some patients regress emotionally. They become like children. Solnit and Green (1963) state that the concern of dying children centers on three questions:

1. Am I safe?
2. Will there be a trusted person to keep me from feeling helpless, alone, and to overcome pain?
3. Will you make me feel all right?

Proper disclosure to the patient during all phases of her illness, close attendance, and pain relief will help answer these concerns. The physician should show the patient his concern for her as a living human being in the process of dying. He can let the patient feel his conviction that even in the process of dying life can be of high quality. He can exhibit his humaneness and care for humanity and the amenities of living even in the midst of the busy tempo of the modern practice of medicine. He can tell the patient, "You will not be alone." "We will give you medicine for your pain." "We will help you." "All of us know how you feel." Heroics are of no avail. He will provide pain relief, preferably in small frequent doses. Let the patient feel secure in the presence of those who love her. We will help—family, physician, nurses, hospital employees, clergymen, and everyone in contact with the patient.

If we live up to these promises, the final death will be easier for the patient and mourning without undue risk of emotional breakdown will be possible for the family. Such a mourning process is also necessary for all members of the health team who regard death as failure and do not properly view it as the inevitable outcome of life, which while never welcome, can be treated like any other disease. The relatives may grieve adequately or inadequately. Gradual unfolding of the news of the death permits them to anticipate death and grieve gradually ahead of time. They go through the same stages of emotional reactions which Kubler-Ross (1969) has outlined for patients. An interesting study by Rees and Lutkins (1967) in Wales studied close relatives after the death of a loved one. They found 5 percent of close relatives died within the year, as contrasted to control incidence of 1 percent. Widowed spouses had a 12 percent death incidence within a year as approved to a 1 percent in controls while 6.4 percent of men died as contrasted to 3.5 percent of the women. The obvious moral is to comfort and care for the bereaved relatives, because they are potential patients.

EMOTIONAL REACTION TO SPECIFIC CANCERS OF THE FEMALE GENITAL TRACT

VULVA

The patient with vulvar cancer is usually in her sixties or older. Generally, an unmarried woman or a widow, her tumor or ulcer is in an advanced stage when it is first detected. Self neglect may be compounded by one or more physicians who have been having her rub salve on a necrotic ulcer. When biopsy is finally done, surgery is extensive and infection or wound breakdown are possible complications. The presence of metastatic lymph nodes worsens the prognosis. Emotional problems do occur in these elderly, isolated, shy women. The hospital experience may be helpful in introducing them to new friends—their fellow patients and medical attendants. It may also foster new habits of living. Otherwise, the patient frequently dies of neglect and inanition resulting from the foul ulcerating tumor which had replaced the vulva.

VAGINA

Fortunately, primary cancer of the vagina is rare. When he suspects a cancer of the vagina, the gynecologist immediately checks the cervix and the vulva, if there is a squamous cancer. He investigates the possibility of endometrial cancer, ovarian adenocarcinoma and hypernephroma, if adenocarcinoma is present. Unfortunate situations like sarcoma botyroides occur in young girls. The studies of Herbst (Herbst and Scully, 1970) and others have shown the presence of adenocarcinoma of the vagina and cervix in girls and young women whose mothers have received synthetic non-steroidal estrogens during pregnancy. The emotional trauma to the patient and the family is considerable, inasmuch as the only therapy is extensive surgery with loss of menstrual, reproductive and hormonal function.

CERVIX

The earliest cancers are detected by routine cervical smears when no symptoms have occurred. The outlook is good. But since definitive treatment consists of total abdominal hysterectomy, menstruation and the potential of childbearing is lost. Both these losses of feminine functions may cause adverse effects in patients, leading to feelings of incompleteness as a woman or depression or even intense psychiatric reaction. The majority, however, adapt, especially if they are surrounded by a supportive environment of physician, hospital personnel and family.

More advanced (invasive) cancers have usually manifested themselves by irregular bleeding, heavy periods, discharge or any combination of these symptoms. In many instances there may have been months of neglect on the part of the patient. If the cancer has not spread too far, radical hysterectomy may be done. The husband may hesitate to have sexual relations for fear of spreading the cancer or the foreshortening of the vagina may lead to less frequent performances or may cause difficulties in the sexual act. This additional emotional burden at a time when the patient's security is already threatened can result in severe consequences. More advanced invasive cancers will be treated by irradiation. The initial reactions to treatment—nausea and colitis—together with the late complications of fibrosis, strictures, and fistulas, disturb the patient. Since cervical cancer is a disease with local recurrence rather than distant metastases, the patient usually survives either in good health or with recurrences. When recurrences occur, usually the irradiation has been given to full tolerance, hence exenterations of bladder or rectum or both with incidental ureterostomies and colostomy must be done. These various artificial openings are offensive enough, but are even worse to the fastidious or the narcissistic patient. If the course is downhill, the ineffectiveness of palliative therapy may cause profound depression. The general principles alluded to before apply to the various phases of the downward trajectory of the disease.

ENDOMETRIUM

Patients with cancer of the uterus have fewer emotional problems. They are usually older, are in frequent contact with doctors and as a rule report promptly if bleeding recurs after menopause. About one-third of these patients have not gone through menopause. Then the symptoms may be minimal changes in menstrual bleeding or the appearance of intermenstrual spotting. Since the cancer is usually detected in an early phase, the cure rate is the best of all the invasive cancers of the genital organs. Therapy consists of surgical removal of the uterus and surrounding organs with irradiation either before or after surgery. Since the patient is older, loss of the ability to procreate is of no concern. Menstrual function has usually been lost long before. Coital difficulties rarely arise. Since the patient is usually in the age where continuing living in reasonable good health is the main objective, she adjusts well to the treatment and to any complications. If soft tissue metastases occur, high dosage progesterone therapy is effective in many instances.

OVARY

Cancer of the ovary is unfortunately detected late after widespread intraperitoneal surface metastases have occurred. Occasionally, good fortune smiles, early cancer confined to one ovary without overt spread is discovered incidental to some other operation. But in most instances the primary operation is incomplete. Metastatic foci are left behind to be treated by abdominal irradiation or chemotherapy. The patient usually gets steadily worse. Paracenteses are done as ascitic fluid reaccumulates. Progressive weakness is due to the hypoproteinemia and intermittent subacute bowel obstruction. Occasionally metastases to the pleura cause hydrothorax and progressive dyspnea. Repeat admissions occur. This cancer is the classic prototype in its slow inevitably progressive consumption of the vital forces of the body. The long trajectory causes intense personal distress to all affected by it—patient, family and doctor—since the realization grows increasingly evident that everything that can be done has been done and that only palliation remains.

TUBE

Cancer of the tube is fortunately very rare. It is like cancer of the ovary in that it is usually metastatic when first discovered. The correct preoperative diagnosis is rarely made. As complete a surgical resection as possible is followed by irradiation. The trajectory and progressive deterioration is like that of ovarian cancer.

SARCOMA OF THE UTERUS

The discovery, surgical treatment, and prognosis are like those of endometrial cancer. Irradiation, chemotherapy, or hormones do not seem to affect this type of cancer

CANCERS ASSOCIATED WITH PREGNANT WOMEN

The joy of pregnancy is sometimes turned into grief by the association of a choriocarcinoma after a hydatidiform mole, an abortion, or even a full-term delivery. Persistence of bleeding, the failure of the uterus to involute or evidence of direct metastases, pain in the liver area, pulmonary hemorrhage or neurological signs indicate the presence of this dread cancer. The woman is especially vulnerable to despair and sorrow since this is happening at a time when life should be joyous.

The pregnant or recently delivered woman may also have cancer of her genital organs or in other parts of her body. This may have occurred in the past, so that for practical purposes she might be regarded as cured. Also, it may have been so recent that pregnancy has been advised against until it is thought that enough time has elapsed to be reasonably sure that the condition has stabilized. Such a woman is filled with regret, fear, uncertainty. She may request an abortion or may continue with the pregnancy. The normal concerns of pregnancy may be greatly increased during the nine months of anticipation. Operations or other treatments may have to be performed. Modification or delays in therapy may be necessary because of the presence of the fetus. Labor may have to be induced or Caesarean section may have to be done in order that definitive therapy may be started sooner. The degree of emotional reaction is increased because of the presence of two patients—the mother and the unborn child.

SUMMARY

Pelvic cancer causes intense emotional reactions in women. The proper supportive attitude on the part of the physician will aid her and her family in all phases of this difficult time in her life.

REFERENCES

Glaser, B.G. and A.L. Strauss. 1968. *Time for Dying*. Chicago: Aldine Press.
Herbst, A.L. and R.E. Scully. 1970. "Adenocarcinomas of the Vagina in Adolescence: A Report of Seven Cases Including Six Clear-Cell Carcinomas (So-called Mesonephromas)." *Cancer*, 25:745-757.
Kubler-Ross, E. 1969. *On Death and Dying*. New York: Macmillan Co.
Rees, W.D. and S.G. Lutkins. 1967. "Mortality of Bereavement." *British Medical Journal*, 4:13-16 (October 7).
Solnit, A.J., M. Green, and S.A. Provence (eds.). 1963. *Modern Perspectives in Child Development*. New York: International Universities Press.

GYNECOLOGIC CANCER: A CASE REPORT

William F. Finn

Marjorie Johnson (a fictitious name, of course, but how much better than M.J. No. 187529) was 48 years old. She had had a happy life and was married to the same man for 26 years. She had 3 children: a son Ralph, 23 years of age, a daughter Linda, 21 and a second daughter, Joan, who was 13 years old. Her husband, Bob, was a textile salesman who had worked for the same firm for 18 years. She was a college graduate, had been an elementary school teacher, and now was active in her church and many ceramic projects, but her life centered upon her husband and her children and her home. Ralph had just earned an electrical engineering degree and was looking for a job. Linda had just finished her third year of college abroad at Grenoble where she studied French language, history and culture. Joan was an active cheerful seventh grader.

Marjorie had never been seriously ill. Her appendix had been removed when she was 14. She had outgrown a childhood allergy to spring grasses. Her menopause had occurred uneventfully two years ago at the age of 46. Marjorie noticed one night that her panties were stained with blood. She was disturbed, but did not think that this was significant as she said to herself, "It isn't enough for a period, but it must be that." When this recurred three times over the next two weeks, she called her family doctor, Dr. Gorham. He told her that any bleeding after change of life should be investigated promptly and further suggested to save time that she see a gynecologist of her choice. Since she did not know a gynecologist, he referred her to Dr. Farber.

Dr. Farber examined her that afternoon. As Marjorie and he sat in his consultation room afterwards, she asked him what he had found. He told her that the physical examination, blood count, and urinalysis were normal and that while he had taken a vaginal smear, a curettage was necessary to find out the cause of bleeding. Marjorie was surprised to learn that bleeding after change of life was not normal but could mean polyps, overgrowth of the lining of the uterus or even an early cancer. This first partial disclosure of the possibility of cancer led to vigorous denials inasmuch as no one in her family had ever had cancer. Dr. Farber explained that cancer was not based on a genetic inheritance, but a sound gynecological axiom stated that any bleeding after menopause required a curettage.

When Marjorie arrived home that night, she promptly told Bob that she might have cancer. He replied that it would have to be early since she had seen the doctor "right away" but in any event she should be admitted to the hospital right away. Although she was still disturbed, she was able to sleep. Fortunately there was no delay in admission, so her anxiety did not increase further. She was heartened by the good reports of her chest x-ray, her EKG and her blood chemistries. As she spoke to Dr. Farber on the afternoon before the surgery, she said, "If you find a cancer, I want you to tell me." Since he did not know her well, he replied, with a noncommittal, "Let's hope for the best." The examination while Marjorie was under anesthesia was normal. Curettage produced endometrial tissue which was abundant but well preserved. Marjorie and Bob waited impatiently for the report the next day. Dr. Farber received a pathology report of "Well differentiated adenocarcinoma of the endometrium." Late that afternoon he met with a tearful Marjorie and a very concerned Bob. He outlined the need for removal of the uterus, both tubes and ovaries and for vaginal irradiation to the vault and maybe lower abdominal x-ray irradiation depending on how deeply the cancer had spread into the wall of the uterus. Marjorie sobbed, "But I'm going to die. Bob and the children cannot get along without me." Bob sat with a glacial expression on his face. Dr. Farber explained, "It is better to know your diagnosis. Since you saw a doctor very quickly after your first symptoms, you have an excellent chance of complete cure. I will give you a headline digest of your treatment now and the time that will be involved, and I will always give you advance notice of a change or possible complication of treatment." Marjorie interrupted, "Then I'm not going to die?" "Of course not," replied Dr. Farber, "Endometrial cancer has the best outlook of all pelvic cancers. You are in a good hospital with all facilities for surgery and irradiation." When Marjorie and Bob sat alone in her room later, he hugged her and said, "Dr. Farber leveled with us. Now we are just going to do as he says. The kids and I will help you." That night Bob phoned Ralph and Linda and later sat down with Joan on his lap. He told them that Mommy had an early cancer of the womb which required surgery and x-ray, but that Dr. Farber said that she would be all right.

The hysterectomy was performed without event the next morning. Marjorie's postoperative course was excellent. Because there was some penetration of the cancer onto the wall of the uterus, Dr. Farber recommended lower abdominal irradiation as well as the application of radium to the vagina. Apart from a moderate degree of nausea and diarrhea she did well. Her fears of death and of separation from her family diminished. Occasionally, she awakened at night and could not go back to sleep (her thoughts dwelling on the cancer "eating her insides"), but gradually she reassured herself that Dr. Farber had told her the truth. For a time Marjorie felt weak and tired easily; but the incision on the abdomen and in the vagina had healed well. Her blood count and urinalysis were normal. She told Dr. Farber that she felt better every day, was able to do most things, and that she was eternally grateful to him. Then she said, "Tell me really how I'm doing." Dr. Farber who regarded medicine as more than a profession but as a lay vocation got out of his chair, walked around his desk, and sat next to her, taking her hand in his. After a minute he said, "Marjorie, we never regard cancer as cured. You had an early cancer of the lining of the womb; this kind of cancer has the best outlook of all cancers of women's organs. You and I are going to get to know each other very well because we will be seeing each other every two months for the next two years and after that every four months for the rest of your life. I will talk to you or see you at any other time if you think that it is necessary."

At six months after surgery Marjorie was tearful. Her examination was fine. Afterwards, Dr. Farber asked, "Marjorie what is wrong?" Her reply was, "It's Bob. He's afraid of me. He's afraid that sexual relations will spread my cancer." This led to a trialog, after which Bob said, "Doctor, you're sure that this won't hurt Marjorie?" "Not in the least," was Dr. Farber's reply. "This is part of the basics of life like fire, bread, soup, and physical contact." With that assurance life progressed smoothly in the Johnson house. Ralph phoned and visited more often. Linda helped with the housekeeping and cooking. Joan remained her ebullient self and drew Marjorie from the slough of despondence when black thoughts encompassed her. Bob remained a tower of strength, both father and husband while Marjorie saw Dr. Farber. Fortunately, she never developed metastases or had a recurrence.

COMMENT

This case report was selected because it is typical. The patient was stable emotionally. She sought medical care promptly and followed advice. She had the normal worries and concerns of a patient with endometrial cancer. Her husband and family supported her, both physically and emotionally.

Her physician was honest in his presentation of facts. He was prompt in treatments; he spoke to both patient and husband together and maintained this contact. He kept the patient informed of diagnostic procedures, treatments, and prognosis. This permitted cooperation and the gradual buildup of trust and confidence.

ARE THERE MIRACLES?

Yvonne M. Parnes

It is Christmas again, evoking bittersweet, poignant memories and hopes for miracles. Hope for those who are threatened is higher; compassion for those who are doomed reaches profound depth. For caregivers there may be holiday depression stemming from what we recognize as our limited ability to provide, continually. There is a compelling need to cushion the sadness for those leaving life at a time of year when mankind becomes rededicated to peace and good will.

One miracle to behold is enough to ponder, enough to provoke belief in something greater, enough to contemplate what can be restored.

He is sixty-three, but a patriarch of three special, grown children and an old world wife. When the call came on a Saturday morning that he had become dizzy and had fallen, I told his sons to bring him to our center. We were almost closing. Others wanted me to send him to the emergency room. "He may have a brain tumor," I said. He did!

After devastating surgery, the pathologist identified the kind of tumor. It was the type described so eloquently by John Gunther in *Death Be Not Proud*. It had taken his son. Now it threatened to destroy a family unit, touching a father. But it united them in an admirable effort to cheat death.

They grieved but used their strength to support a life they refused to surrender. By spring the prescribed course of radiation had been completed. Staff began to plan for terminal care at home of a bedridden and disabled patient.

Love works inexplicable wonders. By summer, the wheelchair was gone and he was using a cane. "Doing remarkably well," the progress note read. Remarkably? What was hoped for with radiation was jubilantly achieved. Cat scan now reads, "Possibility of residual or recurrent tumor cannot be excluded"—or included, we muse. Whatever time radiation has given is appreciated. And so to bargaining! If the maximum number of rads received bought this year, could not another course of radiation do as much? It is to be considered.

It is almost Christmas eve. The younger son summons me. His father leans lightly on his cane, smiling, strong, hair receding from the surgical site and obliterated by radiation. He takes my hand and squeezes it with life. His wife is next to him offering home-made cookies in gratitude. Their faces are glowing with the miracle.

We shake our heads. For all our sophistication, we cannot define the forces that have spared him so that this family will have a blessed holiday.

This must be proper application of radiation therapy at its very best. It is restoration!

MANAGEMENT OF THE PATIENT WITH CANCER

Christie Goeggel Lamping and Sigmund Benham Kahn[*]

LUNG CANCER

Carcinoma of the lung is a metastatic disease in most patients at the time the primary lesion is diagnosed. Only 25 percent of lung tumors are surgically resectable and less than 5 percent of all lung cancer patients will live more than five years after the diagnosis has been made. The median survival is six to nine months from the time of diagnosis, with only 20 percent surviving more than one year. There are approximately ten histopathological varieties of lung tumor with anaplastic and squamous cell types being the most common. The poor prognosis is related to the tendency of these tumors to metastasize widely at an early stage in their development. The organs most commonly involved by metastases are liver, brain, bone, and adrenal glands. However, any organ may be invaded.

The patient most likely to be cured is one with a small peripheral lesion which can be removed completely by surgery. In practice, unfortunately, patients with such lesions are rarely seen. Once staging procedures have indicated unresectability or if following resection recurrence is found, other forms of treatment become necessary. It should be emphasized that all patients should have a tissue diagnosis before any radiation treatments or chemotherapy are administered. This tissue can often be obtained by node biopsy, bronchoscopy, mediastinoscopy, or by cytologic study of the sputum.

The typical patient with carcinoma of the lung is a middle-aged male with a heavy smoking history and often some background of chronic lung disease. He will come to the physician complaining of dyspnea, cough, hemoptysis and sputum production. By this time, the disease is usually so far advanced that signs of

---

[*]This study was supported by USPHS Grant No. 5R25CA 17963-07, NC1.

metastasis may be found on careful physical examination. Adenopathy in the neck and axillae and enlargement of the liver should be carefully sought. Mediastinoscopy should be done before thoracotomy. If any of the above are positive, thoracotomy should not be done.

Once the diagnosis is made and the patient is felt not to be a surgical candidate, radiation therapy or chemotherapy should be used for palliation. Chemotherapy is preferred if there is wide dissemination of the tumor. Recent results utilizing combination chemotherapy in small cell carcinoma of the lung have been encouraging.

Despite the dismal response rate to chemotherapy, symptomatic therapy often helps many patients. The medical problems of these patients are complex and challenging. Dyspnea is the most common and distressing symptom. The physician should not hesitate to provide the patient with a source of oxygen for home use. This measure alone will often ease much suffering. Some patients will be helped by chlorpromazine or meperidine. Cough is another disabling symptom and the use of codeine in liquid or tablet form is recommended as an effective anti-tussive. The most common medical problem that compounds cough and dyspnea is chronic obstructive lung disease. Medical therapy of this condition may help alleviate nagging symptoms. Pleural effusions should be tapped repeatedly if necessary and nitrogen mustard or tetracycline instilled into the pleural space. Congestive heart failure, pneumonia and recurrent pulmonary emboli may occur in these patients and should be treated appropriately.

Patients with lung tumor involving the apical lobes may develop the superior vena cava syndrome due to obstruction by tumor. This condition should be treated by radiation therapy. Patients who have metastatic tumor to the brain should receive central nervous system irradiation. Single lesions in bone should also be treated in this manner. Finally, if the primary tumor is creating symptoms such as pain, radiation therapy to the primary lesion often palliates the patient. Indeed, we often irradiate primary inoperable lung cancer if evidence of widespread disease is lacking and the expected survival is greater than six months.

When the physician judges the patient to be terminal, he should not hesitate to use whatever sedation or analgesia is necessary to relieve anxiety, dyspnea or pain, allowing death to come with comfort and dignity.

The following case illustrates some of the problems mentioned:

A 42-year-old woman with a long history of excessive cigarette smoking was admitted to a community hospital with a three month history of cough and chest pain. A chest x-ray revealed a mediastinal mass. Sputum cytology and bronchoscopy were negative. Because of the suggestion that the mass might be vascular in origin, right-sided transfemoral arteriogram was performed. This clearly excluded vascular and cardiac involvement. Within 24 hours the right leg became cold and pale. The patient was transferred to a major medical center where an endarterectomy corrected the vascular occlusion. Forty-eight hours later mediastinoscopy and biopsy established the diagnosis of oat cell carcinoma of the lung. After consultation with a medical oncologist a course of cyclophosphamide was given. The mass shrunk, and the patient's symptoms were relieved. She returned to work, and chemotherapy was continued. One year later a seizure occurred and brain scan revealed a frontal lobe abnormality. Anti-convulsants and steroids were administered and a course of cranial irradiation was delivered. The patient returned to a normal life. Three months later back pain occurred and a lesion in the lumbar spine was found. Another course of irradiation relieved her. Her disease was obviously unresponsive to cyclophosphamide, and a few newly acquired experimental agents were given. No objective responses were noted. Her terminal picture was that of enlarging intrathoracic mass, which caused cough and chest pain, and nodular hepatomegaly. The terminal illness was pneumonia. After discussion with the family, no antibiotics were given and the patient was sedated with morphine. She died within 48 hours.

The total survival from diagnosis to death was 18 months. While this length of survival is unusual, her life was undoubtedly extended by chemotherapy. During the last six months of her life when chemotherapy was no longer effective, the problems she developed were similar to those encountered by patients with widespread metastatic lung cancer whose tumors fail to respond to drugs. Currently, the use of Adriamycin and methotrerate have yielded even better results.

THE LYMPHOMAS

Lymphomas constitute a heterogeneous group of diseases with varying clinical pictures and prognoses. From a clinical and pathological viewpoint they may be classified as follows:

1. Hodkin's disease (all pathological types)
2. Non-Hodkin's lymphoma (recently reclassified according to presence or absence of nodularity in the node, maturity of cell present and predominant cell type seen on microscopy), but including those entities heretofore described as reticulum cell sarcoma, lymphoblastic, lymphosarcoma, lymphocytic lymphosarcoma, and giant follicular lymphoma.
3. Burkitt's lymphoma
4. Chronic lymphocytic leukemia

While a complete description of the problems encountered by these patients is beyond the scope of this chapter, an outline of difficulties encountered by most patients during the course of their disease would include the following:

1. Adenopathy and tumor masses or both causing pain or impaired organ function. The most pressing problem is spinal epidural metastases since if these masses remain untreated, irreversible paralysis results.
2. Hematopoietic abnormalities including anemia, leukopenia and thrombocytopenia. The primary mechanism is marrow failure but immunohemolytic anemia may occur.
3. Immunological failure (cellular in Hodgkin's disease and humoral in the non-Hodgkin's lymphomas) leading to increased susceptibility to infection.

4. Weight loss, anorexia, fever.
5. Skin lesions including Herpes Zoster, and various dermatitides.

During the last ten years much progress has been made in the therapy of these diseases. Many disorders formerly considered hopeless are now being cured by aggressive radiation therapy and chemotherapy. Therefore, all patients suffering with these disorders should be referred to a major cancer center where staging procedures (i.e., determining the amount and location of tumor involvement in the patient) can be performed. Following these tests, definitive and aggressive radiation or chemotherapy or a combination of both should be given. The possibility of cure (especially in those with limited disease) or of long-term control of these diseases makes an early and aggressive approach imperative. Note well that the initial therapeutic effort is the most important one in ensuring long-term survival.

The only exception to this rule may be in the treatment of chronic lympathic leukemia. This is a disease of the elderly and in some patients runs a benign and chronic course. Many hematologists do not treat these patients unless severe anemia or thrombocytopenia has occurred. Even these complications can often be controlled by low doses of chemotherapeutic agents or steroids. Some patients also respond well to anabolic steroids. It is important to reassure these patients that although they have "leukemia," their prognosis is good. However, they should be observed at fairly frequent intervals, even if they are receiving no therapy, and it should be recalled that there is a very high incidence of second malignancies in these patients. In addition, since these patients are usually elderly (mostly elderly men) they may suffer any of the more common medical problems of the aged. Thus, their complaints should not always be blamed on their leukemia. Other causes should be sought and treated.

The therapy of the lymphomas is a rapidly advancing, complex and changing field. Most patients, even those with advanced disease, will obtain long-term remissions from chemotherapy and irradiation. Patients who suffer relapses following therapy with standard regimens may be treated by newer chemotherapeutic agents with an expectation of response. In view of the development of newer agents and the success of multi-drug chemotherapy and chemotherapy-irradiation therapy, combination approaches, even the therapy of chronic lymphocytic leukemia, is being re-evaluated. New protocols will test whether aggressive therapy of this disorder while the patient is asymptomatic will extend survival.

Death in patients with lymphomas may be due to tumor involvement of vital organs such as the lung and the liver. This occurs after the condition becomes resistant to chemotherapy. Even more commonly, the debility and poor resistance to infections of these patients cause a septic death. Bizarre and opportunistic infections are often encountered. Any signs of infection in such patients should be treated aggressively since both the disease and its treatment impair the ability of these patients to resist infection. Finally, many patients succumb to other illnesses such as heart disease. In these patients the leukemia aggravates a chronic disease.

NEUROLOGICAL NEOPLASMS

Primary brain tumors represent 3 percent of the deaths from cancer in the United States each year. There is a high incidence in childhood, where CNS tumors are the second most common cause of death below the age of fifteen. A second peak incidence occurs in middle age. Morbidity and mortality are high for all types of brain tumors, although recent advances in neurosurgical techniques, chemotherapy, and radiation therapy have improved the outlook.

If one considers all brain tumors occurring in a given population, the majority of tumors in the CNS are metastatic. The most common primary sites of origin are the lung in men and the breast in women. Spinal cord metastatic disease is most often caused by lymphoma or breast cancer.

The most common *primary* brain neoplasm is the glioma which constitutes 31 to 49 percent of cases. All gliomas are considered invasive, but have varying degrees of malignancy ranging from the astrocytoma grade I or II with low invasiveness to the highly malignant Grade III or IV also known as the glioblastoma multiforme. This tumor causes death 7 to 14 months following diagnosis. Other primary brain tumors include meningiomas which represent 9 to 18 percent of tumors and pituitary adenomas which represent 3 to 18 percent of brain tumors. These latter tumors are considered benign, but their location may cause complications and problems similar to those of malignant tumors. Other rarer CNS tumors include sarcomas, hemangioblastomas, craniopharyngiomas, and neurinomas. The medical complications of all brain tumors no matter what their histology are related to their location in the central nervous system since rarely do they spread beyond this area.

The initial diagnosis of a brain tumor may be difficult especially if the tumor is located in the frontal lobe. In this location subtle personality changes may be the earliest clinical sign of disease. More obvious symptoms and signs include headache, vomiting, visual changes, seizures and motor and sensory loss. Initial evaluation of such patients should include a careful history with questioning of family members about changes in personality and a thorough neurological examination including fundoscopy. If the findings are suggestive, the patient should be hospitalized for precise diagnosis. Most commonly the CT scan but also the EEG, brain scan and arteriography allow the clinician to localize the lesion in the majority of cases. No one test should be considered diagnostic, but CT scanning has certainly erased the diagnostic difficulties of the past. Since the largest number of brain lesions encountered in clinical practice will be metastatic in origin, and since this radically alters therapy and prognosis, the search for a possible primary site should not be neglected. This is especially true if there are multiple CNS lesions. Lung, colon, breast, stomach cancer and malignant melanoma are some of the primary tumors that commonly metastasize to the brain.

Surgery is the treatment of choice for most primary brain tumors. Meningiomas and other noninvasive tumors can often be removed completely. Even if the tumor is malignant, surgery can be helpful. In some cases, the tumor can be removed completely; in others, palliation by decreasing intracranial pressure and tumor bulk prolong survival and improve patient comfort. If the tumor is a glioblastoma where complete resection is often not possible, palliative surgery should be followed by radiation therapy. Forty percent of such patients will live one year, although only 13 percent will be alive at the end of five years. This represents a considerable improvement in the survival of these patients, although the long-term prognosis is still poor. In occasional patients surgical removal of a single metastatic lesion may be indicated. In all patients with metastatic cranial or spinal disease irradiation should be given after the diagnosis is established.

Chemotherapy of brain tumors is now possible and promising. The development of drugs that can penetrate the blood-brain barrier has given this therapy a new role in the management of patients with malignant tumors of the brain. Evidence is accumulating that these agents may prolong survival in patients with glioblastomas as well as those with metastatic tumors. These drugs, which are experimental, have significant hematologic toxicity and must be used with great care. However, most major centers have investigators who are familiar with their use.

The major medical problems in patients with CNS tumors are increased intracranial pressure and cerebral edema. Headache, vomiting, status epilepticus and coma are symptoms that warrant emergency treatment. Considerable and rapid improvement can be obtained by the administration of corticosteroids such as dexamethasone 8 to 10 mg. IV followed by 16 to 20 mg. daily (oral or parenteral) in divided doses. Decompression may be used to prolong the improvement following this therapy. In all instances appropriate therapy with anticonvulsants is mandatory.

While in the past, patients with brain tumors were "written off" and given narcotics, the following case illustrates the effectiveness of the newer chemotherapeutic agents in prolonging useful survival:

A 60-year-old salesman was found to have a malignant glioma of the parietal lobe. Following craniotomy a course of x-ray therapy relieved his headaches and despite some sensory impairment he returned to his desk. After six months, signs of increased pressure occurred, and he was treated with dexamethasone and BCNU (bis-chlorethylnitrosurea). His symptoms lessened and he maintained his job. He was given an injection of BCNU every four to six weeks for the next eight months. He died of recurrent disease 16 months following diagnosis. He was capable of maintaining a sedentary but active life for 12 months following surgery.

PROSTATE

Cancer of the prostate is the second most common malignancy causing death in men. It is a disease of the elderly with a median age at onset of 70 and is rarely seen before the age of fifty. Carcinoma of the prostate *in situ* is found with increasing incidence in each decade past the fifth. Many diagnoses are made incidentally at the time of surgery for prostatism. It is unknown whether all these patients have disease that will become metastatic. About 5 to 10 percent of patients with symptomatic cancer of the prostate have disease limited to the gland. These men can be cured by radical prostatectomy. Radiation therapy may also cure these patients. If the success of radiation therapy of limited prostatic cancer is confirmed, this mode of treatment will replace radical surgery. In any event, only those patients with limited disease are candidates for surgery or x-ray therapy. A normal acid phosphatase and negative bone scan should be present. If either of these tests is positive the patient has metastatic disease. Careful evaluation of pelvic nodes is also mandatory since these patients do not have limited disease despite negative acid phosphatase and liver scans.

The majority of patients unfortunately have spread or metastatic disease at the time of diagnosis. The survival of these patients is generally two to three years, while in those patients with localized disease the five-year survival is about 60 percent.

Patients with disseminated disease have many complex medical problems. Local growth of unresectable tumor may cause obstruction of the urinary tract. Palliative surgery or urinary diversion may be necessary to prevent hydronephrosis and uremia. Bone metastases create hypercalcemia in some patients. This problem should be treated with I. V. saline, diuretics, and steroids. The most serious problem these patients face is widespread bony disease which is painful and debilitating. Such metastases are usually evident on skeletal survey or bone scan. Anemia often associated with leukopenia and thrombocytopenia occurs and leads to symptoms. Because these men are elderly, associated cardiovascular or peripheral vascular disease may dominate the clinical picture.

Patients with widespread metastatic disease should undergo orchiectomy or estrogen therapy. Diethylstilbesterol 1 mg. daily is the drug and dosage of choice. Higher dosages are not any more effective and have been shown to produce an increased incidence of myocardial infarction and thromboembolism. Ninety percent of patients will experience marked relief from either hormonal therapy or castration. Local irradiation to isolated bony metastasis or those in weight bearing areas may also be instituted. For those who fail on these standard therapies, some will respond to Prednisone, P-32, or alkylating agents.

It should be stressed that almost all patients with widespread disease may be successfully palliated by the above methods. During this time other diseases may occur and cause symptoms. Each problem (even if unrelated to the malignancy) should be treated aggressively since the overall survival of patients with carcinoma of the prostate is measured in years rather than in months.

SARCOMA

Sarcomas are tumors which arise from the primitive mesenchyme. Their primary site may be from any supporting tissue including fat, blood vessels, muscle, cartilage and connective tissue. Thus, these tumors may arise in any part of the body and may give rise to any symptom complex related to the organs involved. The wide variation in the clinical pictures presented by these tumors makes it impossible to give a typical case report, while the clinical and pathological details of each type of tumor included in this group is beyond the scope of the present chapter.

The sarcomas fall into two clinical groups, those with a high malignant potential which metastasize widely and those which grow by local infiltration. The overall 5-year survival rate is reported to be 40 percent. However, it should be remembered that this figure includes the highly malignant embryonal rhabdomyosarcoma with a 5-year survival of 20 to 35 percent and the dermatofibrosarcomas which grow slowly and have a 5-year survival rate of 88 to 96 percent.

The most common problem presented by the patient with incurable disease includes pain, bulky tumor interfering with function, vascular and lymphatic obstruction leading to edema below the site of the primary and in those patients with widespread disease, renal, hepatic and pulmonary dysfunction. The rate of progression of symptoms varies with tumor type. Slowly progressing retroperitoneal fibrosarcomas, often locally unresectable, may be unassociated with symptoms. In these patients survival is measured in years. On the other hand, radiation responsive and chemotherapy responsive rhabdomyosarcomas often produce many symptoms and may kill the patient in less than a year.

Therapeutic approaches are as varied as the diseases. Localized tumor is best treated initially by surgery in an attempt to cure. Radical surgery is sometimes curative and should be a consideration when the patient first presents to the physician. Amputation may be necessary if the tumor involves an extremity. Even if the tumor is not curable by amputation, palliative removal of an extremity may convert a pain-ridden patient into a useful person for the remaining time of his survival.

Radiation therapy is another line of attack used against these tumors. Some sarcomas will respond to radiation alone, and radiation therapy is sometimes used preoperatively to decrease tumor bulk and ease the surgeons' task. However, it should be remembered that not all types of sarcomas respond to radiation therapy and even if responsive, it is not uncommon for large doses of x-ray to be required.

Palliative radiation or surgery or both may also be of great help even when cure is not a feasible goal. The surgical treatment of bowel obstruction or impaired blood flow is indicated in a patient with slowly progressive disease whose medical condition justifies an aggressive approach. Any therapeutic decision for these patients should be made by the primary physician with the advice of the surgeon, the radiation therapist and the medical oncologist to assist him.

SKIN

Skin cancer is the most common malignancy that afflicts mankind. The majority of cases are basal cell or squamous cell tumors which are locally invasive and readily cured by surgery, radiation therapy, and chemotherapy. The overall cure rate is 95 percent. Those cases not cured by currently available techniques are generally those which have been neglected for a long period of time.

Even in these neglected cases local extension rather than metastasis is the cause of death. Multiple tumors may occur in patients with hereditary predisposition or excessive exposure to sunlight. These multiple tumors may be treated with topical 5-Fluorouracil in a cream base.

The remaining cases of skin cancer fall into a heterogeneous group. Each has a poorer prognosis than does basal cell or squamous cell carcinoma. This group includes malignant melanoma, Kaposi's sarcoma and mycosis fungoides. By far the most common of this group is malignant melanoma. The following case report illustrates the history of a patient with such a tumor:

The patient was a 43-year-old white male. Two years previously a melanoma had been removed from his back. He did well after surgery for a year and a half after which he developed pain and swelling in his right leg. An x-ray showed a lytic lesion of the right femur. The rest of the physical examination was unremarkable. A complete evaluation for metastatic disease was done including a complete blood count, liver function tests, chest x-ray, bone survey, liver scan, and brain scan. He was found to have a positive liver scan. The patient was treated with radiation to the right leg for symptomatic relief and given the experimental drug, Methyl CCNU. On this regimen his pain has improved and he has returned to work.

This case illustrates but one behavior pattern of malignant melanoma. In this man blood borne metastases led to widespread disease within two years. In other patients metastatic lesions might appear five to ten years after initial surgery, while in others the pattern might include local recurrence with extension to regional nodes. In brief, all patients should be followed at regular intervals on a long-term basis even if there is no evidence of disease during the first five years following therapy.

Metastases usually appear in the lung, liver, brain, and bone, and the medical problems that must be faced are a result of tumor invasion of these vital organs. Some patients have an intrinsically slower growing tumor and may live longer than those whose tumors grow rapidly and aggressively. The tumor's aggressiveness can often be estimated from the patient's clinical course. The inherent variability of the tumor's course impairs the clinician's ability to estimate prognosis and alters his ability to evaluate the effectiveness of therapy unless the patient is matched to a similar alternatively treated control group.

BIBLIOGRAPHY

These clinical segments have not been extensively referenced primarily because the busy practitioner rarely has time to seek the core articles relevant to the content of these chapters. The authors recommend the following core texts in which are covered the details relevant to this material:

1. Summary text to be used as refresher:

   Clinical Oncology: A Manual for Students and Doctors.
   A paperback book published by a distinguished committee for the International Union Against Cancer. Springer-Verlag publishers, Berlin-Heidelberg-New York, 1973.

2. Encyclopedic textbook

   Holland, J.F., E. Frei III (eds.). *Cancer Medicine,* Lea and Febiger, Philadelphia, 1973.
   This textbook covers in great detail virtually every aspect of cancer in man.

3. Therapy Reviews

   Brodsky, I., S.B. Kahn, and F. Conroy (eds.). *Cancer Chemotherapy III.* Grune and Stratton, New York, 1978.

   Brodsky, I., S.B. Kahn, and J.H. Moyer (eds.). *Cancer Chemotherapy II.* Grune and Stratton, New York, 1972.
   An up-to-date clinical treatise on the drug therapy of cancer including information about those experimental drugs mentioned in this chapter.

   Kahn, S.B. and I. Brodsky (eds.). *Seminars in Drug Treatment.* Vol. 3, No. 1, Summer, 1973, Grune and Stratton, publisher.
   A problem-oriented review of the problems of the cancer patient.

BRAIN TUMOR

John C.M. Brust

A patient coming to a doctor for headaches often asks if he has a brain tumor, intracranial neoplasms, although less common than many other kinds of cancer, are frighteningly familiar to many people. George Gershwin and Eero Saarinen died of brain tumors, and the inexorably fatal course of John Gunther, Jr., is described in his father's book, *Death Be Not Proud*. Brain tumors, it is popularly believed, cause rapidly progressive paralysis, feeblemindedness, and coma, punctuated by neurosurgery which leads to further brain damage, radiation therapy which causes intolerable nausea and vomiting, and chemotherapy which produces dangerous side effects. While a relentlessly downhill course may indeed be associated with such tumor types as glioblastoma or metastatic lung cancer, it is important for patients and their families to be aware that for many kinds of brain tumor the story is quite different, and that even with malignant varieties there are greater grounds for optimism than was possible even a decade ago.

Brain tumors are either primary or metastatic. Certain cancers, for example those originating in the kidney, often metastasize to the brain. Others, for example prostatic cancer, do not. The most common brain metastases are from lung and breast cancers, reflecting their greater frequency as primary cancers. How metastatic tumors respond to treatment depends in part on their primary sites. Some types of lung cancer, for example, are quite sensitive to radiotherapy, and others are radioresistant. Radiotherapy may produce remissions of months or years in patients with breast cancer, restoring normal neurological function, while metastases to other organs are treated chemotherapeutically or hormonally. Although rare, there are cases of complete "sterilization" of brain metastases by radiotherapy. In some centers surgical extirpation is performed on brain metastases considered "solitary" on the basis of diagnostic tests.

Primary brain tumors are also of different types and prognoses. The most common are gliomas, which arise, not from nerve cells, but from the brain's supporting or glial cells. Within this group is the malignant glioblastoma, which tends to occur after middle age, and, being unresectable and relatively resistant to radiotherapy and chemotherapy, is inevitably fatal, usually within a year. Other gliomas are more benign, however, and while, with the exception of cerebellar astrocytoma, they can rarely be totally resected, their courses can extend over decades, as, for example, in the case of a woman recently seen whose 27 years of well-controlled seizures turned out to be secondary to a cerebral oligodendroglioma. Less malignant gliomas are, moreover, often quite radiosensitive.

The "malignancy" of gliomas refers to their surgical inaccessibility and rapidity of growth rather than, as with other cancers, to a tendency to metastasize to other parts of the body. Other brain tumors, especially those arising outside brain substance, can be cured surgically, and include such common types as meningioma, acoustic neuroma, and tumors arising from the pituitary gland. Even when their location makes total extirpation impossible, subtotal removal may produce symptomatic remission lasting many years.

The symptoms of a brain tumor depend upon location and growth rate. As noted, tumors may present as epileptic seizures without other apparent abnormalities. If the tumor is large enough or critically located, the main symptoms may be those of increased pressure within the cranium, namely headache and vomiting. Depending on its site, a tumor may cause weakness or loss of sensation on one or both sides of the body, visual or hearing disturbance, abnormal gait and coordination, difficulty with swallowing or speech, or perhaps most important, change in mental functioning or personality. A particular feature of brain tumors is their ability to disrupt structurally that organ which is itself the mind. There may be a special disturbance of language (aphasia) in which the ability to speak, to understand spoken speech, or to read and write are impaired, with at least relative preservation of personality or other cognitive processes. The primary problem may be with spatial perception or with memory, or there may be alterations of personality, with mood changes or even psychosis. Loss of mental ability will of course radically alter a patient's reaction to his own illness, depriving him of insight and understanding and isolating him from family and friends. Whether such lack of insight is viewed as merciful depends on one's philosophical view, in any event it makes irrelevant the concept of passing through appropriate emotional stages of terminal illness as, for example, described by Kubler-Ross (1969) in patients with presumably intact intellectual function.

Considerable progress has occurred in the past decade in both the diagnosis and treatment of brain tumors. Computerized tomography, whose inventors won the 1979 Nobel Prize in Physiology and Medicine, is both safer and more accurate than procedures such as angiography or pneumoencephalography, and while it has not entirely replaced these techniques, or, for that matter, diagnostic neurosurgery, the identification of brain tumors today is both faster and safer than in the past.

Treatment of brain tumors includes, variably, surgery, radiotherapy, chemotherapy, and drugs to reduce brain swelling. Brain surgery is understandably terrifying to many, so much so, in fact, that it may be refused even when a tumor is potentially resectable. A woman recently admitted to our hospital with a probable meningioma was fully aware of the consequences of rejecting surgery, yet did so and gradually lapsed into stupor. Her family, respecting her decision, also disallowed surgical intervention, and she eventually died. While neurosurgery is never entirely without hazard, patients and families should recognize that recent advances, including the use of the operating microscope, have substantially reduced risks. For example, the recently developed transphenoidal approach has made surgery on pituitary tumors the treatment of choice in patients who a decade ago would have received only radiotherapy. Modern radiotherapeutic techniques have also become safer and more definitive, and a variety of recently developed chemotherapeutic agents, such as the nitrosoureas and cis-platinum, while still at the experimental stage in larger medical centers, are considered promising advances. Swelling of brain adjacent to tumors may account for both the non-specific symptoms of increased intracranial pressure and the more specific symptoms (e.g., weakness) of local brain compression; corticosteroid drugs reduce this swelling and may by themselves produce considerable symptomatic remission for extended periods.

The grim prognosis of many brain tumors cannot be denied. Such a diagnosis is not, however, synonymous with early death. Not only are many brain tumors curable, with little or no functional disability, but modern medicine may be on the threshold of treating the more malignant variety with an effectiveness unimaginable only a few years ago.

REFERENCE

Kubler-Ross, E. 1969. *On Death and Dying.* New York: Macmillan Co., Inc.

EXPERIENCES WITH CANCER PATIENTS IN PSYCHOANALYSIS

Selwyn Brody

Cancer is a powerful force mobilizing the will to live. The threat of death appears to heighten the challenge for survival and awakens the life-creative drive and the joy of expression. The struggle between eros, or life-drive, and thanatos, or death-wish, is never more dramatically staged than in the psychoanalysis of the cancer patient. Self-reparative and survival mechanisms may prevail over despair and death. The author has observed the determination of cancer patients who have used psychoanalysis to change self-destructive patterns and arrest cancer growth. One exceptional patient with Hodgkin's disease who refused chemo- and radiotherapy and relied exclusively on psychoanalysis is now in her eighth year of complete remission. She may represent a rare instance of spontaneous regression. Other patients have come for analysis after surgery or during the course of radiation and chemotherapy. They all rejected the current concept of "dying with dignity."

Although extreme skepticism prevails against the acceptance of emotions in the "most organic of all organic diseases," emotional factors have been linked to cancer for centuries and more studies continue to appear on the subject. According to Lipowski's overview (1977), several articles on emotional factors in cancer are described, but there is no reference to psychotherapy as a treatment modality. Evidence of stress-induced tumors in laboratory mice has been demonstrated, yet scientific proof for similar factors causative of cancer in humans seems unlikely to be presented in the foreseeable future. Despite the priority accorded tangible carcinogenic entities, current screening projects also include the psychological in their research for predictive factors. Long-range psychosocial studies on medical school freshmen have been correlated with their state of health twenty-five years later. One such survey revealed that those who developed cancer had given a history of family alienation (Thomas and Greenstreet, 1973).

Emotions are in the mainstream of the vast research on brain function. The major psychoses, moods, memories, affects, impulses, dreams, fantasies and even thoughts are associated with biochemical processes. Emotions are no longer regarded as unreal abstractions. Psychic experiences appear to coincide with real neural events at the synaptic junctions. Researchers promise exciting new discoveries in the accelerating field of neurotransmission and neuroinhibition (Chester, 1977). We may hope for a demonstrable informational link between inhibited destructive impulses and the site of malignant transformation at the cellular level.

Impressed by a remarkable interplay between physical symptoms and psychosis, the author was drawn to the psychoanalysis of cancer patients from earlier studies on organic disease. Among the patients observed, not one who developed a psychosis died of the disease and not one who died sustained a psychosis. It appeared that psychosis had had a therapeutic effect which could be life-preservative and which served a survival function by preventing a fatal outcome (Brody, 1956).

Clinical and psychological studies revealed that the personalities of such patients were dominated by the need to control impulses to act destructively against others. Their behavior was evidently based on the fear that they would not be loved unless they concealed and internalized their destructive impulses. It is believed that the child's constitution or parent's personality interfered with the healthy discharge of natural aggressive impulses and forced the use of internally directed self-destructive forms of tension release. The mechanism of turning aggression inward against the self accounted for the striking clinical impression that these patients were actually destroying themselves. Menninger (1938) described organic disease as unconscious suicide. Confirming the observation that psychosis and physical symptoms are interrelated is the statistical finding of lower cancer incidence in hospitalized psychotics. The Mid-Manhattan survey of 1954-1974 also found lower cancer mortality in the nonhospitalized mentally disturbed population (Singer et al., 1977).

The importance of the interface between psychosis and physical disease has gained wider recognition. The obverse of cancer as a defense against psychosis exists in the reported remissions of schizophrenia when physical disease supervenes (Lipper and Werman, 1977). This is referred to as "pathocure" by Fenichel. In "Group Therapy of Terminally Ill Patients," Yalom states, "Cancer cures psychoneurosis" (Yalom and Greaves, 1977).

Three decades of studying the factors in psychosomatic organic disease and cancer supported this author's conviction that there are emotional factors in the etiology and course of these disease states (Brody, 1952; 1957; 1959; 1961a). Clinical experiences with patients who have benefited from psychoanalysis have reinforced my belief in the effectiveness of modern psychoanalysis with apparently "too late" disorders. Trying to prove the existence of emotional factors in cancer etiology may be an exercise in futility, for in contemporary medicine the emphasis on "risk factors" is more pragmatic. Therefore, I am suggesting a "Type C" person may offer a step toward lowering the mortality rate of our society's number two killer.

Beneath the known reluctance of cancer patients to express anger is found a massive repression and denial of destructive impulses. Secret suicidal and murderous wishes emerge in treatment. Resistance to this recognition may explain the reluctance of many cancer patients to accept psychiatric referral (Simonton and Simonton, 1974).

Historically important to a psychoanalytic study of cancer is Freud's compelling analysis of aggression in society. In *Civilization and Its Discontents*, written when he himself was afflicted with cancer, he contended that the aggressive instinct constitutes the chief impediment to civilization. He added, "What a potent obstacle to civilization aggressiveness must be, if the defense against it can cause as much unhappiness as aggression itself." This defense basically consists of the biblical command "Thou shalt love thy neighbor as thyself." Freud believed this to be a "psychological mistake" we do not admit at all. The "mistake" includes the cultural assumption that man's ego is capable of anything that is required of it or has "unlimited mastery over his id."

In our culture, although many individuals thrive on competition, the competitive pressure is an alleged component in the Type A personalities prone to fatal coronary attacks. The popular slogan, "winning isn't everything, winning is the only thing," may be a potential social stress capable of inducing cancer in susceptible individuals, the "Type C" person noted above.

Stress-inducing relationships are also expressed in the popular idiom of one person's being "allergic" to another, or one person's being a "pain" to another, and there are those who give ulcers and those who get ulcers. It appears that this folk wisdom may also apply to cancer. Spitz's term "psychotoxic mother" describes a destructive relationship, with psychosomatic disturbances in infants. Undoubtedly there can be psychotoxic effects in any human relationship (including the iatrogenic). Psychotherapy of groups, families, and marital couples may reveal mental disturbances as well as occurrences of cancer (Brody, 1961b).

The author has found a useful working hypothesis in correlating the physical laws of thermodynamics to the psychodynamics of mental equilibrium. The cancer patient's attempt to preserve his pseudo-orderly mental control is maintained by the simultaneous discharge of destructive energy into the disorderly chaos of cancer. With pathological social conformity man can no more defy the laws of thermodynamics than he can the laws of gravity.

Case Report

Miss D. is an attractive lady of twenty-five. She was referred to me for serious personal problems and reported that she had been unable to talk to her previous analyst. Taking such failure in communication as a cue, I facilitated the patient's talking freely, and a positive working relationship was effected.

During one of the summer breaks from therapy, the patient was found to have Hodgkin's disease involving the neck and abdominal lymph glands. With access to medical literature, the patient made a study of the chemotherapy being offered her and decided to refuse it. She was particularly afraid of the debilitating side effects. In spite of my warnings against a delay in appropriate treatment of her disease, she insisted that we proceed with psychoanalysis and requested a stepped up schedule, ignoring the recommendations of her oncologist. After agreeing that it might be irrational to embark on unconventional treatment, she launched into a furious attack on me for my cautious approach and defensiveness. A full-blown negative transference emerged rapidly and dominated the analysis for several months.

At times the intensity and content were characteristic of a psychotic transference. More remarkable was the observation that whenever the patient freely expressed her negative feelings, her physical symptoms were relieved. She blamed me for taking a summer vacation without having adequately helped her work through her separation anxieties, which she claimed had caused her the traumatic stress that induced the Hodgkin's disease.

An alternating cycle in the clinical picture became manifest. Physical symptoms cleared when she released negative emotions. They tended to recur when she resumed a more reasonable posture or reverted to silence. When the patient's Hodgkin's symptoms reappeared with fever, malaise, and painful abdominal glands, my negative suggestion helped her overcome her resistance against release of her tension. I would remind her that analytic treatment was obviously a mistake and that she should permit chemotherapy. I would go so far as to tell her she was obviously dying. These negative interventions consistently helped the patient to discharge aggressive attacks on me. During one silent session, I sensed the angry tension in her and said, "You make me feel as if you want to kill me." She angrily screamed, "You must be a paranoiac," and other hostile criticisms.

Gradually, the patient's periods of physical improvement became more prolonged. She never missed a day of work and requested extra analytic sessions, including some on week-ends. Even in winter's worst blizzards, she would get to my suburban office more promptly than I did.

In addition to her negative transference the patient also communicated other areas of her life story. She clarified her tension states, which she connected with allergies, separation syndrome and even mononucleosis. She had contracted the latter while away at college and called it a "homesick disease." She explained that when she "clammed up" into tense silences, "I get myself in an uptight tension and hate it; but I'm afraid of releasing it? it is like losing part of me and losing control of myself. I'm afraid anyone I let go at, even you, would get back at me." She found it painful to reveal compulsive anal masturbation and fantasies. The pleasurable release was followed by unbearable tension, shame, and guilt. She also recalled recurrent childhood nightmares in which she saw herself about to die. When she would awake terrified, screaming for her mother's reassurance and asking, "Am I going to die?", the mother's reply was, "I don't know for sure if you're going to die or not." She feels she failed to make her mother and father happy from the time she was born. "What has always made my unhappy and brings my cancer back is my upsetting you. I'd like to enjoy upsetting you, without its giving me cancer." She quoted the English analyst Winnicott who believes, "the child has to destroy the object and the object should not oppose or inhibit it or feel threatened at being so used." This is an aspect of Winnicott's concept of the "good enough" parent (1958).

The patient would exclaim, "I have to cure my mother and you of your hangups." Actually, the mother was antagonistic to the patient's psychological treatment and as she went into a remission, her mother contracted cancer and was dead in a few months.

The patient discontinued treatment approximately two and one-half years after the onset of her disease. Follow-up after ten years indicates she is still in remission. The dramatic remission of Hodgkin's disease without the use of standard medical procedures is exceptional and may represent a rare case of spontaneous regression. The psychoanalysis, with its striking sequence of negative transference states, may be a secondary or coincidental effect of a recovery based on a self-reparative process.

Case Report

Mrs. M. is a 60-year-old woman with cancer of the breast and suspected metastases to the bones of the lower extremities. She had been in and out of psychoanalysis and group therapy chiefly to maintain her defenses against a psychotic breakdown. An acute stress in her life was her elder child's sudden fame in the entertainment field. She had a hostile symbiosis with this child which had begun before her birth when the pregnancy was marked by serious threat of miscarriage. She had had her first consultation with me nearly 20 years previously because of several miscarriages in an attempt to have a second child.

With the diagnosis of cancer, the patient's defense of "continual denial" (Yalom and Greaves, 1977) failed and she returned to treatment as much for anxiety over a threatened breakdown as for a magic cure of her cancer. Although massive defenses of denial and flight of her pre-cancer analysis were again exhibited, the presence of her cancer forced her to remain in treatment and to deal with the painful resolution of her defenses.

An extremely complex and confusing negative transference emerged as a stubborn resistance to communicating words or feelings. Her expressionless, tense, facial appearance accompanied a monotonous, lifeless voice. The patient gave a history of terrifying parental strife and admitted that her mother had probably tried to abort her. She recalled fantasies of a happy life with her self as the mother, which became more real to her than the external reality. She also imagined being her favorite elder sister who was thought to be a childhood genius. The patient experienced periods of panic and depersonalization saying, "I don't know who I really am, myself or my sister." Enjoying the success of her daughter is complicated by her fear of loss of her own identity. The sister had an emotional breakdown in adolescence, becoming seclusive and severely hypochondriacal. She died at age 40 from a lung cancer.

The patient was determined to have a normal life with marriage and children, despite her serious emotional problems. She also abandoned a career in the entertainment and arts world in which apparently she could have become a star performer. Her facade of normality did not entirely conceal bitterness and hostility from her family, who could not discuss this with her at all.

Progress gradually became more definite as the analyst was able to verbalize consistently the hopelessness and hatred induced in him. This "feedback" of extreme verbal interventions enabled the patient slowly to loosen her resistances. She was able to verbalize profound negative narcissistic transference material. She brought out how automatically she blocked and turned off feelings and said, "I find myself clamming up as I talk to you." It clarified why she had rejected therapy so intensely (Brody, 1964). In the past, any success experience or positive feelings in the treatment usually meant emotional or physical flight from the treatment. She said from her childhood on she believed herself to be nothing and believed her therapist to be nothing also. She explained, "I don't have to feel like killing you off or get rid of you because I never let you enter my mind." She did this with her hated father also. She complained, "You aren't real, you don't ever reach me, because I don't let you."

In addition to progress in expressing feelings in words, the patient began to cooperate with reconstruction of her early history and her complicated mental life. Typical of many cancer patients was her extreme shame in revealing family problems to outsiders. The patient expressed the belief that the analysis has achieved continuity, and she was determined to maintain interest in discovering her real self. She stated, "I begrudge telling you, but this treatment is working a little. I am bringing out my terrific negativism, as you've reached my diabolical streak against anything ever working."

Patient and analyst have worked toward the goal of bringing life to the analysis, which appears to be helping the patient recover her health and arrest her malignancy. She has received anti-cancer therapy and although we are aware of the dangers of unwarranted optimism, the patient has gained in physical strength. She is more active in family and social responsibilities and plans a limited return to her artistic career.

DISCUSSION AND CONCLUSIONS

This paper is a preliminary study on psychoanalytic experiences with cancer patients. In the literature there is but scanty reference to psychiatric treatment. Cole and Everson, authors of "Spontaneous Regression of Cancer" (1966), who are surgeons, believe that the remote possibility of spontaneous regression may be of therapeutic value in the cancer patient who is not amenable to surgery, chemotherapy, or radiation therapy. but they warn that it would be foolish to reject orthodox methods in the hope for the extremely rare spontaneous regression.

This paper emphasizes the paradoxical life preservative impact of cancer and the critical role of repressed destructive forces in etiology and treatment in certain patients. One aspect of the aggressive instinct and the defense against it consists of a reciprocal connection between cancer and psychosis. Cancer, commonly regarded as "the most organic of all organic diseases," may actually be the outlet for most violent and negative emotions.

It is important to understand that the problem of aggressive impulses originating in the earliest phases of infancy is distinguished from aggression in milder emotional disorders. Glover (1956) assumes a primitive functional phase of the mental apparatus that is concerned almost entirely with regulating excitations and discharge. He maintains this is the period of original psychic and traumatic stress, when the rudiments for psychosomatic disorders are formed. The defenses involved in "damming up" excitations and blocking perceptions are pre-ego and pre-verbal mechanisms, which precede mental content and conflict. These formulations make the onset of cancer following the stress of object loss more comprehensible. The traumatic period of early infancy parallels the period known as primary narcissism and in modern psychoanalysis the conception of narcissistic transference experienced with such patients has become a cornerstone of treatment.

The author suggests that using the label "Type C" for the cancer personality may help to identify and treat such people. Obviously, such typing is not proposed with absolute or dogmatic intent. The massive defenses against destructive impulses in those predisposed to cancer appear to constitute a serious risk factor. Patients and students over several years have consistently conveyed the idea that keeping their communication channels open, particularly for negative emotions, has made them more confident of physical health, including greater immunity to cancer. However, reminders that cancer may strike anyone, anytime, are frequently expressed.

An authority (Kernberg, 1973) on pathologic narcissism, who avoids the subject of organic disease, recommends preventive analysis for narcissistic disorders to avoid psychiatric disturbances when the prime of life has passed. Optimistic researchers prophesy a serum or vaccine for leukemia and other cancers by perhaps 2000 A.D. In the meantime, preventive radiation treatment or chemotherapy are not feasible. The Mayo Clinic's lung project acknowledged little success in persuading men of 45, the highest risk age, to cut down smoking (Mayo, 1976). Many cigarette smokers say they could only stop smoking once the diagnosis of cancer was made. Other therapy-rejecting smokers reveal that when they do stop smoking, they experience a "psychotic madness" of unbearable hatred for everybody and themselves.

Case material presented suggests that a real negative transference including transference psychosis is associated with arrest of cancer. In one case of Hodgkin's disease a complete remission occurred without orthodox medical therapy. Other patients with less intense negative transference are maintaining their physical strength and well-being. Prognosis must always be guarded with cancer patients. Patients who succumbed to the disease did not bring out destructive impulses through negative transference.

Extreme verbal communications are necessary from the analyst to help loosen the patient's deadly resistances. When Freud stated that transference was a decisive factor in all medical influence, he meant positive elements. Other positive transference forces of belief, suggestion, magic, faith, and even transference of energy are no longer heretic subjects in official scientific psychiatry. Panels on mysticism at the annual American Psychiatric Association meetings have been more popular than sex therapy programs (Dean, 1977). At this preliminary point, it appears justifiable to state that communicating a negative transference may be a life-preserving mechanism.

If verbalization can be an effective therapeutic vehicle for externalizing aggressive emotions in the cancer-prone personality, the term "communication disease" ought to apply to cancer. Organic symptoms or "organ language" can be considered forms of communication resistance to change. Consequently, if transference is a decisive factor in medical influence, then medical resistance to cure may be equally decided by the psychologic resistance to negative transference.

This report indicates that radical verbal interventions may contribute a powerful influence to the reversibility process of cancer patients when their negative transference was fully expressed.

REFERENCES

Brody, S. 1952. "Psychological Observations in Patients Treated with Cortisone and ACTH." *Psychosomatic Medicine*, 14:94.

———. 1956. "Psychological Factors Associated with Disseminated Lupus Erythematosus and Effects of Cortisone and ACTH." *Psychiatric Quarterly*, 30:44.

———. 1957. "Psychophysiological Factors in the Collagen Diseases." *Psychoanalysis*, 5:71.

———. 1959. "Value of Group Psychotherapy in Patients with 'Polysurgery Addiction.'" *Psychiatric Quarterly*, 33:260 (April).

———. 1961. "Simultaneous Psychotherapy of Married Couples." *Psychoanalytic Review*, 48.

———. 1961a. "Effect of Steroids on Mental Processes and Their Treatment." In Mills and Noyer (eds.), *Inflammation and Diseases of Connective Tissues*, Philadelphia: W.B. Saunders Co.

———. 1964. "Syndrome of the Treatment Rejecting Patient." *Psychoanalytic Review*, 51:243.

Cole, W.H. and T.C. Everson. 1966. *Spontaneous Regression and Cancer*. Philadelphia: W.B. Saunders Co.

Dean, S.R. 1977. "A Quest for Purpose in Psychic Research." *Psychiatric Opinion*, 14:2, 17.

Glover, E. 1956. *Functional Aspects of the Mental Apparatus on the Early Development of Mind*. New York: International Universities Press.

Kernberg, O. 1973. "Technique. Prognosis in the Treatment of Narcissistic Disorders." *Journal of the American Psychoanalytic Association*, 21:617.

Lester, H.A. 1977. "The Response to Acetylcholine." *Scientific American*, 236:106 (February).

Lipowski, Z.J. 1977. "Psychosomatic Medicine in the Seventies. An Overview." *American Journal of Psychiatry*, 134:233-245.

Lipper, S. and D.S. Werman. 1977. "Schizophrenia. Intercurrent Physical Illness." *Comprehensive Psychiatry,* 18:11-22.

Mayo Lung Cancer Project. 1976. *Clinical Notes on Respiratory Diseases,* 15:13.

Singer, Garfinkel et al. 1977. "Mortality and Mental Health. Evidence from the Midtown Manhattan Restudy." *Psychiatric Spectator* (Sandoz), Vol. X, No. 11.

Simonton, C.C. and S. Simonton. 1974. "Belief Systems and Management of the Emotional Aspects of Malignancy." Department of Health, State of Florida.

Thomas, C.B. and R. Greenstreet. 1973. "Psychobiological Characteristics in Youth as Predictors of Five Disease States: Suicide, Mental Illness, Hypertension, Coronary Heart Disease and Tumor." *Johns Hopkins Medical Journal,* 132:16-43.

Yalom, I.D. and C. Greaves. 1977. "Group Therapy with the Terminally Ill." *American Journal of Psychiatry,* 134:401.

THE EFFECTS OF RADIATION THERAPY UPON PSYCHOLOGICAL AND BEHAVIORAL FUNCTIONING: A LITERATURE REVIEW

Gene Kopelson

A PRELIMINARY STUDY

Although patients receiving radiotherapy often have underlying psychological disturbances that may contribute to the formation of or are due to their malignant disease, it is certainly true that psychobehavioral functioning can change during or after the course of radiation treatments. It is difficult to distinguish which changes are due to the natural history of the disease process, the single or synergistic effects of the various modalities of therapy (radiation, surgery, chemotherapy, immunotherapy), or the fact that the patient is being placed in the milieu of radiation treatment (with the concomitant experiences of sitting in a waiting room of patients with varying stages of malignant diseases, seeing the large therapy machines, being evaluated and followed by physicians, being set-up by technicians, and finally being treated by invisible radiation beams). This paper will attempt to review what is known about the direct effects of radiation therapy on psychobehavioral functioning in man.

Although the neurological changes produced by radiotherapy are fairly well-known, there is only scant clinical data available about the effects of ionizing radiation on psychobehavioral functions. This information may be divided into reports dealing with radiation applied to three distinct anatomic locations: whole- or half-body irradiation which includes the brain, radiotherapy localized specifically to only the head and central-nervous-system, and radiation delivered to non-central-nervous-system parts of the body.

WHOLE- OR HALF-BODY IRRADIATION

The oldest relevant study in this area dealt with an unspecified number of adult males with advanced neoplastic disease of unspecified types who were given three standardized U.S. Air Force complex coordination tests both before and at 1, 3, 5, 7, 9, and 11 hours after a course of whole body irradiation (varying from 15-50r measured at the midplane via one exposure or five equal fractions at hourly intervals by a 400kv generator; alternating lateral opposed fields were used (Payne, 1959). A continuation of this study used similar patients and treatments, but the doses were increased in some patients to as high as 200 r via 25r increments; and those patients receiving a dose greater than 75r were treated with a 250kv unit. Posttreatment testing was increased to a 9-day follow-up after the therapy in this group also.

When the results from both groups of patients were analyzed, the only statistically significant finding ($p < .01$) was that in one of the three tests used, the higher the dose rate, the greater was the decrement in that patient's performance over the 9-day follow-up. The author attributed this to the fact that the patients who received the higher dose did so because of their advanced disease, and this itself may have contributed to their decreased performance. The basic conclusion of the author was that radiation had no effect on the observed psychomotor functioning.

The only other reported study of this type (Gottschalk et al., 1969) evaluated 16 patients with metastatic solid tumors (plus good nutrition, normal renal function, and stable hemogram) who received palliative partial- or total-body irradiation (50-300r via ^{60}Co teletherapy via two lateral opposed ports). They were evaluated for several complex psychological variables, including cognitive and intellectual impairment, hope, hostility, and anxiety. In addition they were given the Halstead Battery (a test of complex sensorimotor abilities), the Wechsler-Bellevue Adult Intelligence Scale, and several others. After this testing, the patients were sham-irradiated (both for treatment planning and experimental control purposes). The tests were repeated after the sham irradiation, before and immediately after the actual irradiation, and at days No. 1 and 3 plus weeks No. 1, 2, 4, and 6 post-radiotherapy.

Analysis of the resultant data revealed that there was statistically significant ($p \leq .02$) evidence of transient impairment of intellectual functioning appearing immediately after the actual irradiation and lasting for one day. However, this result was obtained only with one of the tests used; the other tests delivered to measure the same functioning did not show these results; and the fact that there was no statistically significant difference between sham and actual radiation results, nor between pre-sham and post-sham irradiation, casts doubt upon the importance of the first result. The authors had insufficient data to determine whether upper-body or lower-body irradiation yielded differing psychological results. They concluded that it was best to be conservative and to accept the probability that radiation could temporarily interfere with intellectual processes in some individuals.

CENTRAL-NERVOUS-SYSTEM IRRADIATION

Whereas the previously-discussed studies were short-term in nature, the literature dealing with irradiation to the head is a series of long-term follow-up studies of patients treated for tinea capitis, leukemia, and brain tumors.

More than 2000 patients treated for tinea capitis, a benign skin infection, by irradiation (the scalp was exposed to 5 fields via 75-100 keV to a total dose of 300-400r with the brain receiving 175r at the surface and 70r at the base) were evaluated 15 and 20 years after the radiotherapy; they were compared for the incidence and type of psychological problems that developed in a similar group of non-irradiated tinea capitis patients (Albert et al., 1968; Shore, 1976).

The 15-year follow-up study (Albert et al., 1968) found a statistically significant higher incidence of various disorders in the irradiated group: 2.5-times (65 cases) as many mental disorders overall ($p<.01$), 4.5-times (19 cases) as many personality disorders ($p < .05$), 3-times (25 cases) as many psychoneurotic disorders ($p<.05$), but a non-statistically significant 1.6-times (21 cases) higher incidence of psychotic disorders.

The incidence of overall mental illness was higher in the irradiated group regardless of sex or race; the greatest contrast was in white females in regard to psychoneuroses and in black males in personality disorders. Of the psychoses reported for both the irradiated and nonirradiated groups, though all cases were schizophrenia, the former group had a higher percentage of paranoid schizophrenia. The average age at diagnosis of the psychoneuroses and psychoses in both groups was 20 years, and this was 12 years after treatment. In the personality disorders, the age at diagnosis was 18 years, and only eight years had passed since treatment.

In both groups, roughly half finished high school and a third entered college. The stability of marital relationships was also similar in both groups.

Interestingly, the 20-year follow-up study (Shore et al., 1976) found an increase in the incidence of mental illness in both the irradiated and nonirradiated groups, but that the relative difference had now diminished and was so small as to be statistically insignificant, with the new finding that whites had inexplicably consistently higher rates for each category (neurosis, psychosis, and personality disorder) than did blacks.

Recent work has also evaluated 30 children with intracranial tumors who survived at least five years after unspecified doses of radiation. They were examined retrospectively to assess intellectual functioning, emotional, and social problems (Bamford et al., 1976). As evaluated by a history of educational attainment and by giving the Revised Stanford-Binet test, 57 percent were classified as from below average to subnormal. Significant emotional problems occurred in 43 percent of the group, with two suicide attempts and many having difficulty relating to peers.

The authors felt that these effects, unlikely to be due to the tumor, were due to either radiation endarteritis or the anxieties produced in the parents and children because of the disease and its treatment, with resultant pathologic overprotectiveness of the child by the parents. The authors suggest that growth hormonal deficiencies owing to scatter irradiation of the hypothalamic-pituitary axis could lead to a plateauing in mental development; the authors are investigating this possible radiation-induced effect further.

Leukemic children are given prophylactic treatment, often consisting of craniospinal irradiation or cranial radiotherapy plus chemotherapy. Two retrospective and one prospective studies have attempted to determine the long-term psychologic consequences of this radiation treatment.

In one tetrospective study (Soni et al., 1975), of 11 patients receiving prophylactic craniospinal irradiation (2400r via ^{60}Co) and chemotherapy, there were no neuropsychiatric differences when compared to a control group which received the drugs only; the comparison was made after a 4-year follow-up. Tests included the Stanford-Binet, the Wechsler Intelligence Scale, and various perceptual and visual-motor tests.

A similar study (Verzosa et al., 1976) examined retrospectively 22 patients with Acute Lymphoblastic Leukemia who received cranial irradiation (2400r via ^{60}Co) with chemotherapy. Five years after the treatment with the radiation, these patients were judged by their school-teachers to be on levels similar to their peers; in addition, neurological examinations were all perfectly normal.

Prospectively, 34 patients with leukemia who received either cranial irradiation with chemotherapy or craniospinal radiotherapy alone (2400r via ^{60}Co in either case) were compared to 27 controls who received noncranial irradiation (Soni et al., 1975). After 18 months, there were no neuropsychologic differences between the two groups except that the group which received the cranial irradiation scored questionably better on the Johns Hopkins perceptual test yet at the same time did not improve on the Wechsler Intelligence test as had the control group (see below); the Stanford-Binet results showed no differences between the two groups. The authors tentatively concluded that this particular course of radiotherapy had no as-yet detectable effect on neuropsychiatric functioning.

NON-CENTRAL-NERVOUS-SYSTEM IRRADIATION

The least explored area is how radiotherapy in which the cranium receives zero or negligible radiation affects psychologic functioning.

Already discussed has been the analysis of leukemic children receiving central-nervous-system irradiation as compared to controls with solid tumors or Hodgkin's disease who received non-central-nervous-system irradiation. The control group had a statistically significant ($p < .05$) improvement on the Wechsler test scores compared to the non-improving experimental group (Soni et al., 1975). Unfortunately, no comparison with normal children was made.

A study of 16 stage I and II cervical carcinoma patients treated by intracavitary and external radiotherapy (details of dose not given) and evaluated five years after therapy found that two patients were divorced shortly following treatment after marriages of 5 and 24 years; these were felt to be related to the radiation-induced vaginal stenosis leading to dyspareunia with resultant decreased frequency of intercourse and eventual divorce. Two cases exhibited loss of libido, and 11 of 15 patients who were pre-menopausal before therapy experienced menopause within one year of therapy. The small number of patients without proper controls made definitive conclusions impossible to draw (Vasicka et al., 1958).

The final study to be examined is a 15-year follow-up of more than 2000 patients treated for menorrhagia by ovarian irradiation (Alderson, 1975). Revealed was an incidence of suicide and self-inflicted injury that was 1.4-times the expected incidence ($p \leqslant .223$) with an expected excess of 2.7-times in a larger sample; but these figures do not approach the conventional levels of statistical significance. Most excess deaths from suicide occurred from 10 to 14 years after treatment, and the authors felt that the very latency of this suicide incidence long after treatment argued against a direct radiation effect. However, this could indeed be a radiation effect whose psychiatric manifestations took many years to become manifest, as do many personality qualities in individuals.

DISCUSSION

The short-term results of whole- or partial-body radiotherapy gave equivocal evidence of a transient decrease of intellectual functioning in only one of several tests employed and a questionable loss of performance at higher doses using different criteria. The doubtfulness of the statistical validity of the former coupled with the fact that the latter result can be explained since only the more advanced cases received the higher doses leads one to conclude that very minimal effects, if any, exist in this situation which depend upon the test parameter used.

Irradiation to the head and brain has produced varying results. Patients with tinea capitis treated by radiotherapy showed a higher incidence of mental disease in general, and of personality disorders and neuroses in particular, compared with nonirradiated controls when examined after 15 years; the results also seemed to be dependent upon race and sex. However, a longer follow-up period negated the comparatively higher incidence of mental disease after radiotherapy and found just a higher incidence of mental disease in whites of both groups. The study of residual problems in brain tumor patients after radiation treatment makes it difficult to sort out the contributions of skewed interpersonal relationships, and their consequences once the diagnosis of cancer is made, from the direct effects of radiotherapy. The authors suggest a possible radiation-induced hormonal deficiency might be the cause of the observed high incidence of poor educational attainment, difficulty with peers, and suicide. The various long-term studies of leukemic children receiving cranial irradiation conclude that, at the five-year level, there are no detectable adverse effects.

Finally, the finding of a higher-than-expected incidence of suicide after ovarian irradiation is questionable because of its lack of statistical significance.

Thus, the few clinical studies related to the topic under consideration have found few, if any, known acute or chronic effects of radiation upon psychobehavioral functioning; those questionable results could be explained by other factors such as extent of disease or the home environment and parental overprotection. Certainly, further clinical trials are warranted to answer such questions as: what are the long-term effects of whole- or partial-body irradiation? Can hormonal disturbances due to radiotherapy account for mental changes after cranial irradiation for brain tumors? What are the synergistic effects of surgery and/or chemotherapy and/or radiotherapy and/or immunotherapy upon psychobehavioral functioning? And can any of the resultant observed effects be prevented? And if these studies, plus longer follow-up studies of those studies discussed here, do demonstrate an important effect of radiation upon psychological and behavioral functioning, then a re-evaluation of current radiotherapeutic techniques would be indicated in an attempt to prevent or minimize, if possible, such long-range sequelae.

REFERENCES

Albert, R.E. and A.R. Omram. 1968. "Follow-up Study of Patients Treated by X-ray Epilation for Tinea Capitis. I. Population Characteristics, Posttreatment Illnesses, and Mortality Experiences." *Archives of Environmental Health*, 17:899-918.

Alderson, M. 1975. "Psychiatric Illness after Ovarian Irradiation." *Lancet*, 1:401.

Bamford, F.N. et al. 1976. "Residual Disabilities in Children Treated for Intracranial Space-Occupying Lesions." *Cancer*, 37:1149-1151.

Gottschalk, L.A. et al. 1969. "Total and Half Body Irradiation. Effect on Cognitive and Emotional Processes." *Archives of General Psychiatry*, 21:574-580.

Payne, R.E. et al. 1959. "Effects of Ionizing Radiation on Human Psychomotor Skills." *United States Armed Forces Medical Journal*, 10:1009-1021.

Shore, R.E. et al. 1976. "Follow-up Study of Patients Treated by X-ray Epilation for Tinea Capitis. Resurvey of Posttreatment Illness and Mortality Experience." *Archives of Environmental Health*, 31:17-24.

Soni, E.S. et al. 1975. "Effects of Central-Nervous-System Irradiation on Neuropsychologic Functioning of Children with Acute Lymphocytic Leukemia." *New England Journal of Medicine*, 293:113-118.

Vasicka, A. et al. 1958. "Postradiation Course of Patients with Cervical Carcinoma. A Clinical Study of Psychic, Sexual, and Physical Well-being of Sixteen Patients." *Obstetrics and Gynecology*, 11:403-414.

Verzosa, M.S. et al. 1976. "Five Years After Central Nervous System Irradiation of Children with Leukemia." *International Journal of Radiation Oncology and Biological Physiology*, 1:209-215.

PALLIATIVE RADIOTHERAPY IN THE PATIENT WITH INCURABLE CANCER

Antonio Bosch and William L. Caldwell

> *To cure sometimes*
> *To relieve often*
> *To comfort and support always.*
>
> Trudeau

Over sixty percent of all patients with cancer will receive radiation therapy at some time in the course of the disease. The primary function of radiotherapy in the treatment of malignant diseases is cure, and modern radiotherapy, properly practiced, can make as great a contribution as surgery in the treatment of many types of cancer. Furthermore, techniques using a radical dosage with curative intent almost invariably provide some palliation, even if treatment fails to cure. Yet in spite of the advances made in the treatment of cancer by surgery and radiotherapy, there remain a large number of cases to whom the physician can offer only relief of symptoms but no hope of cure. The radiotherapist must deal with this ever-increasing number of patients.

Patients seen in a radiotherapy department include those with advanced, incurable neoplasms and those with metastatic and/or recurrent disease who require palliative treatment. Palliation in such cases is not a matter of giving a sufficiently high dose to destroy every tumor cell present, but a dose that will arrest tumor growth and cause clinical regression in a short time. Distressing symptoms such as pain, obstruction, hemorrhage, and others will be relieved with minimal damage caused to surrounding normal tissues and vital organs.

Certain basic principles concerning palliative radiation therapy must be applied: the relief of the main symptom should occur early during the treatment; the disturbance caused by the treatment should be minimal and serious side effects or complications of treatment not be acceptable; the duration of the palliative treatment and stay in the hospital, if needed, should be short; the convenience of treatment should be a major consideration, offering more than other palliative measures; and a painful existence should not be prolonged.

The first and most important thing to realize is that prolongation of life in the presence of unrelieved pain or major distressing symptoms is not palliation, and overtreatment in the last stages of the disease is frequently a disservice to the patient with cancer. The appropriate use of sedatives and narcotics may provide more palliation than aggressive, active therapy.

When palliation is considered, it is important to look at the situation from the point of view of the patient and to evaluate carefully what the palliative treatment might do for his mental as well as physical distress. Radiotherapy should be considered helpful only if, subsequent to treatment, the patient is likely to be aware that he has been benefited. Palliative treatment of the patient with incurable cancer must be directed only to the relief of specific distressing symptoms caused by or associated with the disease.

Pain is usually the most important and distressing symptom for the patient with advanced incurable cancer and may completely disrupt the life of an otherwise functional person. Metastatic tumor in bone is a frequent source of pain, and there are few cases which cannot be relieved by suitable irradiation. If only one or a few sites are involved, local irradiation is the best treatment available, and modest doses delivered in a limited number of fractions in a short time will usually produce rapid and complete relief in at least 80 percent of patients. In rare instances when the metastasis is from a well differentiated cancer such as carcinoma of the gastrointestinal tract, pancreas, cervix, or endometrium, the response may be poor with modest doses, and slightly higher doses may be needed in patients whose life expectancy is good. In patients with extensive disease, the use of higher doses of irradiation to local sites is rarely preferable to neurosurgical measures designed to relieve pain, such as nerve block or cordotomy, which in skilled hands is simple and, when successful, is lasting in its effect. If multiple sites of skeletal involvement are present, the use of irradiation as a palliative measure reaches practical limitations, unless newly developed techniques of single, high-dose, half-body irradiation are used.

When pain is produced by direct involvement of peripheral nerves, as in the case of carcinoma of the rectum or cervix uteri infiltrating the sacral plexus, or extension into the pterygoid fossa in patients with advanced tumors of the head and neck, or involvement of cranial nerves from carcinoma of the nasopharynx, the nature of prior therapy and the general status of the patient influence the approach to palliation. Radiotherapy may be beneficial in certain relatively favorable cases, but in many patients other methods of obtaining rapid pain relief are preferable. Frequently, neurological methods, such as alcohol nerve block, phenol intrathecal injection, root sections, cordotomy, or Gasserian ganglion section are required.

Obstruction of the lumen of the organ is also a frequent cause of severe distress for patients with advanced cancer. Malignant tumors infiltrating the mediastinum may cause compression of the trachea, esophagus or large vessels producing distressing symptoms that can usually be relieved by properly conducted irradiation techniques. Bronchial obstruction with secondary pulmonary atelectasis produced by advanced carcinoma of the lung is frequently palliated by short courses of irradiation that relieve the bronchial obstruction.

The treatment of intestinal tract obstruction varies with the specific anatomical sites involved by the tumor. Intrinsic lesions obstructing the intestinal tract are rarely amenable to radiation treatment, and palliation is frequently best obtained by surgical resection, bypass or intubation. One significant exception is carcinoma of the esophagus. In carcinoma of the esophagus, where by any treatment modality only five percent of the patients survive more than five years, palliative irradiation often is indicated in order to relieve the mechanical obstruction caused by the tumor mass protruding into the esophageal lumen. Establishment of a nearly normal esophageal passage is accomplished with simple techniques of moderate dose irradiation in over 50 percent of the patients, without side effects or complications.

Uretal obstruction is always a grave prognostic sign and is the most common cause of death in patients with advanced or recurrent carcinoma of the cervix uteri; the majority of patients with ureteral obstruction die of uremia, which is Nature's way of putting an end to their pain and suffering. Palliative pelvic irradiation may relieve the ureteral obstruction and restore the normal renal function but will be of no benefit to the patient with progressing and uncontrollable carcinoma of the cervix uteri. Uremia is a more comfortable way for patients to end their struggle with their disease, and this course of events should not be prevented by palliative treatment.

Another major distressing symptom in patients with advanced cancer is visible blood loss. This symptom frequently occurs in patients with carcinoma of the uterine corpus and cervix, tumors of the urinary bladder and kidney, tumors of the oral cavity and pharynx, carcinoma of the lung, and metastatic ulcerated tumors in lymph nodes or soft tissues. Owing to its effectiveness and the minimal associated morbidity, local irradiation of these lesions is the treatment of choice, usually using large fractions in a short period of time, which results in a decrease or cessation of the bleeding.

The duration of the treatment course, when palliation is the aim, should be as short as possible, and treatment should seldom exceed two or three weeks. In some cases a single treatment or a few large fractions delivered in one week is usually adequate. Convenience of treatment becomes a major consideration when palliation is the objective, and use of treatment facilities close to the patient's home or family is advisable. This latter recommendation is made with some reservation. As convenient and seemingly compassionate as it may seem to attempt palliation of patients in their home community, *unless* there are well-trained oncologists to impact on their management, patients may suffer needlessly from inappropriate treatment. Great care must be taken not to use radiotherapy indiscriminately for palliation, and judgment must be utilized to determine whether treatment is having a salubrious effect.

When a patient arrives at the end stages of his disease, usually manifested by profound weakness, sometimes unconsciousness, marked loss of weight and failure of function of one or more vital organs, therapy directed to the cancer itself is a disservice to the patient. Management of the patient rather than the disease, always an important consideration, becomes the paramount feature of care.

The prolongation of life for the patient suffering the distressing symptoms of incurable cancer without relief is not palliation; it is merely a prolongation of the process of dying, always painful to the patient, the family and the attending physician.

CARE OF THE PATIENT WHEN THE DISEASE RECURS

A. Daniel Hauser and Richard S. Blacher

Not infrequently, in the care of patients with cancer, the disease will recur. The recurrence may be heralded in one of several ways, the most obvious being when the patient complains of feeling ill. Usually when a patient who has recently had cancer complains of generalized symptoms of not being well, both patient and physician suspect recurrence of the cancer, and it is usual to embark upon a course of investigation objectively to prove recurrence. This can usually be done by x-rays alone, by biopsy, by blood studies, by radioactive scanning techniques, or occasionally by a combination of these modalities. Since these studies are dramatic and represent an active intervention by the physician after a period of more passive observation, it is always quite obvious to the patient and his family that there is a problem which requires care. The patient's anxiety becomes heightened by these studies.

Occasionally, the recurrence is heralded by no change in the patient's state of well-being, but is brought to the attention of the patient by an obvious and easily apparent physical finding which he can see or feel but which he may not be able to interpret correctly. This may be apparent as skin nodules in a patient with breast cancer who has a local recurrence, or as lymphadenopathy in a patient who has lymphosarcoma.

A third possibility is an objective finding which is apparent to the physician but not so to the patient. This could be an asymptomatic nodule in the lung indicative of metastatic carcinoma or the finding of an enlarged nodular liver.

No matter how the recurrence announces itself, it is obviously of key importance to the patient in the course of his disease. It elicits action on the part of the physician and produces anxiety in the patient. What does one tell the patient when it is suspected that his tumor has recurred? It is impossible to pass off as routine the multiple tests, examinations, scans, x-rays and biopsies that the patient will have to undergo. A patient with even a minimum degree of sophistication will realize that all is not well and that the flurry of activity and interest displayed about him is not routine. In the majority of cases it is wisest to tell the patient that there is a problem that may be related to the underlying neoplasm and that steps must be taken to define the nature of the situation. When given the information the patient will usually become anxious and depressed, but we feel that this is preferable to the charade of doing studies and biopsies under the guise of routine follow-up—a charade which will never really be believed by any patient.

In the event of a reasonably proven recurrence, the next decision is whether to share the information with the patient or not. As with the initial diagnosis, this will depend largely on the style of the physician, the patient, and his family.

In some respects the decision to tell a patient about a recurrence is more anxiety provoking than when the original diagnosis is made because of the ominous implications. The question of what to tell the patient has been long debated (Blacher and Winkelstein, 1968), but since it is usual for the patient to receive either radiotherapy or chemotherapy in the event of a recurrence, one may well wonder what other explanation than the truth can be offered to justify an extensive and often uncomfortable treatment. When the patient is not told, he often knows anyway (Peck, 1972), realizing that he would not be treated if indeed he were well. This may well interfere with his communication with his physician and may serve to isolate the patient from the physician, family, and friends. The patient may know that he is being deceived, but, out of embarrassment and fear of contradicting his physician and family, he may refrain from voicing these well placed doubts. Furthermore, because of these inner conflicts, the patient may become angry and may really not have anybody to whom he can tell his troubles. After all, since he has been told by his physician and family that he is well, it would be pathological for him to express his regrets about his real condition to the people around him. What is there to regret when he has just been given a clean bill of health?

On occasion, this problem eventuates in rather fascinating solutions.

> A 55-year-old woman was being treated for recurrent breast cancer with bone metastases. She had considerable bone pain. Her treating doctor, a radiotherapist, told the patient that she had arthritis which was causing her bone pain and, furthermore, that the cobalt therapy she was receiving was for the arthritis. The woman developed hypercalcemia which required that she be seen by an internist. The internist, unaware that she had been told that she had arthritis, told the patient with suitable explanations, that she had metastatic cancer. After a day or two of obvious depression, the patient was able to assimilate these data and then returned to her usual level of good spirits. She continued to be treated by the same internist and radiotherapist until she died of her tumor and to the end, she discussed her disease with the radiotherapist in terms of her arthritis and its treatment, and she discussed her disease with her internist in terms of her cancer and its treatment. As far as could be told, she was able to compartmentalize these two divergent concepts and yet comfortably live with them.

Another problem may arise when such a patient, if successfully deceived, becomes clinically ill with his neoplasm. Thus, a patient, who has an enlarged liver due to cancer, may have a liver biopsy which shows metastatic carcinoma. He may be told by his physician that the biopsy is negative, but as a precaution, he will be given a series of injections to prevent any problems in the future. The patient feels well and perhaps he can accept the explanation at that time. But six months later, he has become sick. He is anorectic; he has lost weight; he is jaundiced. At this time, it is difficult to explain to the patient what is happening. Not infrequently, by dint of massive denial, the patient does not recognize the changes occurring in his body. Somehow, he does not realize that he is losing weight; somehow he does not recognize that he is jaundiced and that his urine is dark. These patients, the deniers, are in a way fortunate and with them, the withholding of information may succeed up to the very end.

A difficult situation involves the treatment of a patient who has been told he does not have cancer when, indeed, he does. It would be most valuable for the physician to know what he has been told in the past before discussing the matter. Often, the revelation of the diagnosis in such circumstances may lead to an emotional storm, with rage at the lack of honesty of his previous, well-meaning doctors and a concern about everything told to him.

In some circumstances, the patient's family will feel that under no condition should the patient be told that he has cancer and especially recurrent cancer. What they are usually saying is that *they* cannot bear the knowledge. It is of utmost importance that the physician have a harmonious relationship with the patient's family since the two mainstays of the patient in his travail are the patient's physician and his family. It is of great importance that they work together so that the patient can have the benefit of their cooperation.

If the physician can convince the family of the advantage of sharing the knowledge with the patient, a good deal of grief may be avoided. Writing in 1769, John Buchan stated, "It may indeed be alleged, that the doctor does not often declare his opinion before the patient. So much the worse. A sensible patient had better hear what the doctor says than learn it from the disconsolate looks, the watery eyes and the broken whispers of those about him. It seldom happens, when the doctor gives an unfavorable opinion, that it can be concealed from the patient. The very embarrassment which the friends and attendants show in disguising what he has said, is generally sufficient to discover the truth."

At times it would be patently unwise to tell the patient that he has a neoplasm which has recurred. This event usually will arise in very old and infirm people who may have organically impaired intellects to begin with. In these cases, it does not serve any purpose to attempt to clarify the exact significance of what is happening. On the other hand, there will arise situations where it is vital that the patient be told the diagnosis at the time of the recurrence. This will occur in situations where the patient has important personal business or political commitments that require planning. While one would like to give the patient all of the information that one can, occasionally this may have to be tempered by a knowledge of the patient's expected reaction to the news. Thus, at times when one feels that the patient could not bear the burden of the news, it will be necessary to withhold the information from him and simply let his various problems sort themselves out as best they can.

REFERENCES

Blacher, R.S. and C. Winkelstein. 1968. "The Initial Contact with the Cancer Patient." *Journal of Mount Sinai Hospital*, XXXV(4):423-428, July/August.

Buchan, J. 1769. *Domestic Medicine*, Edinburgh.

Peck, A. 1972. "Emotional Reactions to Having Cancer." *American Journal of Roentgenology, Radium Therapy and Nuclear Medicine*, CXIV(3), March.

PALLIATION THERAPY

A. Daniel Hauser and Richard S. Blacher

Palliation therapy is meant to indicate treatment which is not in any way intended to cure the patient of the neoplasm, but which is intended either to extend his life or make his life more comfortable. It is often during this period of treatment that the patient makes, if he can, a transition from a sense of feeling cured to an awareness that his disease is incurable and his life is endangered. His hope for a cure now shifts to a hope for a comfortable, pain-free and extended existence.

Palliation makes greater demands on both physician and patient than curative treatment, since what is gained is less, and, therefore, decisions more difficult. Thus, a patient, who would not hesitate to undergo surgical oophorectomy to cure an ovarian lesion, might be reluctant about undergoing such a procedure for bringing about a temporary remission in breast cancer. Interestingly, such procedures are rarely refused since both patient and physician are usually willing to undertake anything that promises improvement.

In carcinoma of the gastrointestinal tract, surgery is utilized to establish or maintain gastrointestinal continuity even though it may be apparent that cure is impossible because of distant metastases. This permits near normal nutrition and alleviates the severe symptoms of intestinal obstruction with its dire complications and outcome. If distant metastases are present at the time of resection, the patient is still doomed to die of his neoplasm, but his death may occur after a variable period of well-being. Usually when this type of surgery is undertaken, the procedure is more conservative than the ordinary cancer operation and is aimed only at maintaining bowel continuity.

Radiotherapy is frequently utilized as a palliative measure in the treatment of the cancer patient. In cancer which is metastatic to bone, radiotherapy in relatively low dose is used to give prompt, albeit often too short-lived, alleviation of pain. At times, in extremely radio-sensitive tumors such as lymphosarcoma, radiotherapy can be used to treat localized tumor masses which are often annoying to the patient and unsightly. While this is in no way curative, it can give great relief to the patient. Radiotherapy to the ovaries can also be used as an alternative to oophorectomy to produce castration in the treatment of breast cancer.

The physician ordering radiotherapy is often not aware of the emotional hazards of such a treatment. The patient is often terrified. The treatment itself is harrowing, and it may stimulate old, frightening idiosyncratic fantasies. The patient is carefully positioned on a table in a thick-walled room, with a massive piece of equipment suspended over him. He is then left alone for an extended period, communicating only via intercom. Not infrequently, patients worry that they are in danger from the heavy machine.

Some patients suffer a great deal from radiation illness, and since this must be explained as a possible complication, patients, in general, worry about it.

Chemotherapy is assuming an ever-increasing place in the treatment of cancer. Although increasingly used as a curative modality, it is used most often in an attempt to prolong life, and make remaining life more pleasant. Unfortunately, the side effects of chemotherapy are often severe and the frequency of temporary remission is not as great as one would desire.

Adrenal steroids can often produce transient relief of symptoms in cancer patients. They may act to relieve pain, and especially in certain lymphomas and leukemias, they may act more specifically against the tumor. They have fewer side effects and are often easier for the patient to take than chemotherapy.

Just as ablative endocrine procedures are used to ameliorate hormone dependent tumors, administration of appropriate hormones are used in the treatment of hormonally responsive tumors, the hormones having the advantage of ease of administration and minimal side effects.

Occasionally, neurosurgical procedures are resorted to in order to relieve the pain produced by neoplasms. This may involve cooling the spinal cord or actually cutting nerves or injecting the nerves or otherwise interrupting spinal cord tracts which conduct painful stimuli from tumorous areas.

During these various attempts at palliation, the patient struggles with his reactions to the recurrence of the disease. A little appreciated, but quite common reaction is one of resentment. This feeling is usually hidden from the staff because the patient needs his medical attendants now, more than ever. His anger is stimulated by the fact that the doctors and nurses are well and he is ill and may die. In addition, there is a sense of disillusionment in his doctor. After all, if his doctor is so good, how has he allowed the illness to recur? The resentment is often evidenced by a sullen withdrawal, mild depression, and irritability. When the patient is reassured that such a response is expected, and more importantly, that it is acceptable to his medical attendants, he is usually greatly relieved.

Drugs to relieve pain often play a great role in the amelioration of the symptoms of cancer. Usually the physician starts with the mildest analgesics and then proceeds to the more potent analgesics. The necessity for pain relief varies greatly from patient to patient. Some patients do quite well with Anacin and never require any other drug for pain relief, and other patients will not be relieved with morphine for their pain. Unfortunately, all narcotics produce tolerance in a short interval which requires increasing doses of the narcotic to bring about satisfactory relief of pain. As the dose and frequency of narcotic administration are increased, the patient my develop a severe organic mental syndrome which increases the problems in management.

In general, however, there is a tendency to undermedicate, rather than overmedicate patients with severe pain of cancer. Thus, house officers and nurses often fear adequate opiate administration lest such patients develop an addiction. That this withholding of drugs really makes no sense goes without saying. We feel it represents a denial, by the staff, of the impending death.

The duration of action of the narcotics can be enhanced by the addition of other drugs, especially the phenothiazine derivatives. The addition of phenothiazine derivatives to the narcotics results in a lower dose of the narcotics needed and permits the narcotics to have a longer duration of effectiveness. On occasion, the minor tranquilizers such as Valium or meprobamate are useful to reduce anxiety and muscular spasm. In any situation of pain control, if anxiety can be kept under control, less narcotic medication will be needed.

The psychiatrist can often be of great value to the patient at this stage. It may be easier for the patient to express his feelings about the treatment and his resentments to such a member of the team rather than to the treating physician. Psychotherapy is often of great value to the patient with cancer. It often permits him to express feelings and thoughts that he finds difficult if not impossible to express to his doctor and family.

Once the tumor has become incurable, the patient is condemned to an often slowly deteriorating state. His symptoms frequently develop in an alarming profusion of manifestations. As the symptoms present themselves to the patient, he naturally demonstrates increasing fear, depression, and feelings of hopelessness. He cannot understand what is happening to him. A short time before, he had taken his body and his health for granted and now, it is as if his physical resources are abandoning him. It is at this point that the physician must explain clearly to the patient the nature of the events that are occurring.

It is important to make clear to the patient that although the initial attempt at treatment had not been wholly successful, there are still many avenues of treatment available. Furthermore, it is important for the physician to utilize the modalities in an orderly sequence so that the patient can get the maximum benefit from each method of treatment and feel that the physician has further treatment to offer after one method fails. In this way, the patient is able to experience the vitally needed sense of hope that sustains him until the point where he can accept his inevitable fate.

DILEMMA OF THE DYING—
"WHY WON'T PEOPLE LISTEN TO ME?"

Rae Ellen S. Stager

> *When it came to my feelings, an invisible curtain seemed to drop. The behavioral cues from my colleagues varied from lack of eye contact to hovering over my bedside in an authoritarian posture. They talked superficial banter about non-health topics and then made hasty exits from my room. . . . How clear it was: the message sent is not always the message received.*

Out of context, the above thoughts conflict with the reality of the situation, but I propose to give a personal account of how I, as a health care professional as well as a patient with metastatic carcinoma, have reacted to the impact of cancer on my life. My purpose in sharing my observations is not to give an intricate two-year medical history of a cancer patient, but rather to express a personal and professional point of view about the myriad of thoughts, feelings and interactions that one experiences as a person who is terminally ill or who perceives himself as dying. Specifically, I would hope to impress upon readers the importance of communicating with the patient throughout a medical crisis which may ultimately terminate with death and the significance of recognizing the psychological aspects of dying and reactions to death in patients facing a life-threatening illness.

To give some perspective to the impact of a life-threatening disease on my own life, it is perhaps best to give a brief overview as to what has happened during the past two years. In October 1976, at age 29, I had experienced a rather rapid series of significant changes in my life that produced a stressful period of time, albeit positive. A year before I had remarried and found myself enveloped in the growing pains of establishing a new marital relationship. Two years earlier I had accepted a newly created position as an assistant director of nursing at Sheboygan Memorial Hospital, a 250-bed acute care facility, and was intent upon bringing about significant changes in the psychiatric services. Added to these positive stressors was a most critical responsibility affecting my life: raising my six-year-old son. Life was both challenging and fulfilling. The goals that I had set for myself in earlier years, from a professional and personal point of view, were beginning to become a reality. I viewed myself as starting to approach the prime of my life.

In retrospect, I realize that I took my good health status for granted. Inwardly, it amused me that after 11 years of working in a hospital the closest I had ever come to being a patient was being admitted for the birth of my son. I never actively pondered the possibility that as a young woman, I might fall victim to a disease. Even more difficult to comprehend was the possibility of facing a life-threatening disease.

In my role as a health professional, I was accustomed to telling others to practice preventive types of health care (which included self-breast exam). However, it is fair to say that I never anticipated finding any potential abnormality in myself. Even though I consistently practiced the preventive measures that I taught, the shock and disbelief I felt upon the discovery of the nodule in my left breast will never be forgotten. Looking back over the first few days after my discovery of the nodule, I realize that one of the immediate reactions was to deny consciously that the mass could be anything out of the ordinary. Perhaps I was painfully aware of what the worst possible consequences could be: I did not want to bring myself to believe that at age 29 I might fall into the category of "cancer patient." Despite the logical concerns about the mass proving to be malignant and, therefore, challenging my life expectancy, I found myself selfishly rationalizing that I could not have that disease at this point in my life. There just didn't seem to be time "to work it into my schedule" or to tolerate and contend with a disease entity that would interrupt my life so drastically just when things were going so well.

In spite of all the reasons I could conjure up for the nodule not being anything to worry about, I went to see a surgeon who recommended that a biopsy be performed at Christmastime in 1977. Since the procedure was performed under local anesthetic, I was fully conscious when the surgeon told my husband and me that the preliminary results of the frozen section indicated a tentative diagnosis of carcinoma. I will never forget that moment: the three of us sitting so close together that our knees touched; my surgeon hunched over, leaning toward us, and talking in hushed tones. I remember looking at the clock and seeing the hands show 10:06 in the morning. I also remember crying and disbelieving the statement about a positive pathology report. My last thought was that I had just been handed a death warrant and would not live to see the next Christmas.

A period of 12 days elapsed between the biopsy and the modified radical mastectomy which was performed in January 1978. During that time I found myself painfully going through the familiar stages of grief defined by Kubler-Ross (1969). While I did not actively perceive myself as working through the grieving process, in retrospect I feel that the period of time between the two surgical procedures enabled me to be better prepared for the amputation of the breast. It gave me the much needed time to prepare my young son with the thought that I would be in the hospital and would "not be feeling well" for several weeks to come. In addition, at that point I needed time to sort out my own thoughts and to be in better control of my emotions. It was a time for sharing, for crying, and for talking with my husband. It was a time for garnering support from each other, from other family members, and for trying to put some perspective into the nightmare that we were experiencing as a couple.

Subsequent to that surgical procedure, the physical and emotional recuperative phase was relatively uneventful and by summertime I felt physically strong and confident that the immediate crisis of adjusting to cancer had passed. It came as quite a shock to those involved in my medical care, as well as to my husband and myself, when I found a metastasis to the supraclavicular nodes in my neck in September 1978. Considering that I had received excellent follow-up care on a quarterly basis following the mastectomy, it seemed almost incomprehensible to believe that, with negative nodal status following the mastectomy, the nodules had not been found earlier. As a result, I became a patient in the oncology service at University of Wisconsin hospitals and have been followed there since October 1978. Chemotherapy was initiated in November 1978 and continues to be the ongoing treatment plan at this time.

One cannot imagine the depth of growth experienced by a patient and his family when undergoing a medical crisis. The past two years have yielded many insights into myself as an individual and as a nurse. It is because of some of the frustrations experienced by my family and me in dealing with a life-threatening disease that it seems appropriate to speak to the issues of communication with terminal patients or those patients who have concerns about dying.

One of my first observations is that most health care professionals seem to be very uneasy in approaching patients who are concerned about their mortality or, indeed, are dying. It seems that we are raised with the concept that only old people die and that young people do not have to consider the possibility of their mortality until they have lived a long life and have succeeded in achieving the goals and milestones of a lifetime. Likewise, rarely have we as parents spent time with our children relating to issues concerning death and dying (Kubler-Ross, 1969); subsequently, a child perceives that there is some mystique surrounding death and dying which fosters the notion that death is to be feared. Therefore, it is not difficult to understand why a young woman would find it extremely difficult to accept the notion of a life-threatening illness and possible death. The health care professional is not exempt from the difficulty of relating to someone who is dying or perceives herself as about to die. Each of us as human beings carries a complex collection of thoughts, ideas, and preconceived notions about death and dying. We have carried these thoughts from our early years. Perhaps it is because we struggle to find the right words, or perhaps it is because we do not accept the idea of death at a young age, that it is difficult for us to communicate with patients.

And what do patients see in the health care professional throughout their involvement with the health care system? I have experienced a wide range of reactions from individuals that have left me feeling empty, angry, frustrated and, occasionally, pleased about the support I have received from them. Most frustrating are the many assumptions made by health care professionals in dealing with terminal patients or those facing a life-threatening illness. Because of my expertise in psychiatric nursing, it was not unusual for me to receive cues from colleagues indicating that I should be able to cope with my situation. The rationale for this erroneous assumption was based on the fact that I had been engaged in psychotherapy with patients for 10 years and had assisted patients with problem-solving during the crises in their lives. The fact that I was a nurse apparently exempted me from having feelings. I can say with certainty that after being admitted as a patient, one takes off one's "nursing cap" and lives a different role.

I was angry when people assumed that I would be able to cope with this crisis in my life and not have the need to talk about it. Rather, I interpreted some covert expectations of others that I should internalize my feelings and somehow work out a solution which would keep me from "falling to pieces." Not until I literally shouted at one of my colleagues, "Why aren't you people talking to me? Why don't you sit down and listen to me?" was I confronted with the response, "But we thought you could handle this, especially since you are a psychiatric nurse. We just didn't know what to say."

Another assumption frequently made was that I would have other people to talk to about my feelings. This may be true in many cases. There are those patients who do not care to share their feelings with health care professionals during a hospitalization and those wishes must be respected. But not to provide the opportunity to the patient to share how he feels is tantamount to not insuring quality care. He must know that resources exist for sharing and acceptance of his feelings. Although a patient may not be terminal, he may still be concerned about dying and be going through the same grieving process as a patient who is terminal.

Another pitfall into which health care professionals fall is assuming that patients are going to react in a predictable fashion regarding the loss of a body part. Since my mastectomy I have had the privilege of being asked by physicians to see a variety of cancer patients within the hospital where I work. A 49-year-old woman was referred to me by the attending surgeon who had performed a bilateral mastectomy on her. The nursing staff on the unit and I conferred about this woman's ability to cope with her situation during her inpatient stay, and it was suggested to me that the patient was having a difficult time adjusting to the fact that she had had both breasts amputated. However, in face-to-face dialogue and communicating with this patient on a daily basis over a period of two weeks, it was apparent to me she was not as concerned about the loss of her breasts as she was about the fact that she did not know what was going to happen in the future and was afraid that she was going to die. How clear it is, then, that the message sent is not always the message received.

A similar erroneous assumption was made during a panel presentation in which I was involved. The panel's cancer specialists indicated to the audience that women with mastectomies should be encouraged to ask their physicians about the possibility of breast implants following surgery. Those panelists assumed that women with mastectomies would be so devastated by the disfiguring operation that "naturally" they would want to have the breast implant. In speaking with many women who have had mastectomies, I have not generally found that their greatest need was to have a breast implant. Again, health care professionals need to be wary of transferring their personal opinions and concerns to the patient with respect to after-care plans. In fact, the majority of mastectomy patients have made a successful transition from the preoperative to the postoperative state and do not feel a need to go through additional surgery which would, presumably, give them a more normal appearance. Only the patient knows what is important to him or her. Until we take the time to inquire what he or she is thinking and feeling, we cannot make assumptions in terms of what is important.

What makes it so difficult to communicate with the patient who perceives himself as dying? During my initial inpatient stay, I noticed that nurses and physicians feel very comfortable talking about non-health related issues or about giving me the results of my pathology report and laboratory tests. When it came to emotions, however, an invisible curtain seemed to drop. The behavioral cues that I picked up from my colleagues varied from lack of eye contact to standing or hovering over my bedside in an authoritarian posture. They talked superficial banter about non-health related topics, and then made hasty exits from my room. Most bothersome, however, were the statements made in an effort to reassure me, but which certainly fell short of making me feel any better. Well-worn cliches as "Things will be better tomorrow" or "You're doing just fine" or "You don't need to worry about that now" serve as sources of irritation to a patient with concerns about her life expectancy. I did *not* know I "would be better tomorrow" and while finding myself in the midst of a medical/emotional crisis, I did not perceive myself as "doing well." If patients feel their time is limited, they do not want to hear that they "don't have to worry about that now." The present and the future are important to them.

Perhaps the most contagious and pervasive fear for patients is fear of the unknown. How often do we as health care professionals promote the growth of this kind of fear? Some professionals tend to think that information about the patient and about his life-threatening illness should be shared only in certain circumstances. It is noted that the assumption is made that the patient cannot cope and, therefore, information is shared with family members or only very sparingly with the patient. We underestimate the capabilities of individuals to handle "bad news." All those facing a life-threatening illness whom I have met in the past two years have said loudly and clearly that the worst thing that has happened to them is not being told the information they need to know in order to make responsible decisions about their life. Fortunately, the majority of health care professionals realize the negative impact of withholding information from the patient and recognize the patient's right to be informed of his health status (Erickson and Hyerstay, 1979).

Another negative stressor imposed on the patient by health care professionals is the loss of control the patient experiences during the medical crisis. The loss of control, readily evidenced by the minimal involvement we traditionally allow the patient in decision-making regarding his care, yields feelings ranging from anxiety to helplessness to anger. The opportunity for the patient to function as independently as possible in his care is taken away. The patient feels that he has no control over his life and, therefore, feels very hopeless and helpless about his future. Even the smallest decisions that are left up to the patient can be meaningful. Letting him know that he has the right and the responsibility to participate in his care can be of tremendous therapeutic benefit and can ultimately assist the health care professionals in providing the necessary treatment. Those decisions may be as trivial as when the patient wants to have his bed bath to as important as to whether or not he wants to have additional surgery as a result of a biopsy.

Another way to improve our communications with patients, in addition to providing an open atmosphere in staff/patient relationships, is to look at our non-verbal communication. How many times have we been guilty of looking down at a patient who is lying prone in a hospital bed and saying, "And how are we today?" Have you caught yourself *standing* at the side of a bed with your arms folded across your chest and telling a patient what is going to happen? The covert message is one of defensiveness and lack of openness in inviting a sharing of thoughts. I submit that the humanistic way of approaching a patient (which, incidentally, does not take any more time) is to be at eye-level with that patient and to communicate through eye contact, as well as through body language (Fast, 1970, pp. 117-123), that you are concerned about him. Without uttering a word the patient "reads" your body language cues and knows that the time being spent with him is the time that you are devoting *solely* to him.

Years ago, student nurses were taught never to sit on a patient's bed. It is unfortunate that such an old philosophy has carried over into the 70's, because it enhances the patient's feeling of loneliness and makes him hesitant to reach out and say, "I'm hurting, I'm scared, I'm frightened, I do not know what is happening." Not only does our body language deliver very distinct messages to the patient, but similarly we need to sharpen our skills and tune in to the patient's non-verbal behavior. When we approach a patient and find him curled up in his bed with his back to those in the room or staring out a window, do we do the task that we went in to complete or do we take a few minutes to respond to the patient's feelings? Too often we are satisfied to take the path of least resistance; we fall into that old habit described by the cliche, "Let sleeping dogs lie." Is it because we are afraid that the patient is going to ask questions, such as "Am I going to die?" or "How much time do I have left?" and because we are unsure of how we should respond to such questions that we ignore the opportunity to reach out?

Those of us who work with dying patients or those patients facing life-threatening illnesses need to consider how our verbal responses can affect the patient's attitude. Several incidents experienced over the past two years illustrate examples of insensitivity toward the crisis situation. Throughout the course of the chemotherapy regime there have been predictable days when the side effects of the medication prevent me from being at work. Because I can anticipate the illness following the chemotherapy injections and therefore "schedule" my sick time, I have several times heard colleagues tell me, "Well, enjoy your days off; it must be nice to have a vacation." Another statement made to me is what I call that of the eternal optimist, which is "Well, cheer up, things could be worse." *What could be worse?* Saying this to a cancer patient who is concerned about a potentially short life expectancy and the fact that he cannot predict the future in terms of his disease is a rude and insensitive attitude. Most cancer patients would gladly relinquish their diagnosis to anyone willing to take it. A statement that "Things could be worse" evokes very strong feelings. Perhaps the remark is made in the spirit of being supportive and genuine, although unconsciously it is used to deal with personal inadequacies and ambiguity related to coping with feelings about death and dying.

The most genuine type of response, one which patients seem to appreciate and which yields the best climate for interaction between the patient and staff, is that of providing a listening ear and being accepting and nonjudgmental of the patient's feelings and attitudes. Those feelings may include anger, frustration, denial and bargaining. It is not all right to reassure the patient that he is going to be better, but it is our responsibility to respond to the patient's concerns and questions and reassure him that these concerns are normal and important. Some of the most meaningful statements have been made by friends who have indicated their concern for my wellbeing by being honest enough to say, "I don't know what to say but I care and I am concerned about you." There need not be answers to questions, but there does need to be a willingness to be open, to share and to accept.

Health care professionals often underestimate the power of touch as a form of communication (Fast, 1970, pp. 78-93). It cannot be emphasized enough that a momentary holding of a patient's hand, a touch on the shoulder, or a supportive arm for a patient who is walking can communicate genuine caring and concern. The patient feels the openness and will probably venture the sharing of feelings with this individual rather than with someone who rushes in and out of his room to do only routine or technical tasks.

One final thought about communicating with the dying patient is that we, as health care professionals, need to let the patient know that we accept his feelings at any given moment. It is normal for a dying patient, or one who perceives himself as facing death, to feel "down" at times. We cannot and should not expect a patient to "put on a happy face and smile" when he does not feel that way. Perhaps it is because of our own inherent need that we find it necessary to have a patient respond in a positive fashion and conclude that he is not making the adjustment if he, at times, seems to feel hopeless and helpless.

Lack of control, fear of the unknown, and erroneous assumptions made by health care professionals are only a few factors which contribute to the anxiety and frustration experienced by a dying patient or one who perceives himself as dying in response to a life-threatening illness. We, as health care professionals, need to realize that we can greatly eliminate these components by improving communications through verbal and non-verbal means. When we realize that we need to give of ourselves and communicate at a more feeling level with dying patients, we will indeed improve the quality of life for those whom we serve.

REFERENCES

Erickson, R.C. and B.J. Hyerstay. 1979. "The Dying Patient and the Double-Point Hypothesis." In Garfield, C.A. et al. (eds.), *Stress and Survival,* St. Louis: C.V. Mosby Company, pp. 298-306.

Fast, J. 1970. *Body Language.* New York: J.B. Lippincott Company.

Kubler-Ross, E. 1969. *On Death and Dying.* New York: Macmillan Publishing Company, Inc.

PROFESSIONAL ROLES IN PATIENT CARE

RELEGATION OF RESPONSIBILITY FOR TOTAL PATIENT CARE

A. Daniel Hauser and Richard S. Blacher

Two heads are not as good as one in the management of any medical condition. In life-endangering illness, this is especially true, with even minor differences of opinion over small matters being experienced by the patient as major crises. It is, therefore, of paramount importance that the care of the patient be in the hands of *one* physician. Depending upon the situation and the patient's preference, this may be a general practitioner, surgeon, radiotherapist, pediatrician, internist or almost any medical practitioner who is prepared to undertake the responsibility. Having a single physician in charge is important for several reasons. The treatment of cancer usually involves many medical modalities. Often treatment begins with surgery. Thus, a patient may present with a carcinoma of the colon which is resected and cured in short order. On the other hand, a case may involve surgery, followed by radiotherapy and chemotherapy. During this period of treatment, other consultants may be called in—cardiologists, urologists, hematologists, for example. It is important that during and after this bewildering parade of physicians, a single central figure can accurately, honestly, and directly interpret to the patient, what is happening. The patient, who is often too sick and anxious, cannot deal himself with all of the opinions expressed. Even *apparent* disagreements are terribly anxiety-provoking, and the one physician in charge can serve as the patient's guide through the consultations. Even differences of opinion can be presented in such a way that they are useful rather than worrisome.

In addition, there are usually major decisions to be made during therapy, and these ultimately must be made by the patient. Yet the patient with his lack of medical and statistical knowledge, and hampered by his anxiety, may be in no position to choose rationally. Obviously, the final outcome of cancer treatment is borne by the patient. Mutilations such as mastectomy, laryngectomy, colostomy or castration are never lightly undertaken, even if considered lifesaving. A physician who knows the patient and whom the patient knows and trusts can discuss such procedures from the patient's point of view; the consulting specialist may only be able to discuss them from a statistical viewpoint. Thus, decisions made and imposed by consultants may be eminently correct and obviously for the patient's benefit, yet arouse considerable resistance and resentment.

The fact that there is a doctor who is the central focus for the patient serves as an anchor with reality and a strong defense against the mounting fear and anxiety which so often occur even before the diagnosis is made. The patient consults his doctor, perhaps because of a lump or abnormal bleeding. He is told he has a tumor or that he needs a biopsy or operation. After diagnosis, he may be told he needs a mutilating procedure. With each of these steps, there occurs a rising sense of fear and anxiety. The severity and manifestation of the anxiety will be determined by the patient's pre-morbid personality, but the reality of the situation is such as to elicit primitive fears of death and mutilation from anyone. The physician with the temperament to deal with these reactions serves the patient as guide, adviser, translator of the medical situation, and center of hope.

The treatment of a lesion by a mutilating procedure is often followed by what has been termed as "post-operative depression." In our experience, most patients go through a grief reaction, during which they mourn the lost part, their bodily appearance or integrity, just as they would a lost love object. These reactions are relatively short-lived, and if they persist, usually reflect a depressive reaction involving other problems than the immediate procedure. They often require psychiatric consultation, but may be overlooked by the physician who feels that the reality of the loss is awful enough to evoke a prolonged emotional storm.

The one-physician-in-charge concept is important for the family as well as for the patient. Having one source of information allows for a consistent fund of shared information and a unified approach to the patient. The family of the patient needs information, reassurance and hope also, and like the patient, a sense of someone in charge.

Often, an important person in the patient's life, such as a clergyman, attorney, or friend, can serve as a central figure for the patient and his family and often as a valuable ally for the physician. Many clergymen are medically knowledgeable and intimately acquainted with the emotional life of their parishioners. Their role, from a practical vein, may be that of a pillar of strength for patient and family. Yet even in such a situation, the physician-in-charge must assume the role of leader; such figures in the patient's life almost always cooperate eagerly in assisting the doctor in any way.

A MULTIDISCIPLINARY APPROACH TO CANCER CARE

Gordon A. Braatz and Arnoldus Goudsmit

It has been the concern of generations of health care practitioners to provide the best possible care for all of their patients. Quite naturally, this includes providing optimal care for the patient with advanced disease and for the dying. In former times such an explicit inclusion of the terminal patient would not have been necessary, for the task of the physician was intimately interwoven with the care of the very ill and the dying. Rarely did anyone grow to adulthood without firsthand observation of serious illness and death. Society in general and the medical profession in particular recognized that the physician was expected to be a major source of comfort for those who could not be cured. In addition, social supports for the dying and the bereaved were an established part of the rituals and the mores of the culture. However, as technology advanced, the great cultural changes of the past seventy-five years brought also a disintegration of these social mechanisms. Medicine moved more exclusively toward the biomedical and the "scientific," and dealing with death became practically a lost art. With the concentration of practice in the clinic and hospital, and not in the home, even the information needed to provide optimal support was often lost. It is hardly surprising that through the middle of this century sensitive observers noted an increasing tendency for physicians to avoid or deny the frustrations of caring for those for whom cure was beyond hope.

Recognition of this unfortunate situation came through the observations and insights of a number of outspoken practitioners. Most notable among them was Kubler-Ross (1969), whose call for openness in facing issues of death and dying received widespread attention. As a result, recent years have seen a renewed focus of attention on the needs of the patient with advanced disease.

Over the years persons with widely varying training and experience have had a part in providing service to the patient with advanced disease. Beginning with the physician and the clergyman, later to be joined by nurses, social workers, dietitians, psychologists, and a host of others, these health care professionals have applied their knowledge with skill and dedication. However, in the opinion of sensitive observers, even these many professionals, when providing services in an uncoordinated manner, may fail to meet the needs of the patient. Dunphy (1976) notes that even with many resources still at hand the patient with advanced cancer sometimes comes to be regarded as a kind of non-person for whom nothing can be done. Simpson (1976) has enumerated a great many reasons why the experience of the dying is made unnecessarily wretched in modern hospitals.

Every practitioner is familiar with the unfortunate situation that results when the physician has chosen not to divulge a terminal diagnosis to the patient or family. A wealth of anecdotal evidence indicates that the patient is often aware of his condition and becomes perplexed by this evasion of the truth. In such cases the physician is usually compelled to provide only medical care, and the patient is deprived of the opportunity for honest dialogue with family, nurses, clergy, and others.

We are convinced that a properly coordinated multidisciplinary treatment approach is the most promising vehicle for providing optimal care to the advanced cancer patient and his family. In the field of cancer treatment the term "multidisciplinary" has been used to describe two related but distinct approaches. The one usage may be designated as "intra-professional," and emphasizes the need to include surgeons, diagnostic and therapeutic radiologists, pathologists, medical oncologists, and other physician specialists in joint efforts toward diagnosis and treatment. The other usage refers to an "inter-professional" endeavor jointly undertaken by medical doctors, nurses, social workers, psychologists, clergymen, and other health care professionals. Indeed, there is almost no one in the health care establishment whose particular skills cannot be used to advantage in this multi-professional approach. It is the latter form of multidisciplinary enterprise that we are primarily concerned with in this presentation.

For the past four years the Minneapolis Veterans Administration Hospital has been developing a multidisciplinary approach to treatment on its cancer chemotherapy unit. The development of such a team approach has been a gradual, evolving process, changing to meet the needs of patients and to take advantage of available resources. At present, six disciplines are consistently represented on the treatment team: medicine, nursing, social work, psychology, chaplaincy, and dietetics. Since the clinical situation with few exceptions does not incorporate the expectation of cure, the treatment goal becomes that of enhancing the quality of survival. Through the involvement of these disciplines, an attempt is made to provide the patient with coordinated care and balanced support in both the biomedical and psychosocial arenas.

It is important to note that our multidisciplinary approach does not involve an officially constituted body. It is not separately funded, nor is it administratively organized. Rather, it involves a group of professionals with varying responsibilities within the hospital who have come together to provide this coordinated effort toward the total support of the advanced cancer patient. Thus, the team is not a static entity, the existence of which is determined by administrative decision far removed from the level of patient care. The team persists and evolves only to the extent that it demonstrates some value to the patients it serves and is rewarding to the professionals involved.

Perhaps a Veterans Administration hospital is especially suited for this kind of integration of health care. Because the VA employs health care professionals representing many disciplines it was possible in our setting for these individuals to come together on an ad hoc basis and to identify themselves as members of a multidisciplinary treatment team, having the support of their respective superiors.

At the outset, our multidisciplinary team met weekly for a case presentation and discussion. A chemotherapy patient selected from the in-patient population was evaluated from the perspective of each professional discipline involved, and information was shared and discussed. Because some members of the team were relatively unfamiliar with functions of the other disciplines and had little prior involvement with cancer chemotherapy patients, one meeting each month was devoted to a didactic presentation of a topic. Each discipline in turn assumed responsibility for a presentation of some aspect of his specialty and its relationship to the common task. This weekly multidisciplinary conference has become a valuable opportunity for teaching through the regular attendance of students of various disciplines.

It soon became apparent that having identified ourselves as participants in a common endeavor, we needed also to make the patient realize that we were working together as a team. We have sought to accomplish this by making ward rounds together once each week, meeting all new patients, discussing progress and problems, and supporting one another in a way that would show mutual respect among the disciplines. Presently these weekly rounds regularly include a physician, nurse, social worker, dietitian and psychologist. A chaplain joins the rounds when not prevented by other duties.

Neither of these team involvements met the need for an in-depth discussion of treatment plans and management problems of new or particularly challenging patients. Under the leadership of the nurses, weekly multidisciplinary "intake rounds" have been established. These are essentially "chart" rounds in which the head nurse on the unit presents patients to the multidisciplinary team, with particular focus on those patients who present management or disposition problems. The resulting discussion often points up the need for special attention on the part of any one of the participants to address the identified problems.

In an effort to promote patient education and minimize social isolation among our patients, we have offered a weekly discussion group to patients and their families. These sessions are conducted by a clinical nursing specialist, with other professionals attending as resource persons. The sessions are largely unstructured; over the course of time no topic of importance to the cancer patient or his family has been excluded from searching explorations.

Through these regular formal exercises and also through frequent informal consultations and discussions, the multidisciplinary treatment team has grown to become a cohesive unit. The feeling of commonality which has developed as team members confront problems ranging from the molecular biomedical to the existential psychosocial has made for a sense of openness and understanding along many dimensions. The net result has been an effective and efficient approach to health care.

It is well to note that the separate disciplines which together constitute our multidisciplinary team are by no means sharply demarcated according to areas of knowledge or methods of treatment. Practically all of the disciplines show some blurring of customarily accepted boundaries so there is obvious overlapping of experience, knowledge, competence, and practice. This would be true for medicine and nursing, medicine and psychology, nursing and dietetics, psychology and social work, social work and chaplaincy, and so on, through almost every combination. These are not only academic considerations; they also find expression in everyday practice. The nurse, for example, is consistently involved in areas of diagnosis and treatment, indication and contraindication, symptoms and signs, reaction and response, which superficial tradition and accepted dogma have assigned exclusively to the domain of the physician. Similarly, in the area of counseling, nurses, physicians, social workers, psychologists, and clergy find wide overlap in competence and expertise. This kind of role diffusion can be effectively pursued only in an atmosphere of openness and trust. It is also helpful to maintain flexibility and good humor.

An important benefit derived from our multidisciplinary treatment approach has been the facilitation of decisions about the care of the terminal patient. Every treatment setting which cares for the advanced cancer patient must seriously face issues of how much active treatment shall be afforded the terminal patient when that treatment will serve only to prolong dying. Press reports of dramatic cases, promotion of the so-called "living will," and discussion of euthanasia in all of its forms have repeatedly brought this issue widespread attention. It has been our experience that because we regularly look at the patient from all perspectives we can learn much about his wishes for this last phase of his life. Through this broadened understanding of the patient we begin to see a mandate as to how vigorously to pursue treatment in each particular case. This has left the patient, family and treatment team comfortable in decision making. It is noteworthy that the persons who have tended to be least comfortable with decisions arrived at in this manner are those who have had the smallest exposure to the multidisciplinary appraisal of the patient—in particular, newly assigned nurses and rotating surgery residents—but even these expressions of discomfort about procedures are useful. The questions and challenges raised by students force a frequent re-examination of issues which keeps team members from becoming too comfortable with themselves. This is, of course, an advantage of a health care setting which is part of a teaching community.

Our positive appraisal of the multidisciplinary approach in the treatment of advanced cancer has been reinforced by recent experiences. With the establishment at our hospital of a Regional Medical Education Center for a geographical sector of the VA system, our multidisciplinary team designed and presented a two-day program for health care professionals from other hospitals. The program, entitled "Medical Management of Advanced Solid Tumors: From Biomedical to Psychosocial," was conceived as a means of sharing our experiences and insights with professionals facing similar challenges. Approximately one-half of the conference was devoted to biomedical topics, with presentations ranging from "Chemotherapy for Solid Tumors of Women" to "Immunology and Cancer." The other half of the conference was devoted to psychosocial topics, with presentations such as "The Psychologist and Chemotherapy: Shrinking Something Besides Tumors," and "Group Process for Maximizing Inner Resources." Participants in the conference represented nine hospitals and included physicians, nurses, social workers, dietitians, psychologists, and chaplains. A post-program evaluation carried out by the Education Center staff showed enthusiastic acceptance of both the multidisciplinary approach to treatment and this means of teaching about it. Within the limits imposed by time, even quite technical topics were presented in such a way as to include relevant information for the nonspecialist. Thus, there was no evidence that presentation of, for example, immunology was less interesting to the social workers than to the physicians. Physicians, in turn, participated actively in discussions of the psychosocial topics. Of course, we realize that those who attended were volunteers who knew in advance the nature and purpose of the conference. Yet even recognizing this self-selection factor, it appears that professionals with widely differing training and experience can benefit from this overview of a multidisciplinary approach.

As a complement to this two-day program we have been offering a week-long tutorial in advanced solid tumor chemotherapy. Selected participants from other hospitals spend a week in our setting, participating in our ongoing treatment program under the tutelage of the multidisciplinary team. Provision is made for the participant to spend blocks of time with a professional counterpart on our treatment team with a view toward adapting methods and procedures for his own hospital setting.

The management of the patient with advanced cancer has all too often been hampered by a lack of openness. This has seriously interfered with the relationship among all concerned—patient and family, patient and health care professionals, professionals among themselves, and certainly between each individual and his own feelings. There is abundant documentation of this, much of which appears in the growing body of literature concerning death and dying. In our multidisciplinary approach we have attempted to deal with these problems through an atmosphere of openness and honest communication, with an accompanying shift of the focus to life and living.

As with other health establishments, our multidisciplinary team's contact with the patient has been limited in time, depth and breadth. The aim of treatment is to enable the patient to spend as much as possible of his residual life span in customary settings—at home, at work, and involved in favorite activities. In our multidisciplinary approach, we try to provide concentrated effort, making treatment as effective as possible during the shortest period of the therapeutic encounter.

We are persuaded that our multidisciplinary treatment approach has achieved desirable effects to a very promising degree. One indication of this may be the complete absence of suicides among those cancer patients who have been treated by this multidisciplinary approach. Similarly, it appears that other rash decisions on the part of patients and families have been minimized to a considerable extent. As we have prevented withdrawal and regression on the part of the patient, we have also promoted a sense of belonging and rewarding involvement among members of the health care team. We have always sought to recognize that life involves a succession of decisions, and that as long as life lasts, human beings must have opportunity to seek and embrace their most acceptable alternatives. Thus, life may continue in freedom and dignity to the end.

REFERENCES

Dunphy, J.E. 1976. "On Caring for the Patient with Cancer." *New England Journal of Medicine*, 295:313-319.
Kubler-Ross, E. 1969. *On Death and Dying.* New York: Macmillan Co.
Simpson, M.A. 1976. "Planning for Terminal Care." *Lancet*, 2:192-193.

GENERAL PRINCIPLES OF NURSING CARE

Jeanne Quint Benoliel

There is probably no more difficult problem in clinical practice than the provision of care to dying patients and their families. This chapter considers the special position held by nurses in the delivery of services to these patients and outlines some general principles underlying sound nursing care on their behalf. To identify clearly the actual and potential functions of nurses when patients are dying, there is need to define the term *dying* as it is used in this chapter and to clarify the basic assumptions that underlie the viewpoint presented.

BASIC ASSUMPTIONS

Although many persons are diagnosed to have life-threatening injuries, diseases, and syndromes, they become dying patients only when someone defines them as such. In Western societies, the mandate to decide when someone is dying has generally been granted to physicians, although nurses and other members of the health-care disciplines are also in a position to make judgments about this matter.

In the world of medical practice, the term "dying patient" usually refers to those who are in the terminal stages of illness and whose disease or condition is not amenable to cure. In other words, a patient can live for years with a fatal illness such as cancer or heart disease, but he becomes a "dying patient" when nothing more can be done to promote recovery and only palliative treatment remains.

In a profound sense, the dying patient is an affront to physicians because he challenges their power to heal and to cure. Cogently reminded of the limits of their capabilities as medical practitioners, many physicians quite understandably feel helpless and hopeless and frustrated by a patient's forthcoming death. These feelings can trigger a range of responses—denial that they exist at one end of the continuum, a sense of giving up at the other. Denial of the feelings may result in a continuation of active recovery-oriented treatments regardless of their worth. Giving up, on the other hand, may result in withdrawal from active involvement in the case. When the latter pathway is chosen, much of the terminal care of dying patients is left to the nursing staff, sometimes with and sometimes without effective communication among members of the medical and nursing staffs. As a consequence of inadequate communication with physicians, nurses in certain settings find themselves faced with serious social and psychological dilemmas in the implementation of sound nursing care to dying patients.

The physician's relationship with the patient is a singularly important component of care and contributes to the patient's sense of well-being above and beyond any medical treatments that are given (Balint, 1972). Yet the physician alone cannot implement an effective program of services during the final stages of life. The reality must be faced that any person's dying takes place in a sociocultural context and hence becomes a group experience. In essence, the social process of dying for any patient is heavily dependent on the choices and actions of other people, and these other people may or may not agree on what is proper for the occasion. Furthermore, the setting of care—for example hospital or home—heavily influences the kinds of service that can be offered and the persons who will be involved in the decision-making process and the care-giving activities. Fundamentally, however, the nature of terminal care rests in a philosophy—a system of beliefs about the rights of patients—that provides a basis for identifying general principles of nursing care.

A PHILOSOPHY OF CARE

To translate the concept of care into guidelines for nursing practice, one needs to differentiate between the concepts of cure and care as fundamental components of clinical practice. To begin with, the concept of cure centers on the diagnosis and treatment of disease, whereas care is concerned with the welfare and wellbeing of the person. Cure deals with the objective aspects of the case. Care is concerned with the subjective meaning of the disease experience and the effects of treatment on day-by-day living. Cure has many origins in science and instrumentation and "doing to" people. Care has its roots in human compassion, respect for the needs of the vulnerable, and "doing with" people (Benoliel, 1972).

The central premise underlying this philosophy is that each human being has value and worth in his own right and thereby is entitled to dignity in death. Extending the premise further, each human being has a right to dignity in dying, including the opportunity to share in decisions affecting how he will die. Respect for the person means that each individual has the right to be informed about his illness and about what is happening around and to him. Respect for the person also includes a recognition of each individual's special needs and areas of vulnerability. That is, each individual has the right to care and comfort—both physical and psychosocial—in keeping with the disabling and limiting effects of his illness or injury and in accord with his own cultural, religious, and social values and beliefs.

In a very real sense, all health-care practitioners must find a balance between the cure goal of practice and the care goal. Changes in medical technology have brought new procedures and unusual techniques of treatment, and the options available to practitioners have increased in complexity. As Van Rensselear Potter (1973) has noted, deciding when to intervene in the life of another person and when not to do so is fundamentally an ethical problem, and the society needs guidelines for the ethics of intervention involving the use of technology so as to avoid dehumanizing people.

Making choices on the basis of morality in combination with sound clinical judgment is a necessary component of ethical practice if the human rights of patients facing death are to be protected. In addition, however, the reality that patient care is a *team effort* must be openly acknowledged, accepted, and practiced by all of the health-care occupations concerned if the goal of personalized care for these patients is to be achieved.

As used here, *personalized care* for the dying patient contains three essential components. Each patient has *continuity of contact* with at least one person who is concerned about and interested in him as a human being. Each patient has *opportunity for active involvement* in social living to the extent that he is able—including participation in decisions affecting how he will die. Each patient has confidence and trust in those who are providing his care (Benoliel, 1972, p. 153).

By virtue of the positions that they hold in the health-care system, nurses can—if they choose—provide leadership in the provision of personalized care of this nature. Stated differently, nurses are often in position to coordinate team efforts toward finding a proper balance between care and cure and to serve as a primary communication link among the many persons involved. To do so, however, they need a clear understanding of the psychosocial and cultural dimensions of dying, as well as a sound background of clinical knowledge and judgment and a belief in a patient's right to direct his own destiny. (The latter belief must of necessity be balanced against another matter of equal importance—society's right to set and implement rules and regulations for the common good of collective man.)

GUIDELINES FOR PRACTICE

Nursing contributions to the care of patients facing death are of two general types. One set consists of the many supporting, coordinating, teaching, and caring activities provided within the context of outpatient and ambulatory services—including those services made available directly in the patient's home. The other set consists of similar activities provided within the context of inpatient services and modified to meet the varied goals and purposes of different types of institutions, i.e., hospitals, extended care facilities, nursing homes, and other institutions. In both types of nursing, the creation of services designed to meet the special needs of dying patients and their families requires a framework within which to plan, to organize, and to implement programs of care.

Such a framework must be built on a conceptual system that takes account of: (1) the psychosocial dimensions of dying, and (2) the physical and physiological limitations and disabilities imposed on the patient by the illness (or injury) and the accompanying regimen of medical and other treatments. Such a framework must also take account of the reality that *continuity* for patients as well as *care* must be built into the system when multiple numbers of health-care workers—including physicians—are involved.

PSYCHOSOCIAL DIMENSIONS OF DYING

Over the past few years, studies of death and dying by social and behavioral scientists have created a set of terms that provide useful language for conceptualizing dying as a psychosocial process and for describing its salient characteristics under different sets of conditions. Glaser and Strauss coined the phrase "dying trajectory" to refer to the course of a person's dying as it is perceived by the various persons involved—the patient, members of the family, doctors, nurses, and others (Glaser and Strauss, 1968). According to this conceptualization, the dying trajectory has two outstanding properties: *duration*, meaning that dying takes place over time; and *shape*, referring to the graphic picture of the patient's state of wellness or illness as it is *defined* by individuals on the basis of their expectations as to how and when the dying will take place.

The concept of the dying trajectory can serve as a useful framework within which to *locate in time* the major changes and adaptational tasks that patients and their families face as they live through the experience of terminal illness. For practical purposes, the dying trajectory can be defined as follows: living with a terminal illness is a temporal process characterized by critical events, shifts in roles and role relationships, and other major social changes affecting not only the person who faces death but also the social groups of which he is a part. To conceive of dying in this way provides a structure within which to view and understand the psychosocial dynamics of personal reactions and interpersonal relationships as they are influenced and modified by the threat of death and/or the actuality of death.

As Glaser and Strauss perceive the situation, definitions of dying (or expectations of death) are based on a combination of two defining terms: *certainty of death*, meaning the degree to which people believe that death is definitely forthcoming; and *time of death*, referring to expectations as to the point in time when death will occur or when the uncertainty about death will be resolved (Glaser and Strauss, 1965). Combinations of certainty of death and time of death provide a categorizing system for distinguishing some general types of the dying trajectory based on differences in length of time required to die and in patterning of physical signs and symptoms indicative of movement toward death.

Because the indicators of change in the patient's physical condition vary a good deal depending on the type of illness or injury, the shape of dying trajectories (patterns of dying may be a term preferred by some) can show wide variations. One pattern, such as that seen in fulminating septicemia, is marked by an abrupt onset and a rapid downhill course. Another pattern, sometimes associated with serious burns or multiple injuries, is also marked by an abrupt onset but may have a slow downhill course toward death.

Chronic diseases of all kinds produce what can be termed lingering patterns of dying. Sometimes, as with certain malignancies, the lingering pattern can show periods of apparently complete remission before the disease process returns. In other chronic problems, for example, obstructive pulmonary disease or congestive heart failure, the lingering pattern of dying continues without remission—often extending over a period of several years with slow progression toward death. A quite different pattern is that associated with unexpected and sudden death—not uncommonly produced by accidental injuries, myocardial infarction, or suicide. Although death of this type is not always a "dying trajectory" for the patient, the death does serve as a critical event in the lives of his family and often for the health-care personnel involved in his care.

The concept of the dying trajectory offers a tool for analyzing patterns of dying characteristic of different work settings to use as a basis for planning and implementing programs of nursing care based on the psychosocial as well as medical needs of patients, families, and staff at different points in time. Since nurses often work in settings providing services for specific types of clinical problems, the concept can be especially helpful as a way of identifying problems of care that are recurrent to the setting and typical for the illness being treated. The problems of nursing care delivery can be very different depending on whether the cause of the patient's dying is cancer, chronic renal disease, emphysema, diabetes mellitus, or multiple sclerosis.

A sound knowledge base in the social and behavioral sciences and a clear understanding of the critical points for patients and families living with terminal illness provide necessary background for the development of services which can provide the kind of help that is needed at the times when such help is probably most appropriate. Nurses to be maximally effective in assisting patients and families as they live through the experiences produced by fatal diseases need to have a clear understanding of psychological reactions to forthcoming death and of the stages of grieving in response to anticipated or actual loss. They need to be cognizant of different cultural patterns of behavior in response to death and dying and to plan programs of care that take account of differences in cultural and religious beliefs. They need to be sensitive to the importance of time and timing in their interactions with patients and families and to experiment with ways of utilizing contact time as helping time. Hoffman and Futterman, for instance, describe how time spent in a hospital clinic waiting room can be effectively organized to help families of children with leukemia cope with the adaptational tasks which they face (Hoffman and Futterman, 1971).

In addition to understanding stages of personal adaptation to life-threatening illness, knowledge about the impact of terminal illness on the family as a functioning unit is also essential for planning adequate helping services. Life-threatening situations introduce many different kinds of stress and strain into the social system of family relationships. In cases of sudden death, families face immediate adjustment to an unexpected and unforeseen loss with no opportunity for preparation through anticipatory mourning. In contrast, families that must live with a life-threatening disease such as cancer over long periods of time face a variety of adjustments, some of which are associated with different stages of illness. Clearly the stresses and strains for these families that are living with malignancies are different at the time of initial diagnosis, during periods of exacerbation of illness, and at the point when death actually arrives. Essentially, any family that must live for years with a chronic, life-threatening disease in one of its members must learn to live with uncertainty and ambiguity and a continuous undercurrent of tension.

The introduction of life-threatening disease into a family adds to whatever stresses and strains already exist within that group. It is probably fair to say that fatal illnesses can never be completely forgotten by those involved. The experience of living with such an illness, however, can serve as a means for drawing people into a close relationship, or it can add to their already strained problems of daily living. In my judgment, knowledge about the many psychological and social adaptations required of individuals and groups in response to fatal disease is clinical information of key importance for planning and providing nursing care services—whether in doctors' offices, outpatient clinics, oncology wards, nursing homes, or other settings. Recognition of the special vulnerabilities of "high risk" groups (those with limited personal, social and economic resources required for meeting the serious problems posed by the threat of death) is also essential if the services provided are to be effective in helping those with the greatest needs for assistance (Benoliel, 1971). Examples of high risk groups are families with dying children on hospital wards in which death is a frequent occurrence.

PHYSICAL AND PHYSIOLOGICAL LIMITATIONS

Just as knowledge about psychological and social responses is essential for planning, so also is knowledge about the physical and physiological limitations associated with different patterns of dying. Although coming to terms with forthcoming death is probably the central problem faced by persons with fatal illnesses, many of them must also learn how *to live with* the physical disabilities imposed by their diseases. Nurses are often in position to help patients with chronic, life-threatening illnesses, and find constructive adaptations to the physical limitations imposed by the disease and treatment. To do so, however, nurses must be knowledgeable about the signs and symptoms of disease, its expected course and clinical complications, the treatment modalities available, and the type of medical management in progress.

By way of illustration, nurses who provide services for patients with serious heart and lung conditions need to be conversant with the various causes of their breathing difficulties and the steps that they can take to find suitable relief from certain types of distress. Nurses who work in settings where terminal cancer patients are housed need to have a clear understanding of the relationship between pain and cancer (including the fact that roughly 50 percent of those with malignancies have relatively little pain) and to be well informed about drugs and other measures that can be used to provide relief from the many discomforts that these patients experience (Crowley and Benoliel, 1973). In a similar way, nurses who provide services to any group of patients with specialized clinical problems can be maximally effective only if the planned program of services is soundly grounded in clinical knowledge. Needless to say, such programs also depend on a mutually respectful working relationship among the nurses, physicians, and other health-care workers involved.

Just as clinical knowledge provides direction for helping patients to adapt to progressive disabilities imposed by terminal illness, this same clinical knowledge is also essential for helping the same people to learn *to live with* their diseases. In certain types of chronic disease the treatment regimen can be such as to require major adaptations by a family in its ordinary style of living. In the case of juvenile-onset diabetes mellitus, for example, insulin must be taken at the proper times and food eaten at proper intervals to avoid hypoglycemia and to prevent the onset of ketoacidosis. In effect, the implementation of a workable diabetic regimen in insulin-dependent young diabetics requires a time-bound way of living and social adjustments by all members of a family. Empirical evidence obtained in a study of young diabetics and their families showed that parental styles of behavior as agents of delegated diabetic treatment was a principal factor affecting the adaptation of the young diabetic to his disease and the family's adaptation to him (Benoliel, 1970).

The delivery of effective nursing services to patients with life-threatening or terminal illness depends on nurses who can combine the fine art of physical care with the various types of psychological support needed during different stages in the living and dying process. Such services require nurses who are able to talk with patients and families about the threat of death and other critical issues at those points in time when open talk is indicated and wanted. The provision of care also depends on nurses who recognize that a patient's pattern of not talking openly about death is not the same as denial of death; open conversation about forthcoming death is not something that everyone has to do, and some do their talking through symbolic behavior rather than through words (Weisman, 1972). To offer this kind of help, nurses must be knowledgeable about the psychosocial dynamics of personal and group responses to terminal illness. They can also profit from training in the practice of crisis intervention.

FUNCTIONS OF NURSING CARE

Because nurses occupy intermediary positions in organized systems for health care, they have a good deal of influence over the quality and effectiveness of the services that are available to patients and their families. Whether in inpatient or in outpatient settings, nurses provide assistance to dying patients and their families mainly through implementation of four important functions: support, instruction, coordination, and care.

The provision of support takes place in several ways. The ability to listen with sensitivity and concern to the emotional as well as verbal messages of dying patients and their families is central to the supporting function. In addition, however, support is provided by helping them to identify the problems they face at different points in time and to locate community and other resources useful for finding solutions appropriate to their situation. A third way by which the supporting function is implemented is through competent performance of the technical tasks of nursing, including delegated medical activities and physical ministrations of many types.

The purpose of the teaching function is to provide patient and family with information about the disease and treatment and to assist them in understanding the changes which they face. An important part of instructional assistance takes the form of teaching the patient self-care activities and delegated medical treatments to be done at home. Helping patient and family to clarify their understanding means taking the time to answer their questions and to interpret the physician's orders and explanations. The latter activity can be very important when a family has had contact with many medical specialists and is confused by differences in technical language and medical recommendations. Misunderstandings and misinterpretations can often be clarified if opportunities for discussion are regularly included in the nurse's plan of care for a patient and communication between doctor and nurse is open.

Activities that are central to implementing the function of coordination include at least two: the arrangement of regular conferences with all members of the care-giving team as needed to plan the care for and with the patient and his family; and referrals to other social and health-care facilities and services as needed by the patient—with adequate followup and evaluation to make certain that the services desired were in fact given. The coordinating function is centrally concerned with the goal of *continuity of care,* but achievement of the goal of continuity depends on clear designation of one person to serve as coordinator of patient-care services.

The caring function consists of nursing activities that assist the person who is dying to cope with the subjective experience of his terminal experience *on his own* terms. The purpose of care is to personalize the experiences encountered by the patient through allowing him opportunities to maintain control over his own dying and to intervene on his behalf when his wishes and desires are not being heard. The function of care looms large in importance during the terminal stages of illness, and especially in those illnesses that cause the patient to find himself completely dependent on others.

COMPONENTS OF TERMINAL CARE

During the final period of dying, the patient's need for supportive nursing care are high. Of primary importance to both the patient and his family are physical ministrations which ensure comfort and cleanliness to the extent that they are possible. The need for nurses to utilize a variety of measures to relieve undue and unnecessary pain and distress has already been mentioned. Supportive nursing care, however, does not mean cutting the patient off from the pain of his own grief or from opportunities to bring closure to his life through open contacts with those dear to him. Indeed, supportive nursing care requires the judicious and thoughtful use of medication for pain and avoids drug dosages that cut the patient off from his final human experience.

A vital component of effective terminal nursing care is the maintenance of open communication with the dying patient for three general purposes: to ascertain his wishes, to serve as a sounding board, and to intercede on his behalf if necessary. Effective planning during the terminal period also takes account of the family's wishes and desires and attempts to facilitate open communication between the patient and his family.

If the patient's dying takes place in a hospital or other institution, provision for group planning in the implementation of patient-care services is essential if continuity is to be maintained effectively over the twenty-four hours a day of coverage. Equally important, the nurse who serves as primary caretaker must have regular and open communication with the medical staff concerning plans, priorities, and goals for each of the patients. Coordination of medical and nursing plans and activities must take place if the goal of care is to be realized.

Perhaps the most important component of terminal nursing care centers in the concept of advocacy. The goal of personalized care for the terminally ill person depends on his having *continuity of contact* with someone who is concerned about him as a human being and who encourages his participation in social living for as long as he is able. Implementation of the caring function means giving the patient opportunities to let his wishes be known. It carries with it responsibility to intervene on behalf of the patient with members of his family, physicians, and others when the patient's wishes and desires have not been heard. Nurses are often the persons in best position to help the patient achieve dignity in dying, but to do so, they must be willing to function as his advocate in helping him bring closure to his life in his own way.

REFERENCES

Balint, M. 1972. *The Doctor, His Patient and the Illness* (rev. ed.). New York: International Universities Press, pp. 239-251.

Benoliel, J.Q. 1970. "The Developing Diabetic Identity: A Study of Family Influence." In *Communicating Nursing Research: Methodological Issues*, vol. 3, Boulder, Colorado: Western Interstate Commission for Higher Education, pp. 14-32.

————. 1971. "Assessments of Loss and Grief." *Journal of Thanatology*, 1:190-191 (May-June).

————. 1972. "Nursing Care for the Terminal Patient: A Psychosocial Approach." In B. Schoenberg et al. (eds.), *Psychosocial Aspects of Terminal Care,* New York: Columbia University Press, pp. 145-161.

Crowley, D.M. and J.Q. Benoliel. 1973. "The Patient in Pain: New Concepts." presented at the American Cancer Society's Conference on Cancer Nursing, Chicago, September 10-11.

Glaser, B.G. and A.L. Strauss. 1965. *Awareness of Dying*. Chicago: Aldine Press, pp. 16-26.

————. 1968. *Time for Dying*. Chicago: Aldine Press, pp. 5-7.

Hoffman, I. and E.H. Futterman. 1971. "Coping with Waiting: Psychiatric Intervention and Study in the Waiting Room of a Pediatric Oncology Clinic." *Comprehensive Psychiatry,* 12:67-81 (January).

Potter, V.R. 1973. "The Ethics of Nature and Nurture." *Zygon,* 8:40-41 (March).

Weisman, A.D. 1972. *On Dying and Denying.* New York: Behavioral Publications, Inc., pp. 56-78.

THE PHYSICIAN'S ROLE IN CATASTROPHIC DISEASE

William Regelson

APHORISMS

1. You are there to preside over the living not the dying!
2. You have a shamanistic role to battle the forces of death with all the science (magic) you command! Your lab coat, stethoscope, chemotherapy, house staff and nurses are part of your magic!
3. Honesty with patients should never take precedence over kindness! It is not a question of absolutes, but a balance between reality, therapeutic hope and emotional and societal needs.
4. Negative thinking of nurses and house staff can dissipate your magic. The position of your supporting staff must be affirmative!
5. Do not be afraid of the negative thinking of family or referring physicians as they can actually strengthen your role if you believe in what you are doing and are effective!
6. Therapeutics are more important than diagnosis in terminal disease. However, look out for the surprising disease or complications that make a fool of your therapy.
7. Failures in therapy or worsening of prognosis are not your fault! Always have an optional treatment ready when one fails!
8. Do not give any drug or treatment unless you believe in it!
9. Do not conceal problems but provide positive (optimistic) balance to negative experience or prognosis!
10. Do not be afraid to touch or caress your patients! I.e., feeding or wound dressing are also simple acts which can convey strength and concern.
11. Do not be afraid of emotional involvement or empathy. Contrary to what most people think, a loving commitment to a patient's needs strengthens your resolve and your capacity to cope with death and catastrophe. Remember, unlike others in contact with the patient, you can provide therapeutic help, even if it is only an increase in narcotics.

12. You can, on occasion, give meaning to catastrophe. "If we succeed with your treatment or even if we fail, we will learn from it."
13. Where possible, work with a partner who can cross-cover or take over responsibility when the patient or relatives become too much to bear. However, patients, particularly the terminally ill, should not be burdened by too many doctors or new faces. Beware of too frequent physician rotation which bureaucratizes patient care and one-to-one doctor-patient responsibility.
14. Sometimes, it is impossible to tolerate a patient's or family's personality or the impact and the agony of the patient's disease. It is obvious that the onset of catastrophe or the process of dying does not necessarily strengthen a patient's character or your own. In the face of patient petulance, self-absorption, boredom, and fear, you are, on occasion, justified in sharing responsibility, provided others can be involved.
15. Narcotics are to be used; do not fear addiction in advanced disease! Beware of drug-withholding nurses and house staff! Do not hesitate to use "stat" narcotics to produce immediate pain relief, relaxation or pleasure. This is good positive conditioning in association with your visit.
16. Be careful of anti-depressants! They rarely work and can produce disassociation. Steroids are useful but should be hoarded as the usual gain is short-term.
17. Be honest with appropriate close family members, but not overly pessimistic, on the mistaken assumption that a "true" appraisal properly prepares the family! Families are never "adequately" prepared for death, so don't waste too much time preparing them.
18. Do not hesitate to use chaplains, nurses or family who feel ordained to discuss death and the future with the patient. Remember, you are the Shaman who restores the element of hope!
19. Appropriate social and economic concern to immediate or post-mortem needs frequently does more good than the "chaplain."
20. Do not hesitate to discuss your therapeutic approach with family, chaplain, and friends. Medical staff should always be thoroughly briefed on what your programs are. Those who surround the patient need "optimistic massage" as well as the patient. (The chaplain needs faith in science also!)
21. Many dying patients need a whipping boy! Support the family member or medical staff member who is whipped! However, don't permit a patient or his family to whip you! (Shamans are too busy and whipping them defeats their magic!)
22. Pessimism is worse than artful optimism. While risky to cajole or lie therapeutically, it may be useful for short-term patient benefit. Even with failure in the face of reassurance, the patient should be able to see the kindness and therapeutic intent in the reassurance given. However, this approach should be used sparingly.
23. Remember that your refusal to accept defeat can be sustaining. You can keep patients alive by reassurance and cajoling, but always remember that one

will run out of assurances when a new complication develops. Remember that sympathy and narcotics can be better than artful lying.

24. Find excuses (social and medical) to bring you into the patient's room to develop supportive relationships. There is nothing wrong with "chit-chat" provided that you show concern.

25. Don't hesitate to use consultants! If a family refuses to go along with a therapeutic program (experimental or standard), try to see it from their position. If you feel that strongly that some form of treatment is essential—as short-term gains are in the patient's best interest and the family objects—it is frequently better to ask the family to find another physician than to preside over the dying while the patient still expects that you are there to change his fate.

26. When death is inevitable, do not run! The patient's responsibility is yours. You and you alone have the responsibility for withdrawing life support and/or increasing narcotic intake to obliterate consciousness. The patient or the family must be aware of your withdrawal from sustaining life and concur with your decision.

27. At the time of death or better, prior to the terminal state, ask for a contribution (in lieu of flowers) to your research fund. Fight back!

28. No routine autopsies! Any post-mortem you ask for requires your presence at the autopsy. It is your learning experience, and only the gain of knowledge hallows the dissection. Complete autopsies are not always necessary; families understand this. Ask for a limited post ("like an operation") and go where the question lies. The family is entitled to a verbal autopsy report the next day.

29. If an autopsy causes longstanding pain to any member of the family, forget it! Only rarely are autopsies that meaningful, and the guilt or conflict engendered by them can overbalance the good.

30. Only under rare circumstances go to funerals! They are to be avoided! Exceptions are those colleagues and close friends or family whom you have treated.

31. Encourage the bereaved to come back and talk. The essence of dealing with family and friends is to indicate that all has been done that could be done, and one can have no regrets as to treatment failure! This knowledge is good for you too! Guilt has no place, and do not permit this to remain with family or friends!

32. If you treat the dying, get involved directly or indirectly in basic or clinical research! Only there can one clearly see positive gain developing from human loss.

33. "Living Wills": Under no circumstances are these documents to represent an excuse for euthanasia! Regardless of the patient's intent, depression and despair are not reasons for dying.

34. If you decide to withdraw life support or increase narcotics to hasten death, you are the final arbiter! Your decision has to be clearly indicated in the chart, to nurse, house staff, family, and peers. You must feel medical-legally liable (i.e., "can this be murder?"), no matter what the law permits!

35. "Euthanasia" is more a concern for packaging death (i.e., convenience) than it is a concern for suffering! Beware of the bureaucratization of the dying process that accelerates the patient's demise in the name of "mercy."

36. Never forget that the physician's primary role is to support life! His secondary role is to be kind and merciful!

When a patient is referred to our Division of Medical Oncology he has advanced incurable disease and he is coming for new treatment programs that have in them the element of hope. The patient and his family come to us for treatment; our goal is to bring relief and return the patient to some semblance of normal life or provide supportive therapy.

My role as a physician is, therefore, not to spend my time reconciling the patient to death but, on the contrary, it is to "wrestle with death" and provide the patient with an option which means more and decent life. It is my responsibility to present the patient with an option other than that of dissolution and death. It is my job to restore hope for life and to convince the patient that good life is possible. My task is not to reign over death but to sustain and add quality to existence, and that makes my job, while not simple, at least clear and well defined.

In this role I become less the scientist and more a "Shaman" or "Witch Doctor," who is wrestling with the forces of death and who has ready magic potions and formulae which will allay the inevitable. I take this position because the problem with the vast majority of my patients is that the moment the diagnosis of cancer is given, dying frequently starts—with depression and despondency taking over. No matter how much lipservice we, in our culture, give to the mature understanding of the inevitability of death, for the great bulk of patients faced with this outcome, despondency and anxiety are ever-present companions. Many of our patients with months and even years of survival find hardly a moment of peace because of the despondency associated with the contemplation of death.

For this reason, I rarely, except under special circumstances, confront my patients with statements regarding the finite nature of their survival. Very few patients ask for this information and only under certain very exceptional circumstances is it necessary to deal with predictable dates or events that require a finite time of survival to be estimated for the patient. There are unfortunately many physicians and individuals, whom I call "the death warranters," who love to tell a patient that he is going to die ("six months" is a favorite figure). There is in this a certain morbid pattern of transferring anxiety or achieving pleasure from the power that one has on indicating to patients the mortal nature of their existence. This is unnecessary and a needless cruelty.

In regard to economic or social needs, the importance of time can be conveyed by indicating to a patient that "he or she is seriously ill and that certainly you should put your affairs in order." However, this can be counteracted by indicating that there are drugs or programs that can conceivably help you and, therefore, we shall try them and not despair. You remind the patient that tuberculosis was, only 30 years ago, often a fatal disease but even then it could be arrested and frequently could be compatible with a normal survival. You talk of the discovery of insulin and how it led suddenly to life for millions. Some of the newer gains associated with the programs that you intend to institute or that may be available within a short period of time can be mentioned. Your role, as a physician, is to emphasize the positive and your job is to balance despair and negativity with hope and positive steps toward definitive treatment!

This doesn't mean that the fear of death or the anxiety related to invalidism or conversations about the seriousness of the illness should not be engaged in by others in the family, the medical community, or the ministry. However, my prime role as a physician is to provide the element of hope!

I agree with Maimonides that the essential role of the physician is "to be kind!" Everything beyond this is extraneous to the role of the physician. It is usually not given to us to see the moment of death; to do this deliberately can be an act of cruelty. The clues and the signals that result in the narrowing of a dying patient's world and the closing of resources and opportunity that characterize terminal disease become adequately self-explanatory to the patient soon enough within the framework of his hospital room. Too often I have seen physicians or family apply self-activating prophecy to patients who have considerable viability remaining and in this manner distort the quality of that life which remains.

You frequently read in the popular or professional articles dealing with "the need to be honest with the dying," anecdotes of those who have reconciled the period of life they have left and of how they made an adjustment and took a last "trip" or did something that they had always wanted to do. In my experience, these cases are extremely rare and in most cases the awareness of impending doom is associated with disappointment, the need for constant reassurance, and patterns of ambivalent hatred and love for those left behind.

The popular concept of the mature acceptance of death, while something that represents an ideal which can certainly be achieved, is something that is a rarity in relation to people's attitudes in our society. Death is frequently akin to the rapist who forces his will on the resisting. What the energetic popularizers of this "honest approach to dying" want is a philosophy analogous to the advice that "if rape is inevitable, relax and enjoy it!" However, it is obvious that the rapist's enjoyment is no index of the victim's pleasure. Just because God ordains death does not make the event any more pleasant or acceptable. While some level of philosophic acceptance has to be developed as man is not immortal, it is my job within the range of what I can accomplish to extend life one week, one month, one year for those patients who are in my care. In relation to the quality of survival, who is to say that one week or one month or one year more of existence is not worth the effort?

In the philosophical sense, one can look at death as returning to the womb. Some philosophers relate death to a heavenly rebirth or reincarnation, and Freud has given us Thanatos appropriately mixing thoughts of death with our libido, thus giving it pleasant overtones.

One thing is certain: death is frequently unjust! When children die of leukemia, or a 16-year-old loses a leg and later suffocates from metastatic disease to the lung, it is difficult to find God's justice. Because of the weakening of faith in a just God and in our ability to interreact with God, the majority of people in our society are very seriously crushed and/or angered by being singled out for lethal disease. In relation to this, I feel that the technology and advances we have developed to put us on the moon and other material evidences of our society have set up levels of expectations that make the onset of death or mutilation even more poignant to the individual who suffers this fate. The attitude of the patient is "Doctor, if we can go to the moon, why can't you rid me of this disease?" We have harnessed the powers of creation in control of atomic energy, extended ourselves exobiologically into space, and are now probing biologic inner space relative to control of gene function and human behavior. There are no taboos! Hearts are transplanted, the foetus is fair game, sex is good conversation. The advances of science and technology make it all the more difficult to reconcile those who are dying with the inevitable. To the patient and his family "maybe the miracle that will bring life or health back is in the next formula, the next laboratory, perhaps tomorrow's news will bring it!" Our expectations are great! It is, therefore, my role as a scientist or symbol of rational effort to answer this need for miracles. God is not only a destroyer but a creator and as his symbol I, therefore, rally to the needs of my patients—treating the disease as an evil and death as an enemy. This is shamanistic and I am a "witch doctor!" With my potions and my white coat and all the myriads of glittering instruments in my armamentarium, I set out to apply my magic to the needs of those who want it.

My ability to succeed in this task reflects in a belief in my role. Problems regarding the socio-economic impact of the prolongation of life, the need to limit population, the role of grief in molding society, demographic considerations, and so forth will have to be decided by our society. In the meantime, my responsibility is one of sustaining and improving life of my individual patients. As a Shaman, however, I never give a drug or recommend a treatment to a patient unless I believe in it.

My philosophy is this: I feel that it is man's role to see adversity as a challenge to himself in relation to God. If one assumes that the pursuit of knowledge is the pursuit of God, then one asks the question as to why this is happening to man? And, in asking this question, seeks the answers. It is this pattern of challenge and response that leads to the development of new drugs and programs and, at the same time, permits a personal involvement with your patients, with emphasis on the fact that even illness can have a positive gain. Illness and the struggle against death and/or debilitation provide us with answers to fundamental questions in relation to why we are here and what our role must be in regard to our existence. What really counts is that one can get satisfaction in thwarting death, and in the cancer field, although we have a long way to go, we do achieve striking individual victories.

The aphorisms provide a fundamental outline of both the practical and philosophic as I see it in dealing with the patient and his family. Please understand that my role is that of a therapist and, therefore, the emphasis I present is appropriate for what I think is asked of me. The treatment of cancer not only calls for measures directed against the disease but, even more important, requires the development of supportive drugs and environments as well as psychosocial and rehabilitative interaction to sustain the entire patient. I am involved in trying to develop all these as well. Ideally, the patient should be approached in the team effort that involves a multiplicity of supportive programs which relate to one another. What is presented here is the concept that I feel makes the medical oncologist most effective for the role he has to play.

TERMINAL CARE AND BEREAVEMENT

TREATMENT OF A DYING PATIENT

Charlotte Nadel and Trikante Rajapaksa

The authors present this case report as an example of an unusual way of coping with death. The patient tried to obtain immortality by continuing to control her family, even after death, by giving her husband instructions in minute details as to the conduct of his own life and how to raise their children for many years to come. Because she would continue to "live" after death, she did a minimal amount of mourning for her own death.

First Admission. Mrs. A.B., a 40-year-old married white Jewish housewife, mother of three children (ages 8, 11 and 14 years), was hospitalized at the State University Hospital of Downstate Medical Center in June, 1975, with a diagnosis of metastatic breast carcinoma. In the past she had had three operations—a mastectomy, a hysterectomy and bilateral oophorectomy.

During this hospitalization she was referred to the Medical-Psychiatric Liaison Service because of crying spells and depression. She was initially seen by T.R. who referred the patient to C.N., who then became the primary therapist. T.R. continued to see the patient on daily rounds and played a supportive role. C.N. saw the patient three times during this admission and seven times during a second admission in August, 1975, during the last two weeks of the patient's life. The sessions lasted between 20 to 50 minutes, according to the patient's needs.

When admitted first, the patient was an attractive woman sitting in bed in no acute distress. She spoke spontaneously and freely; at the same time, she appeared depressed and anxious. Mrs. L. related that until recently, although she had known of her metastatic breast cancer, she had felt that she had some more years to live and would be able to see her children "grown up." But now she had the premonition that she would die within a year. She expressed deep concern about her "unfinished duties"; how could she die when she had small children who needed her so badly? She said that she had had a good marriage and that her husband was a reliable and compassionate man as well as a good father, but:

"the children need *me* too." Mrs. L. described how much involved she was in her children's activities, how much she participated in their lives and how much time she devoted to raising them.

During the second session, Mrs. L. expressed great concern about her husband. She felt that he was "very depressed and ready to break down, and then who would be there to take care of everything?" Meanwhile, the husband was told by the attending physician that the patient had liver metastases and that she would probably die much sooner than had been anticipated.

The husband appeared to us an intelligent, articulate, self-sufficient individual. He spoke of their good marriage, having shared with his wife all responsibilities at home and of not feeling overburdened by his present double responsibilities. For example, he did not mind cooking for the children when he came home from work. He felt that he would be able to accept the patient's death; he knew that he would "suffer" and he would mourn when she died: however, he would be strong enough to continue fulfilling his duties as the head of the household. He realized how important it was that his wife understand that he was a strong person who would not be overwhelmed by her death.

As the patient's platelet count was very low and she could not receive chemotherapy, she was discharged to her home where she remained approximately two weeks—bedridden, very weak, depressed and doing close to nothing.

Second and Last Admission. She was readmitted to our hospital at the beginning of August, 1975 because of bleeding from the gums, hematuria and extensive bruising. She was jaundiced and had ascites. She wanted her husband to remain with her and asked him not to leave her alone. He slept on a recliner in her room and left only for a half hour at a time, for lunch and dinner. During the last hospitalization the patient's husband also needed support. He was seen 10 to 25 minutes at a time, usually after C.N. had seen the patient. C.N. pointed out to the husband the importance of his making clear to his wife that he would, indeed, be able to carry on after her death; this would help her die in peace. The husband cried only in the presence of the therapist, then composed himself and continued to take care of the patient effectively, without crying or showing distress.

During the second admission, Mrs. L. started to discuss with her husband in detail the future of their children: how to raise them, how strict he should be with them, which school they should attend and even what clothes they should wear at the funeral. She discussed the family's future, planning for many years ahead. He understood the patient's need to project herself into the years to come and he was able to accept it. He commented, "My wife gives me so many instructions, I know exactly what I shall have for lunch in 1995."

The patient refused to see friends and other relatives, except for her sister and one close friend. It was very painful for her to view her mother's anguish and would see her only sporadically, for 10 minutes at a time.

At the beginning of her second admission the patient had acute anxiety attacks during intravenous steroid infusions; these attacks subsided when the steroid dose was reduced.

However, one week prior to her death the patient began to have anxiety attacks again. After having dozed off she would awaken with a start, hyperventilating and being restless. During one of these attacks she was seen by C.N. who commented, "You look very frightened today—I wonder why." The patient answered, "I am frightened to close my eyes. I don't want to lose control." The physician then made the interpretation that the patient was having difficulty relinquishing her hold on her family, perhaps the most important aspect of her life. After a pause the patient answered: "It is not easy at all." The physician then told the patient about her own grandmother who had died many years ago and said, "She was a wonderful person and I still remember all the good things that we did together." After another pause the patient said, "In a way we don't die." After that day the patient did not have anxiety attacks, appeared less frightened, was not restless and was able to doze off freely.

The patient became progressively weaker; she could spend only short periods of time with her children and felt guilty about this. The therapist alleviated the patient's guilt by telling her that in her present state of health she *should* spend only short periods of time with the children. Shortly before she died, the patient wanted to be alone with the therapist before seeing her children. She cried and expressed much concern about the children's future. Then she composed herself and faced the children with relative serenity as she did not "at any cost" want to create a "death bed scene."

During the last five days of her life Mrs. L. dozed off from time to time. She still felt the need for the continuous presence of her husband who would hold her hand, but she spoke no more with him about the future. She had little to say to either author. When she was last seen one and a half days prior to her death, she held C.N.'s hand and said, "I wish it would be over soon—take care of my husband."

Discussion. The patient established from early on a positive transference to C.N.—a woman somewhat older than the patient. In contrast to the patient's mother who demanded that she fight her illness, the therapist was a mother figure who allowed the patient to regress as much as she needed. The patient did a minimal amount of mourning; she did withdraw only partial cathexes from her love objects, but used the defense of projecting herself into the future through her husband. The treatment of this patient can be summarized as a process in which the therapist supported the patient's coping mechanism—unrealistic though it was—of expecting to have her minute orders carried out by her husband for years to come, thus continuing to "live." This process was possible in the context of a positive transference, which was regressive and archaic and of a strong identification with the therapist. It seemed to us a turning point in the patient's ability to accept her approaching death, when the therapist told the patient her clear and very pleasant memories of her own grandmother, 30 years after the latter's death. This comment gave the patient the feeling that she too would be remembered and that her wishes would be carried out.

The therapist strengthened the patient's coping mechanism also by encouraging, successfully, the husband to show to the patient his strength in their difficult situation and, thereby, to give her the feeling that he would be able to carry on after her death.

Eissler and others (1955) postulated that mourning eases the plight of dying by accomplishing a decathexis of objects. Our patient did seem to go through a minimal process of decathexis. With a loving and supportive husband who remained very close to the patient to the end, the patient was able to accept death believing that her hopes and wishes for her children would be fulfilled through him, their father. The patient's last words to the therapist "take care of my husband" expressed her desire that a source of strength to which she had had access during her illness would be available to her husband and that he, therefore, would be able to remain strong in meeting his children's needs, in accordance with her wishes and instructions.

REFERENCES

Eissler, K.R. 1955. *The Psychiatrist and the Dying Patient*. New York: International Universities Press, pp. 2-3.

A HOSPICE AT WORK

Madalon O'Rawe Amenta and Janet Hamnett

The hospice concept originated during the Crusades when religious orders—most notably the St. John's Hospitalers—set up way-stations for dying travellers or pilgrims where physical care, food, cleanliness, prayer and spiritual counseling were provided. In the mid-nineteenth century, the Irish Sisters of Charity in Dublin established clean places for the dying poor to receive loving care. The idea spread to England and throughout the empire. The modern hospice movement, which has taken this work out of the exclusive domain of the religious and placed it in the secular mainstream of scientific medical practice, is generally agreed to have started in England with the opening of St. Christopher's in London, in 1967. Now in England there are over 25 hospices supported by the National Health Service. In this country there are upwards of 200 in various stages of development.

The pain of the final good-bye to a loved one; an irrevocably changing relationship; dying—like birthing—needs help. These are family affairs—both social and solitary. In an attempt to deal with this emotionally charged paradox, to bring physical comfort and enhance the quality of life remaining for all involved—things which critics claim our health care system has been notably remiss in doing as it has advanced technologically—Pittsburgh's Forbes Hospice opened its doors to the terminally ill in January, 1979.

A contemporary hospice is defined as a multidisciplinary approach to the palliative management of terminal illness symptoms through individualized psychological support of both the patient and family—as well as bereavement follow-up. The Forbes Hospice, the first self-contained unit in western Pennsylvania, spent two years in planning, fundraising and renovation before it became operational. Although the hospice has a completely separate staff and administration, it occupies a wing of the Pittsburgh Skilled Nursing Center, part of the Forbes Health System, a non-profit three-hospital system. The unit consists of eight private rooms leading off a common central carpeted living area furnished with couches, easy chairs, end tables and plants like a comfortable living room. Fresh cut flowers add color, and a vegetable garden growing outside the dining room is visible through floor to ceiling window-walls. Each bedroom has two large curtained windows—one to the outside and the other opening on the central space—so the patient may see and choose whether or not to be a part of the surrounding world or to have privacy. With the exception of portable oxygen apparatus, maintained as a comfort measure, there is no "medical heroics" equipment. There are no monitors or oscilloscopes and no "public address or electronic intercom system" for disembodied, authoritative voices to communicate with patients. All room lights are responded to immediately and in person. All communication with patients and families on the unit is face-to-face.

The general social atmosphere in the unit common area is one of calm and cheer, the latter contributed to by two finches whose cage may appear anywhere it has been decided their presence will help. Music is sometimes heard either through the piped in music system or from live players, the music therapy interns who play guitars and records as patients and families wish. Depending on the time of day, there will be professional staff, volunteers, families, indistinguishable except by function—as all are dressed in street clothes—entering and leaving rooms, getting chores done, delivering food trays, bringing medication, removing soiled linen. There are invariably pairs or small groups engaged in conversation. Sometimes it is brisk, deliberate—content is picked up in passing—necessary information is being transmitted about the patient's condition or needs. Sometimes it is obviously solemn. Two people with intent and serious expressions will be seated closely, their voices low, inaudible—without strained effort—to the close passerby. Even getting within listening range makes one feel like an intruder. Men and women are dying here and others are about to be bereaved. They are often profoundly sad.

Sometimes there is laughter. Families and patients mingle with each other, staff and volunteers. Visitors come to make music, plant gardens, participate in something deeply significant and authentic with patients and families. In the bright dining area, at one end of the common room, patients and families take meals together when possible. Patients have had bridge parties and there have been buffets and teas for the whole hospice community: patients, their families, staff, volunteers and families of patients who died while on the service.

A patient can be referred to the Forbes Hospital by physician, family, hospital or any other agency in the community. In order to be considered for the program, it must be determined that the patient is terminal, that is to say, according to prevailing medical judgment—without the use of acute life support mechanisms—the patient has six months or less to live. There must be an identified caregiver who will be the responsible person to give not only physical care but also to act as liaison with hospice staff when and if the patient goes home. Patient and family must be aware of what the total hospice program is, desire it, and be willing to turn over medical responsibility for the patient to the hospice physicians. When possible, a patient/family meeting is set up with a hospice staff-member either in the hospice, home or hospital to explore these issues. If, after all the information is gathered and studied by the total team, it is felt this patient and family can benefit from the program, they are admitted.

On admission to the unit, active planning and assessment for the maximum individualization of care begins. This individualization is the core of the concept. It is the armature which gives shape, inner structure and strength to the whole service. Individualization of care operates at all levels to help the patient live his own unique life as fully as possible until he dies.

Patient assessment starts with physical symptoms and palliation, or comfort and relief measures, as the nursing and medical interventions employed. Until someone has experienced an easing of such totally consuming distresses as nausea, constipation, shortness of breath and pain, they cannot begin to be concerned about their individuality. Team meetings with physicians and staff focus on discomfort and pain. Not only what kind and what part of the body or psyche it is affecting, but why? Why this distress now? These questions are asked over and over. Every manifestation, its possible source, and relief tactics already tried are examined. Then palliation is prescribed. It might, in some cases, be pain-relieving radiation. It may be the famous Brompton's cocktail, with Morphine or Levo-Dromoran replacing the heroin of the original British formula or it might be any other pharmacological agent that could possibly help. It is tried, the patient's response noted and the dose altered, in collaboration with the patient until the adjusted "mix" of the right medication at the right time is attained. The "right" time is in anticipation of the return of the pain as the patient experiences it—not when the pain has begun or on some arbitrary schedule. The anxiety resulting from the certain expectation of pain and constant fear of its return can so alter people's personalities that they become strangers to their families. Only when the correct balance of pharmacologic mix and schedule that works for them is attained, do many patients "become themselves" again.

Only then can further comfort measures be devised and appreciated. These might be the use of other drugs, such as steroids, to create and enhance a sense of well-being and improve appetite. When people begin to feel a "little better," they can enjoy food and drink. Alcohol is allowed in the hospice for everyone—patient and family. When physical comfort, and whatever sense of well-being is reasonably attainable, are provided, patients are then able to consider their social and emotional needs. From the beginning the hospice team will have been dealing actively with the specific emotional needs of the family. The patient's maximum participation in decision-making for his care and comfort is encouraged at this time. He sees whomever he wishes, and the hospice staff helps the patient, family and friends take care of the "unfinished business" among them.

When possible, unresolved problems and relationships are tackled through honest communication. The counselor and staff (nurses, nurses aides, clerical and cleaning help) pool their sensitive observations and do what they can with active listening and gentle guidance. This helps to make these most important days meaningful, so that as few "regrets" (unresolved guilt and anger) as possible will plague the lives and undermine the health and well-being of the survivors. The staff responds to whatever the patient and those close to him raise as desires, wishes, even whims. If the patient prefers a shower to a bed bath but has difficulty standing that long, an aide will get into the shower with her. The staff has satisfied a wide variety of patient requests. One patient wanted to give away her jewelry as personally given gifts. A nurse and a volunteer drove her around town until her wish was fulfilled. Another wanted to attend the symphony once more. He and his family were helped in the management of it. Yet another desired to see her dog, and the animal was brought to the hospice.

Is the patient railing at his wife for never having done or been enough, and is she so distracted with worry and grief she cannot begin to talk to him? The staff try to help them reach each other before it is too late. Does the visiting family need food as much as the patient? Trays are brought for them, and they eat in the dining room. Does the patient "forbid" his wife to cry in front of him? She can find the relief that shared tears may bring with a staff member in the conference room or nurses' office. Is the patient emotionally accepting his own death and disturbed by a family member's anger or denial? Each can talk to the hospice staff who try to help them get to a point where they can talk to each other. Are patient and family both so accustomed to communicating through bitterness and bickering that they appear not to be able to reach each other in what staff feels are reasonably sensitive and tender ways, no matter how much help is provided? Then the staff must remember and accept that people die the way they have lived. The staff can only help them find the best way for them to do it.

Hospice staff-members must be able to work well with each other as an interdisciplinary team. No one profession or person can manage this complex of physical, emotional, social, spiritual and financial crises alone. While the physician knows most about chemical and metabolic imbalances, the dietitian knows most about kinds of foods that carry greatest nutritional value and palatability in an effort to alter them. While the physician knows most about causes and relief of physical pain, the nurse specializes in round-the-clock adaptation of this knowledge into physical and emotional comfort measures. She synthesizes all of this into a program of patient and family education and home care. The counselor knows best how to talk with people—patients, family, friends and staff—to help them recognize and deal with their feelings. Music therapists know best how to bring artistic and spiritual comfort through their art. Clergy, on call for members of their congregation who are hospice patients, help with the inevitable confrontation of the spiritual questions that often surface at time of death. Volunteers in the Forbes Hospice work at anything they do best, frequently, as companions to patients and families, helping out wherever needed. The secretary is as adept at listening to and bathing patients, as she is at clerical work. Because there is so much empathy between patient, family and staff, everyone must support each other emotionally. The Director of Education and the Home Care Nurse have found themselves weeping together. The Director of Patient Care and a volunteer cried together in the coat room, when a patient they had both come to care for very much, died, and they realized simultaneously that all the patients would eventually die, and they would grieve over and over.

The Staff support each other practically as well. When the Home Care Nurse feels a case is becoming too hard for her to carry alone, the physician agrees to make a home visit with her, and the counselor helps her express and examine her feelings. She proceeds then to shoulder it by herself—even though the patient deteriorates rapidly—for weeks after that.

Because this kind of cooperation, on a team so large and diverse, does not happen automatically, there must be structures built into the organization to develop and maintain it. All staff and volunteers are selected according to established criteria. All undergo the same introductory orientation and ongoing educational courses. There are team meetings with the physicians in which total patient/family care is assessed and planned; and, with a counselor facilitating, support sessions in which the staff's individual emotional concerns are dealt with. This "care team" also gets to know each other through the usual sharing of common tasks and goals that contribute to camaraderie in most work settings, and through the previously mentioned social events—teas, concerts, pot luck suppers—that are held for the entire hospice community.

The supportive relationship established between family and staff carries over into the bereavement period. Grief for a loved one can create a harrowing inroad on the personality, and may put the sufferer at great emotional and physical risk for at least a year. A formal bereavement program is an integral part of any hospice. Members of the Forbes staff often visit mortuaries and attend funerals. They report on how family members and friends are bearing up. The family is contacted by telephone within the week. Needs and reactions are noted and follow-up is provided either by phone or in person for at least 18 months. There are also weekly group meetings of bereaved families held at the hospice, in which commonalities, differences and subsequent reactions are discussed. Since these people have known each other during one of life's most profound experiences, in a setting that uncritically fostered discovery and expression of true feeling, they are uniquely capable of providing the mutual support that self-help groups so satisfactorily supply. They also, because families of current patients are invited, serve as examples for those anticipating imminent bereavement. They demonstrate that others "manage and survive" and continue to benefit from program support.

That the program is appreciated is beyond question. Families overwhelmingly make statements of gratitude for the extraordinary care, humanity, and concern extended to them and their dying member. And they express this gratitude tangibly. Although distributed across the entire income span, they and their friends have made unprecedented (in the history of this hospital system) gifts of money toward the furtherance of this work.

GENERAL CONSIDERATIONS IN THE TERMINAL CARE OF PATIENTS WITH INTRA-ABDOMINAL CANCER

Frank Glenn

The major proportion of individuals with intra-abdominal cancer are in the 50 years and older age group. They have lived in comparatively good health; few have ever had a serious illness. The insidious onset of symptoms often indicates to them very little that is seriousness associated with their complaints. Only a small number among them have thought about the life process other than to be aware of births and deaths that have occurred since they first began to recognize these events. Death is regarded from over a wide range of effects for other individuals but seldom is it thought about regarding its application to themselves.

These individuals enter a hospital or clinic for a complete evaluation of various aspects of their physical disability, with which we are not concerned here other than to say that the results indicate to those in medical attendance the nature and extent of the lesion. If it is small, it is probably resectable and the prognosis is favorable. On the other hand, findings may be rather equivocal as to the degree of involvement, and this must await operation to be definitely established. Then there are those patients for whom any curative procedure is most unlikely and even palliation may be quite limited. These findings may be suggested to the patient and/or the next of kin. They are seldom dwelt upon because it remains for the operative procedure to reveal the true status of the lesion.

As a result of the evaluation, the patient's physician and surgeon usually confer with him and emphasize the necessity of the surgical procedure. Depending largely upon questions from the patient both reflect an optimistic attitude as to what will be found and that it will probably be adequately dealt with. In discussion with the next of kin they usually tend to be less optimistic but still without emphasis upon the possible inability to remove the lesion. The acceptance of the operation on the part of the patient and family and the preparation for the procedure pinpoint the crucial occasion in the course of the rapidly developing events that have taken place since the symptoms first began.

At operation the surgeon is in the key position to evaluate evidence of extension of the tumor. The feasibility of completely removing it, or being unable to do this, and embarking upon palliative procedures that will prolong the patient's life readily become evident. The internist, who is present and observes these findings, realizes perhaps as well as the surgeon what the findings indicate. Depending upon their clinical experience they can be optimistic to the patient if the primary lesion is removed completely and there is no evidence of any extension. If there is extension that cannot be removed, then what is done is palliative in nature. The prognosis so far as the patient and his next of kin are concerned should be guarded. If, however, little can be done even in a palliative procedure, then the urgency of relating this to those who are immediately concerned becomes apparent. Much is dependent upon the pathology demonstrated by a study of the cellular structure of the tumor providing information that is of greatest value to the clinicians who are in attendance. If it be a slow-growing tumor, naturally they are optimistic. On the other hand, if it is "wild" type of cellular proliferation that is observed, pessimism is quite likely to be well justified.

It is the common practice of the doctors, internists, and surgeons to tell the next of kin what the findings were at operation while the patient is in the recovery room. Diagnosis, something that will require perhaps 48 hours, and the verification anticipated by microscopic examination of the tissue removed are described. The next of kin with rare exception after being so informed make the request: don't tell the patient what you have just told us and please do something—try something such as x-ray therapy, cancer cure, and don't let him suffer.

The next of kin, one or more persons, are usually adamant in the demand to keep the facts as they know them from the patient by the divulgence of additional discouraging information from the pathologists. In some instances they are militant and insist that they have the authority to determine what the doctor tells the patient.

The physicians have an obligation not to deceive or lie to the patient. To this extent the patient is legally entitled to know his diagnosis. The terms employed by the physician and surgeon to inform the patient should be commensurate with the patient's knowledge so that he understands the seriousness of his illness. The great difference in patients and their reaction to such information precludes any rigid detailed method of procedure; rather, those in attendance are best guided by general principles.

To render the subject amenable to the acceptance of truth begins with the direct and frank discussion by those responsible. In general, such responsibility is assumed by family, friends and the medical profession. The recognition and evaluation of an intra-abdominal cancer is the domain of the medical profession. Thus, the doctor or doctors are the first in what may become a large and indeed rather diverse group. The facts, the truth as the doctors see it, should be presented to the patient, and no truth should be withheld, including all doubts or questions of the diagnosis. Few people will receive such information with equanimity or satisfaction. Many will seek confirmation or refutation and then bring together their abilities to best meet their problem in their own way. Some will refuse to believe what they are told and still others will be rebellious of their lot blaming it upon their fellowmen, doctors, or God and sometimes "fate." They are often surprised, angered and belligerent. Such reactions may indicate that, previously, they had been oblivious to death as pertaining to themselves.

Established medical diagnosis revealed to the patient by the doctors in attendance becomes the basis for the role of family, friends, and associates in the patient's future and remaining life span. The ideal objective is to be obtained by an appreciation of what this interval holds for the patient and the assistance of those who attend him, both lay and professional. As in all endeavors man's intelligence, understanding, and kindness are required to attain success. When these are lacking, failure is common and blame is useless and, indeed, tragic. The medical profession cannot predict the life expectancy and they should refrain from estimating it in time and explain to the patient and family why this is not feasible.

There are many approaches in relaying to the patient the true situation which he is so entitled to have without delay. There are two extremes in these approaches. Merely to emphasize the differences, they may be stated with exaggeration. First, tell the patient that he has a cancer which is incompatible with life, and that death is inevitable and to be anticipated. The second approach is to describe briefly with minimal detail the findings at operation and then portray to the patient the ordinary differences in life span and how they differ from individual to individual. At this juncture the lack of specific knowledge for estimating life expectancy is readily emphasized. It may be inferred that in all probability, as far as the physician can discern the existing condition, his tumor will be the cause of death. There are two elements that are important to the patient. One is that his disease is generally fatal, and two that the length of survival is unknown to those in attendance.

One may supplement these by adding that just as we are born, so we eventually die. These phenomena are as constant as the force of gravity. One may embark upon a discussion of the weather—how it is variable but equally consistent as to pattern of sequence. The reception of such information varies from patient to patient. In my experience few ask questions.

Regardless of the approach, an awareness of a sudden turn of events in their life implicating a short survival time is shocking and devastating. Those with many responsibilities and with others dependent upon them seem to rise to the greatest degree of activity and become concerned with them. Opposite to those are those who have lived unto themselves, who have become dissociated from responsibility because of age, socio-economic shifts, and deaths of their associates. The reaction is dependent not so much upon these circumstances as upon the interpretation of what death means to the individual.

I have had considerable experience with patients who are awaiting death and who are reasonably knowledgeable about its proximity. Some are quite rebellious thinking that life has treated them badly; repeatedly, they raise the question, why does this have to happen to me now? But the majority, regretting that they must die, express feelings of disappointment or satisfaction for events of the past and the opportunities they seem to have had. In any wasting disease, fatigue, suppression of mental alertness, and pain tend to obscure the emotional reaction. Pain, if severe, on the other hand is difficult to control with or without medications and leads to agitation, mental confusion, and sometimes is associated with outbursts that some psychiatrists consider release of suppressed feelings.

Psychotherapy is of value when a patient has something he wishes to discuss or talk about. He wants to be listened to by someone who he feels can understand him. In the course of this type of discussion or expression, it often becomes obvious to the patient that the questions he has raised he can best answer himself. Because his internists and surgeons do not take time to provide the patient with this opportunity for decompression of pent-up emotion, the psychiatrist plays an important role. It is, I think, of great importance that the institution, as well as all involved personnel, recognize that it is the attention that the patient receives and the opportunities he has to continue in participating in his own welfare and in settling his own problems that provide the greatest satisfaction.

The mechanics of dying are variable and emphasize the role of extreme illness, physical discomfort, mental agitation, as distinct from the actual process of lowering of blood pressure, cardiac failure, toxic state due to absorption of broken down tumor, and so forth. The majority of patients actually die in an unconscious state, with little or no apprehension of approaching death. On the other hand, there is untold apprehension for those who are anticipating death, particularly during the early hours of the morning or late at night in the quietness of either a hospital room or a bed at home. The feeling of loneliness, perhaps greatest among the aged, is comparable to the fear and apprehension of childhood when left alone. The keynote to management is indeed summed up as being embodied in the golden rule: What would you want done if you were in the patient's position?

Many patients in terminal disease are aware of factors that render them objectionable, such as odor, ghostly appearance, seizures, complaints of pain, inability to eat sometimes associated with vomiting and incontinence of urine and feces. Because of this realization a patient may actually look forward to death as a release from an intolerable situation that has brought him into being deserted by those with whom he has long been closely associated.

The recognition of rejection leading to neglect, of course, prompts resentment. This resentment varies dependent upon the feeling of wellbeing on the patient's part. The completely debilitated are unable to do anything about it and find some relief in medication which they increasingly depend upon. Those who have periods of reasonably good sense of wellbeing remonstrate, complain, and do all they can to attract attention. In many instances this is well conceived on their part and carefully planned. On the other hand, perhaps an equal number are examples of reflexes that they are unconscious of to fulfill their desire or need.

Planned participation of the patient in his surroundings and within his capacity is important. There is great need for the profession to counsel patients fairly, honestly, and with patience so that they will not be attracted to quack cures so common among those with cancer. Devastating is the effect of the statement that there is nothing additional that can be done by the medical profession. This encourages individuals to seek a "quack" cure, to spend the substance of the family, to be benefited not at all. Finally, we may refer to the different methods prevalent in practice in different cultures with great diversity throughout the world. The death hut of the primitive tribes of Africa, the euphanasia of the Oriental, and the starvation of those in the terminal phase of life on the basis of preservation of food for the young and active emphasize the wide recognition of the problems that confront every people. Assistance during the termination of life seems to have little reward for those in attendance because the burden is mental, physical, financial, and social. The greatest and most prevalent defect rests in neglect. Whether or not this neglect is remedied is dependent largely upon the particular culture in which it occurs. Certainly, the exploration of these problems and their revelation to those who are younger and in the robust period of life promises to accomplish more than the writing of directives for hospital or home care programs.

A few patients are concerned about the vital processes that are going on. Among those who know that they have a tumor or cancer an interest in the mechanism of how it causes death is common. Many of the concepts that evolve are based on photographs or pictures they have seen of cancer and its extension in the body. Extension of the tumor and its pain are anticipated among individuals who possess some knowledge of anatomy and physiology. It is in this same group that anticipated death tends to be well-defined. Examples of this are encountered among the medical profession and those participating in the care of the terminally ill.

In the minds of many death is associated with a loathesome change in which the body becomes livid, mottled, cold, and inert. To others, there is the rather indistinct visualization of the soul or spirit which leaves this dead body behind and enters into the ethereal realm which is the ideal and eternal existence of that individual. Religion plays a great role in this, for a visual picture of a world hereafter is usually based on a small amount of imagery that has been provided by the clergy most often in early life. Superimposed on this are the fantasies of eternal existence that, according to Freud, are exceeded only by those of the sexual drive. For the most part, however, one can seldom elicit from a patient a reasonably distinct picture of what they anticipate after death. Sometimes a patient who holds no religious belief expresses his rationale by stating that as he recalls nothing before his early childhood, he is equally sure that he will remember and encounter nothing when he loses consciousness prior to death. Questions directed to the patient by relatives, close friends, and physicians, even in a state of mental clarity, seldom elicit convincing answers to what they expect. One may observe this frequently with patients who have lived long and close together as a family and who are indeed very dependent upon each other. The questions concerning what will occur after death are most often answered by something relative to what they hope will occur and take place. In other words, if they have given it great thought, the tendency is to express hope for continuation of being in some form. They are reluctant to admit or even speak of oblivion. Occasionally, hallucinatory effects of medication lead the patient to perceiving mental pictures that are described in a rambling manner, though the confusion is quite evident to those who listen to him. On the other hand, these are sometimes interpreted as a visualization of a life hereafter. Regardless of the feeling that the individual may have, or their interpretation, the administration of last rites to a patient, particularly among Catholic patients, has an astoundingly soothing effect and indicates, superficially at least, an acceptance beyond that ordinarily accomplished by other means.

BEREAVEMENT SUPPORT: AN ESSENTIAL PART OF COMPREHENSIVE CANCER CARE

Elizabeth J. Clark

Comprehensive care for patients with life-threatening illnesses includes not only optimal medical care, but also addresses the social, emotional, spiritual and occupational needs of the patient and family. Using comprehensive care as the goal, a Cancer Care Program was begun at a 450-bed community hospital. The main components of this program include: 1) the patient *and* the family seen as the unit of care; 2) emphasis on living rather than on dying; 3) use of a multidisciplinary team approach; and 4) comprehensiveness and continuity of care provided from diagnosis to rehabilitation or to death and through the subsequent bereavement process of the family.

It is the fourth of these components, that of bereavement support, that this paper addresses. Whenever a program is designed for persons who have life-threatening diseases, there must be some planning for those whose lives will be lost due to the disease. Over an 18 month period, approximately one-half of all the patients referred to this Cancer Care Program have died.

As mentioned above, the emphasis of this Cancer Care Program is on living and coping with cancer, not on dying. The goal is to help persons live as well and as fully as possible, whether until rehabilitation or until death. In addition, an attempt is made to help them and their families maintain hope throughout the disease process because hope is essential to optimal functioning.

A particularly relevant concept is proposed in Doyle's "Changing Mosaic of Hope" (Doyle, 1972). Every day the hope of a patient with a life-threatening illness changes. Initially, patients hope for cure. If this is not forthcoming, they hope for control of the disease. If control is not possible, they shift the hope to something such as a return to work one final time or to relief from pain. Hope persists throughout the illness, but the mosaic of hope changes as reality closes in.

Ideally, the patient and the family have been supported throughout the entire disease course and have been helped to cope with the grief reactions that accompany different stages of the illness. These might include reactions to the loss of a bodily part or function or they might include reactions to loss of a role or family function that occur when a man can no longer perform the role of the breadwinner or when a mother can no longer assume total care of her children.

When it becomes evident that a patient's illness is terminal, other aspects of grief have to be considered. Kutscher (1973) has discussed the continuum of anticipatory grief, death and bereavement. A comprehensive program for life-threatening illnesses will need to address each of these areas and will attempt to facilitate anticipatory grief, provide support during the crisis of death, and expedite the bereavement process.

FACILITATION OF ANTICIPATORY GRIEF

According to Weisman (1974), bereavement encompasses the entire process of accommodation to specific loss. In its broadest outline, there are four stages of bereavement: 1) anticipatory grief; 2) mourning; 3) resolution; and 4) restitution.

The first stage of bereavement, anticipatory grief, is alleged to possess natural adaptational value (Lindemann, 1944). It is a rehearsal of what to expect after an impending loss. There is a distinction between prematurely thinking of the family member as already dead and no longer a part of the family and to planning for life after the inevitable death has occurred. Families and patients must gently be encouraged to think about future plans and the necessity of getting their affairs in order. Practical matters, such as wills, cemetery plots, and funeral arrangements, need to be considered and acted on. Often the terminally ill patient is more capable of discussing these areas than is the family who feels this kind of discussion to be disloyal or a sign of relinquishing hope. It should be emphasized that these decisions, like those of the treatment process, should be made jointly and openly. If painful decisions and plans can be made even while the patient is in the final stages of life, some of the trauma and difficulty of decision-making at the time of the death when grief is most acute is relieved.

Robbins (1974) noted that "the early development and continued maintenance of meaningful two-way communication between health professionals and the family unit provides a structural means of tolerating, accepting and utilizing anticipatory grief." Similarly, intervention at the time of death fosters continuity of care for the family. It facilitates emotional expression and catharsis, and it provides the opportunity for education about the normality of the grief process. Additionally, it enables the health professional to identify those family members who might be at high risk to extended or pathological grief.

INTERVENTION AT TIME OF DEATH

If at all possible, it is desirable for a member of the Cancer Care team to be present at the time of death. This not only fosters continuity of care and continued support for the family, but also enables the health professional to later answer those questions about the death and related events that family members often have. It also helps to facilitate the aftermath of the death when necessary arrangements, such as the decision about which funeral home to use, need to be made. In addition, a health team member who has had intimate contact with the patient and family is able to encourage the family to grieve openly and to help allay many of the guilt feelings that arise at such a time. The professional can reassure the family that they did all that was humanly possible, that their loved one received the best care, that they made their decisions together, and that they will be able to cope with their grief. An early relationship with the family also affords the health care worker the opportunity to observe the family's reaction and coping abilities and to anticipate future problems which may be grief related.

If a member of the Cancer Care team is unable to be present at the time of death, a contact is established with the family as soon as possible thereafter. Preferably, this should be done in person. The family will often want to discuss the last hours of the patient's life in detail, and allowing for this and encouraging the family members to express their grief (which includes anger and guilt) are vital.

BEREAVEMENT SUPPORT

Attendance at the viewing or funeral has also proven useful in the Cancer Care program. This has many variables and is determined not only by the family's needs and the depth of attachment that the Cancer Care team member feels for the family, but also upon other factors such as the worker's ability to deal with her own reaction to the loss. It has been our experience that families welcome this attendance and often continue to seek our support during this time. Caution is used on these occasions not to intrude or to usurp a role that a family member should be fulfilling.

The second bereavement contact is made a week to ten days after the funeral. This is a time when most of the relatives will have returned to work or to their normal routines and the protective numbness and shock of the death will have begun to wear off for the bereaved. The reality of the situation then begins to become more evident for the family, especially for the remaining spouse. This contact is made by a telephone or home visit.

The next two bereavement contacts are made at monthly intervals. At the three-month contact an assessment is made to determine the need and timing for future support. It is ideal for the contacts to be made around significant anniversaries or birthdays—if these dates are known.

If, at the end of three months, the family members appear to be coping well and adjusting appropriately to their loss, no further contacts are indicated until a telephone call at six months, and one again a year after the death. In addition to these contacts, it is also imperative that the family members are aware that they can contact the Cancer Care team at any time that they have difficulty. If the team has been available at crisis points throughout the illness and death, the family has generally already established a pattern of using the team for needed support.

Using this program, bereavement support is offered to the family for the entire first year of bereavement in order to include the anniversary grief reactions which occur on significant dates such as holidays, the date of the patient's birth, wedding anniversaries, and finally, the one year anniversary of the patient's death.

SUMMARY

This paper has described the bereavement support component of a Comprehensive Cancer Care Program at a medium-sized community hospital. It is an essential component for any program dealing with life-threatening illnesses, and it is based on the framework of the continuum of anticipatory grief, death, and bereavement. It attempts to be facilitative and supportive throughout the patient's illness and death and to expedite the bereavement process for the family members so that they may resolve their grief and proceed to a healthy restitution.

REFERENCES

Doyle, N. 1972. *The Dying Person and the Family*. New York: Public Affairs Pamphlet.

Kutscher, A.H. 1973. "Anticipatory Grief, Death and Bereavement: A Continuum." In A.H. Kutscher and M.R. Goldberg, eds., *Caring for the Dying Patient and His Family*, New York: Health Sciences Publishing Corp.

Lindemann, E. 1944. "Symptomatology and Management of Acute Grief," *American Journal of Psychiatry*, 101:141.

Robbins, G. 1974. "Anticipatory Grief and Cancer." In B. Schoenberg et al. (eds.), *Anticipatory Grief*. New York: Columbia University Press.

Weisman, A. 1974. "Is Mourning Necessary?" In B. Schoenberg et al. (eds.), *Anticipatory Grief*. New York: Columbia University Press.

THANATOLOGY AND THE FOUNDATION OF THANATOLOGY

Austin H. Kutscher and Lillian G. Kutscher

WHAT IS THANATOLOGY?

Derived from *thanatos*, the god of death in Greek mythology, "thanatology" has been defined as "the description or study of the phenomena of somatic death" (Webster's Third International Dictionary). In its current usage and interpretations, however, thanatology refers to far broader concepts that include psychological aspects of death as these relate to life-threatened or dying patients and the significant individuals in their environment. Stated in a medical context, it is a discipline whose focus is on the art of enhancing humanitarian caregiving for patients who are critically ill or dying, with equal concern expressed for the well-being of their family members.

Emphasizing life and living (even in the presence of death and dying), the broadened perspective of thanatology includes psychosocial elements that have made it imperative and possible to create a temporal framework with readily identifiable characteristics. Therefore, parallel to the phenomena of somatic death are stages of psychosocial evolution related to death "events" that are designated as follows: 1) *anticipatory grief*, that is initiated by the unfavorable diagnosis of the patient's illness and continues through the pre-death period; 2) the actual process of *dying and death;* 3) *acute grief* that is precipitated by the death of the patient and that can continue for a period of two to three weeks (or longer) after the death, 4) *bereavement*, the period during which grief symptoms are present among the survivors and when the multitude of practical and emotional adjustments to the loss are begun; and 5) *closure* or *adjustment to the loss*, a time when the bereaved individual has been able to complete the work of mourning and re-establish a stable and productive pattern of living.

Thanatology has established these facts of living with death and has recognized and stressed the importance of the psychosocial aspects of caregiving for the terminal patient and his family; thanatology is deeply concerned that all aspects of clinical treatment of the terminal patient be monitored and initiation of medical heroics be questioned to avoid dehumanization of the patient; thanatology proposes a philosophy of caregiving that reinforces alternative ways of supporting the positive qualities of the life of the dying patient; thanatology strives to introduce methods of intervention on behalf of the emotional support of the patient's family members and bereaved survivors.

In the still most commonly understood context, those involved as "thanatologists" include professionals, paraprofessionals, and all others who can offer therapeutic intervention for the critically ill or dying patient, his family, and staff both before and following the patient's death or during those instances or contexts when the patient may continue to survive, though in a life-threatened status. It is evident from the above, that the work of thanatology extends far beyond the earlier and confining dimensions of providing care only for those who are terminally ill and during only their very last days. Moreover, in fact, it is increasingly being perceived that "supportive" efforts for the family and caregivers and their respective support systems must be accorded concern equal to that involved in caring for a dying patient no matter when, during terminal care, needs arise.

However viewed, the ultimate phases of living—terminal illness and death—spare no one. Clearly, death—whether sudden or after long suffering—is part of the pattern of life's design and those emotional affects stemming from it—loss, grief, mourning, bereavement, sadness, loneliness—cannot be avoided. The professionals and others affiliated with The Foundation of Thanatology have tried to clarify the consequences of life's tragic events and to broaden perspectives through conscious efforts that can permit changes in the ways our society cares for its dying and its bereaved, thereby tempering the negative forces of tragedy. When living and dying are surrounded and often controlled by mechanical devices and biological advances that border on the miraculous, accepted ethical and moral values need to be subjected to questioning and doubt. Decision-making about how care should be given and what care should be given becomes a sophisticated process whereby both the professional caregiver and the lay person can become enslaved by and victims of the very instruments that have been created to be beneficial. The programs of The Foundation of Thanatology have been conceived to examine these dilemmas and to propose solutions to them.

Within the temporal scope of "medical" thanatology are the events leading to and coming to pass at the termination of a life and when survivors pursue adjustment to new roles and new circumstances. However, viewed over the span of a lifetime, thanatology appears to encompass: the normal concerns of all healthy individuals who wish to deal with their own mortality as part of living; the concerns and obligations of those who would serve as caregivers, educators, and conceptualizers, and the development and elaboration of information for integration into our systems of education, starting even from kindergarten and continuing through grade school, high school, college, professional schools, and thereafter through adult education programs. Death is thus affirmed in a positive sense as a part of the living process—and The Foundation of Thanatology's position in all of its educational programs has been to support such affirmation in principle and to articulate and disseminate the ways in which it can be achieved.

Those in sympathy with the goals of thanatology give equal value to the art of medicine without denying the imperatives of the science of medicine. They have espoused the concept of the multidisciplinary caregiving team—internists, surgeons, psychiatrists, psychologists, clergymen, nurses, social workers, lawyers, dentists, sociologists, funeral service counselors, volunteers, and so forth—whose every member has a commitment to the patient's welfare. With most deaths occurring in hospitals the patient's need for such a team is apparent. It has been thanatology's function to stimulate those in the clinical and social sciences to an acknowledgment of expanded concepts and to promote certain ideals: 1) a commitment to unceasing care of the dying patient and his family and his supporting staff to the very end, and for those survivors, family, staff, friends, and members of the community who may be in distress thereafter; 2) a commitment to only the highest of ethical and moral codes, barring compromise for any reason; and 3) a commitment to assigning as high a value to "care" as has been assigned to "cure"—when cure becomes impossible but when care may yet achieve those crucial goals, freedom from pain and abandonment and reduction of fear.

THE FOUNDATION OF THANATOLOGY

Purposes

THE FOUNDATION OF THANATOLOGY was established to initiate, stimulate, and organize educational, scientific, and humanistic inquiries into the psychological aspects of: dying, reactions to death, loss, and grief; and recovery from bereavement. More broadly and clearly stated, The Foundation is dedicated to promoting vastly improved psychosocial and medical care for patients critically ill or dying from cancer, heart disease,stroke, and diabetes (among other diseases); and for their families.

Directly affiliated with the activities of the Foundation are professionals in the allied health sciences and the humanities—psychiatry, more than 13 other specialties of medicine, psychology, dentistry, nursing, social work, law, religion and theology, social sciences, funeral service, communications, volunteer service, geriatrics, history, philosophy and so forth—who give care and counsel to the dying patient and his family. The Foundation of Thanatology is served by a multidisciplinary Professional Advisory Board of distinguished individuals from many disciplines.

THE FOUNDATION OF THANATOLOGY is a public, tax exempt educational and scientific organization. The Foundation received its Certificate of Incorporation from the Supreme Court of the State of New York, County of New

York; was chartered by the Board of Regents of the University of the State of New York; this non-profit organization has received tax-exempt status as a public foundation from the Internal Revenue Service. All contributions to The Foundation of Thanatology are tax deductible.

Founded in 1967, The Foundation of Thanatology was the first such institution to develop on a national scale and to enlist the support of multidisciplinary professionals on all levels of the health care hierarchy and in the liberal arts. As a result of the interest of these professionals and others who joined out of humanitarian concern, information about death and dying, for too many years suppressed or expressed only in euphemistic terms, began to be communicated to the public at large in a more effective and healthy fashion. The psychological consequences of concealing the facts of death-related phenomena became evident, and The Foundation of Thanatology rose to the challenge of educating health professionals and the public to the emotional hazards inherent in the trauma of death and dying, loss, bereavement, and unresolved grief and to ways of intervening that would facilitate coping with loss and grief.

Through a series of symposia The Foundation of Thanatology has focused on specific issues involved in the extension of health care in a humane way to those patients afflicted with cancer, cardiovascular diseases, and other life-threatening illnesses. These symposia have involved, both in their planning and presentation, professionals and paraprofessionals in many disciplines, and they have been attended by concerned others who have found no other source from which to obtain information and no other similar series of conferences at which they can participate with colleagues in their own particular field or confer with recognized leaders who have dedicated their careers to educational, clinical and research efforts of a thanatological nature.

Symposia and Books

The Foundation has encouraged research on, and introduced a comprehensive and coordinated approach to, continuing discourse on and discussion of the subjects encompassed by the above parameters of the field of thanatology. Its sponsorship of symposia has been a means of generating a current and innovative literature of thanatology in the form of papers, research reports, monographs and books. The resultant group of publications constitutes the largest collection of recently accumulated knowledge in this field. This aspect of the Foundation's program has produced a series of major, national interdisciplinary symposia: "Psychosocial Aspects of Terminal Care" (1970); "Death and Bereavement in Chronic Lung Disease: Cystic Fibrosis as a Model" (1971); "Oral Care of the Dying Patient: I" (1971), "Psychopharmacologic Agents in the Care of the Terminally Ill and the Bereaved: I" (1971); "Psychosocial Aspects of Anticipatory Grief" (1972); "Ministry to the Dying and Bereaved" (1972); "Communications (including Interpersonal Approaches of All Kinds) and Thanatology: I" (1972); "Philosophical Aspects of Thanatology" (1973); "Bereavement" (1973); "Acute Grief and the Funeral" (1974); "Role of the Community Hospital in the

Care of the Dying Patient and the Bereaved" (1974); "Living, Dying and Those Who Care: A Nursing Symposium" (1974); "The Family and Death: A Social Work Symposium" (1975), "Oral Care of the Critically Ill and Dying Patient: II" (1975); "The Role of the Volunteer and Volunteer Director in the Care of the Terminally Ill and the Bereaved" (1975); "Death, the Press and the Public" (1976), "Home Health Care and the Quality of Life" (1976); "Psychosocial Aspects of the Life-Threatened Cardiovascular Patient, The Family and the Staff" (1976), "Psychosocial Aspects of Radiation Therapy: The Patient, the Family and the Staff" (1977); "Education of the Medical Student in Thanatology" (1977); "Acute Grief II: Counseling and Care of the Bereaved" (1977); "Use of Psychopharmacologic and Analgesic Agents in the Clinical and Psychosocial Care of the Dying Patient and the Bereaved: II" (1978); "Thanatology and Geriatrics" (1978), "The Child and Death" (1979); "The Bereavement of Body Loss: Recommitment to Life, Health and Function" (1979); "The House Staff and Thanatology" (1979); "The Role of the Community Hospital: II" (1980); "Acute Grief: Counseling the Bereaved" (1980); "Veterinary Medical Practice: Pet Loss and Human Emotion" (1981); and others. Research reports or position papers now usually numbering 100-125 for each symposium, written specifically for presentation at these symposia, have provided in each instance the substance of one or more textbooks (bearing names similar to that of the symposium) on thanatology (over 40 already published, with others currently in press) for practitioners of medicine, nursing, psychology, dentistry, social work, as well as for many other professionals and paraprofessionals and for students. Participating in these symposia have been world-renowned medical and allied health scientists, social scientists, theologians, philosophers, and representatives from a large number of disciplines who have responded to an unequalled opportunity for the exchange of ideas and the formulation of new approaches, procedures, and programs for their own hospital/university/academic/intellectual or professional environment. Symposium Planning Committees of the Foundation meet regularly to explore sensitive areas on which to focus in future conferences.

Reports on the above and other Foundation activities have received widespread coverage in leading newspapers throughout the country (including *The New York Times,* the *San Francisco Examiner, Boston Globe, Houston Chronicle, Philadelphia Bulletin, New Orleans Times Picayune,* and the *Washington Post*), in magazines and newspaper magazine sections, via university press releases, via wire services, on nationwide and local television and radio programs, and in other media. This kind of publicity has been welcomed as a means of not only calling attention to The Foundation of Thanatology's efforts at its base in New York City but also as a means of encouraging the efforts of others who are trying to raise the standards of care for the life-threatened patient and his family members in other areas of this country.

Education, Conferences and Courses

The Foundation is engaged continually in the planning of conferences for medical, nursing, and allied health students and has begun to play a wide liaison and planning role as a consulting agency for those organizing the courses on thanatology being introduced into curricula, often under The Foundation of Thanatology's encouragement, on college campuses across the United States, in secondary schools, and, especially, in medical and nursing schools. Models for medical and nursing student/faculty conferences were established by programs held for the students of Tulane Medical School, New Orleans, Louisiana (1971) (published thereafter as a textbook); New York Medical College at its New York, New York and Valhalla, New York campuses (1973); and for Columbia-Presbyterian Medical Center students (1973-1975). Elective courses are being offered all classes (first through fourth) at the College of Physicians and Surgeons, Columbia University, New York, New York, under the direction of members of the Foundation who are also members of various Columbia-Presbyterian Medical Center faculties. A postgraduate course for medical and other practitioners has been offered through the College of Physicians and Surgeons, Columbia University.

The Foundation places primary emphasis on the use of its multidisciplinary symposia as an unexcelled avenue for continuing education. In this context, continuing education course credits have been available to such disciplines interested in applying for same, and in the future, this policy will be followed and expanded.

Research

The Foundation has developed, in whole or in part, plans for and is either itself working on, attempting to obtain funding for, or encouraging the inauguration of, extensive research programs which include, among many others, the following: surveys of an curriculum planning for professional education (medical school, nursing school, dental school, and divinity school curricula—including student interest— as these relate to thanatology, surveys of attitudes towards death of both faculty and students at similar institutions; pioneering projects on an aspect of thanatology heretofore largely neglected—the study of anticipatory grief and the development of methods for providing emotional support and guidance to the family of the dying patient; the establishment of a permanent facility for the treatment of anticipatory grief; the advancement of studies focusing on the use of psychopharmacologic drugs for the dying patient and the bereaved; the effects of unresolved grief; the development for the first time of a multi-faceted approach to premalignant disease resulting from in-depth studies relating to the thanatologic concerns of this stage of life-threatening disease; placement of thanatology oriented personnel in community agencies and/or development of such agencies; intensive involvement of the elderly and volunteers in Foundation programs; establishment of the areas of death, dying and bereavement as public health hazards; the semantics of thanatology; training programs for "clinical associates" and others who would coordinate patient and family care; studies of the feasibility of "life conferences" preceding death to determine what steps should be taken to assist the patient, family, and hospital personnel in managing their painful feelings of grief, guilt, depression, anxiety, and anger; approaches to bereavement, detailed approaches to education at all levels, from kindergarten to high school and continuing into college, graduate school and postgraduate and continuing education courses; and, of crucial importance, concerted impetus towards the development of an effective research methodology for these most sensitive areas.

Examples of Specific Projects

1. Geriatrics.

The aging of our population represents a major health care issue as well as a major social problem. The elderly, those 65 years of age and older, are the heaviest users of health care services. Further, because of the multiplicity of health and other problems afflicting the elderly, their care frequently involves decisions and judgments about the individual, his life situation and his potential for which health care professionals have received little preparation. Finally, the many issues involved in the care of the terminally ill patient are, sooner or later, issues in the care of the geriatric patient.

No one argues against providing our elderly with sensitive, humane and cost-effective as well as quality physical care. But without some reasonably explicit model of what such care implies, one which has been shown to be feasible in actual practice, those concerned with the care of the elderly can only exhort and the practitioner must, in the midst of a host of pressures, develop his own model.

The Foundation of Thanatology is proposing to undertake a four-year effort to develop a preliminary Audit Model for the care of the geriatric patient. This will be one of the most complex and ambitious programs in the history of the Foundation. Even the most superficial consideration has led us to conclude that separate models must be developed for the geriatric patient per se as opposed to the declining geriatric patient. It is also apparent that different models will ultimately be necessary for hospital based care, ambulatory care, home care and nursing home care.

2. Peer Review Studies (Psychosocial Approaches)

The words "Terminal Patient Care" invoke a myriad of images, emotions and misconceptions in the minds of health care professionals and laymen alike. The purpose of this study is to begin an evaluation of terminal patient care as it is currently manifest and to explore the need for a new conceptual framework within which such care can be both rendered and documents in a hospital, nursing home, or even at home, etc.

In a retrospective study of terminally ill lung cancer patients, the psychosocial components of terminal patient care, as indicated in their charts, were considered. A concerted effort was made to incorporate the principles of peer review of medical care in this initial evaluation. It was found that there was an information vacuum in such chart entries.

We feel that this approach to a review of terminal patient care will facilitate the elucidation of new, ordered criteria for treatment and subsequent documentation, and that psychosocial care will be emphasized in the future commensurate with need. Substantial benefits will accrue, to the primary physician and patient, to the consulting physician, and to peer review investigators, and hopefully will outweigh certain risks inherent in such an approach. Ultimately, our hope is that the guidelines established for peer review will be also the guidelines followed in the education of the medical student, resident and professional with regard to the responsible care of terminally ill patients.

Further Goals

The Foundation has sought successfully and hopes to stimulate further the coordination and dissemination of current knowledge and efforts in the field of thanatology among all disciplines; to serve as a catalyst for more humane care, assistance, and treatment of the dying patient, the survivor-to-be, and the bereaved; and to foster communication among the various groups studying these problems. An effort is now underway to establish a nationwide network of Foundation newsletters and chapters (centers) to: provide information and initiate local conferences in hospitals, academic institutions, churches, etc.; provide local speakers; and offer counseling services for those professionals needing a referral service for those suffering from the psychosocial and emotional problems of prolonged lethal disease, loss, and grief.

Current Information Services of The Foundation of Thanatology

Foundation funds are employed not only to sponsor and bring these projects to fruition, but also to establish, by various approaches (i.e., symposia, workshops, advisory resources for the media, continuous intercommunication with thanatologists) a network of communication with and among investigators throughout this country and abroad.

In an ever-expanding role, as a service organization, The Foundation of Thanatology responds constantly to group and individual requests and inquiries. Hospitals, schools, churches, civic organizations, and professional societies have been provided with speakers, panelists, or information regarding programs on subjects germane to the issues of thanatology. Mass media, including television and radio stations, newspapers, and magazines, routinely have utilized the Foundation as a source of specific and/or general information, as well as a source for referrals to those who are engaged in highly specialized investigations or projects. Such requests have come from groups and individuals throughout the country.

In order to provide often requested guidance and assistance, definitive listings of books and monographs, particularly suited to professional school or medical center hospital, and public libraries, are now being compiled with the assistance of members of the Professional Advisory Board. These will be distributed upon request to such institutions and facilities.

Individual requests, often urgent, by mail or telephone or otherwise, are received daily seeking general information, supplemental support, or the identity of physicians, psychologists, nurses, dentists, or others who are sensitive to the psychological and psychosocial environment of terminal illness or bereavement and are able to suggest better management. In specific situations, information has been provided by appropriate members of the Foundation's Professional Advisory Board to persons before and after the death of a spouse, parent, or child, especially when psychiatric referrals have been sought, and a Referral Panel of qualified professionals is being organized to assist those seeking guidance.

Periodical Publications

The *Archives of The Foundation of Thanatology* is a quarterly publication of The Foundation of Thanatology. Regularly included in the *Archives* are *abstracts of all* (if available in time for publication) *manuscripts prepared for each symposium* and selected manuscripts which are published in full. The *Archives* is designed also to provide details of the ongoing program and activities of The Foundation: to serve as an outlet for prompt publication of original reports of a research, philosophical, observational, or editorial nature, to notify readers of and/or describe new Foundation of Thanatology publications including books, monographs, periodicals, reprints, etc.; and to serve as a reference source of the Foundation's Professional Advisory Board, programs, symposia, research, educational efforts, lay activities, etc.

Advances in Thanatology publishes full-length manuscripts derived from investigations throughout this country and others as well as those reporting on our Foundation's own research and investigations. *Advances* is an outstanding academic periodical.

A monthly Foundation periodical, *Thanatology News,* has been planned to assure the prompt, interdisciplinary dissemination of information relative to all the allied health sciences and other study areas included in the field of thanatology.

No other journals provide these multidisciplinary channels for publishing the literature of thanatology.

Foundation Texts and Books

The books already published under Foundation sponsorship include the following: *But Not to Lose: A Book of Comfort for Those Bereaved,* edited by Austin H. Kutscher with 49 contributors (Frederick Fell, Inc.), First Edition; Second Edition, 1981, edited by Austin H. Kutscher et al. (ARNO PRESS/A New York Times Company, 3 Park Avenue, New York 10016); *Death and Bereavement,* edited by Austin H. Kutscher with 49 contributors (Charles C. Thomas, Publisher, Springfield, Illinois); *Loss and Grief: Psychological Management in Medical Practice,* edited by Bernard Schoenberg, Arthur C. Carr, David Peretz, and Austin H. Kutscher (Columbia University Press, 136 South Broadway, Irvington-on-Hudson, New York); *Psychosocial Aspects of Terminal Care,* edited by Bernard Schoenberg, Arthur C. Carr, David Peretz, and Austin H. Kutscher (Columbia University Press—see address above); *Psychosocial Aspects of Cystic Fibrosis: A Model for Chronic Lung Disease,* edited by Paul R. Patterson, Carolyn R. Denning, and Austin H. Kutscher (Columbia University Press—see address above); *The Terminal Patient: Oral Care,* edited by Austin H. Kutscher, Bernard Schoenberg, and Arthur C. Carr (Columbia University Press—see address above), *Psychopharmacologic Agents for the Terminally Ill and the Bereaved,* edited by Ivan K. Goldberg, Sidney Malitz, and Austin H. Kutscher (Columbia University Press—see address above); *Anticipatory Grief,* edited by Bernard Schoenberg, Arthur C. Carr, David Peretz, Austin H. Kutscher and Ivan K. Goldberg (Columbia University Press—see address above); *Religion and Bereavement,* edited by Austin H. Kutscher and Lillian G. Kutscher (Health Sciences Publishing Corp., 443 Greenwich Street, New York, New York); *Caring for the Dying Patient and His Family,* edited by Austin H. Kutscher and Michael R. Goldberg (Health Sciences Publishing Corp.—see address above); *Bereavement: Its Psychosocial Aspects,* edited by Bernard Schoenberg, Irwin Gerber, Alfred Wiener, Austin H. Kutscher, David Peretz and Arthur C. Carr (Columbia University Press); *Grief and the Meaning of the Funeral,* edited by Otto S. Margolis, H.C. Raether, A.H. Kutscher, R.J. Volk, I.K. Goldberg, and D.J. Cherico (Arno Press—see address above); *Death and the Ministry,* edited by J.D. Bane, A.H. Kutscher, R.E. Neale and R.B. Reeves, Jr. (Seabury Press); *Acute Grief and the Funeral,* edited by Vanderlyn Pine, Austin H. Kutscher, David Peretz, Robert Slater, Robert DeBellis, Robert Volk, and Daniel J. Cherico (Charles C. Thomas); *A Comprehensive Bibliography of the Thanatology Literature,* edited by Martin L. Kutscher, D.J. Cherico, Austin H. Kutscher, Amy E. Hanninen, Stephen Johnson and David Peretz (Arno Press); *Communicating Issues in Thanatology,* edited by Thomas P. Fleming, Austin H. Kutscher, David Peretz, Ivan K. Goldberg and Daniel J. Cherico (Arno Press); *The Nurse as Caregiver for the Dying Patient and His Family,* edited by Ann M. Earle, Nina T. Argondizzo and Austin H. Kutscher (Columbia University Press); *Grief: Selected Readings,* edited by Arthur C. Carr, Bernard Schoenberg, David Peretz, Ivan K. Goldberg and Austin H. Kutscher (Health Sciences Publishing Corp.); *Oral Care of the Aging and Dying Patient,* edited by Austin H. Kutscher and Ivan K. Goldberg (Charles C. Thomas), *Pastoral Care of the Dying and Bereaved: Selected Readings,* edited by Rev. Robert P. Reeves, Jr., Robert E. Neale and Austin H. Kutscher (Health Sciences Publishing Corp.); *The Role of the Community Hospital in the Care of the Dying Patient and Bereaved,* edited by E. Gerchick, Dorothy Huttunen, Austin H. Kutscher and Daniel J. Cherico (Arno Press); *Social Work with the Dying Patient and Family,* edited by Elizabeth R. Prichard, Jean Collard, Ben A. Orcutt, Austin H. Kutscher, Irene Seeland and Nathan Lefkowitz (Columbia University Press); *Death, the Press and the Public* (Arno Press); *The Role of the Volunteer Director and Volunteer in the Care of the Terminal Patient and the Family,* edited by M. Newell, H. Naylor, M. Moritz, Betty Marcus, Austin H. Kutscher et al. (Arno Press); *The Mouth in Critical and Terminal Illness,* edited by Austin H. Kutscher, Bernard Schoenberg, Arthur Carr, Sydney Rappaport, Robert DeBellis et al. (Arno Press); *Suicide and Bereavement,* edited by Bruce Danto and Austin H. Kutscher (Arno Press); *Psychosocial Aspects of the Life-Threatened Cardiovascular Patient: The Family and the Staff* (Columbia University Press); *Nursing and Thanatology,* edited by Elsa Poslusny, Marjorie Sears, Carol Farkas, Mary Mueller and Austin H. Kutscher (Arno Press); *Social Work and Thanatology,* edited by Ben Orcutt, Elizabeth Prichard, Jean Collard, Austin H. Kutscher et al. (Arno Press); *Home Care of the Dying Patient* (Columbia University Press), *National Thanatology Directory; Philosophical Aspects of Thanatology* (in two volumes), edited by Florence M. Hetzler and Austin H. Kutscher (Arno Press); *Perspectives on Bereavement,* edited by Irwin Gerber, Alfred Wiener, Austin H. Kutscher, Arthur Arkin, Delia Battin, and Ivan K. Goldberg (Arno Press); and *Acute Grief: Counseling the Bereaved,* edited by Otto S. Margolis et al. (Columbia University Press).

Future booklength texts will include: *Psychosocial Complications in the Care of the Dying Patient and the Bereaved: Cases and Comments,* edited by Austin H. Kutscher (Columbia University Press); *Education of the Medical Student in Thanatology; Education of the Medical Student in Thanatology: II; Psychosocial Aspects of Radiation Therapy: The Patient, the Family and the Staff; Home Care of the Dying Patient: II; A Cross Index of Indices of Books on Thanatology,* edited by Martin L. Kutscher, Daniel J. Cherico, Austin H. Kutscher, Stephen Johnson and Robert DeBellis (Arno Press); and *Psychosocial Aspects of the Life-Threatened Cardiovascular Patient: The Family and the Staff: II.*

The title of Foundation of Thanatology texts, the dates of publication, and the order of their publication are subject to change owing to publishers' schedules, editorial judgments as to urgency of academic needs, promotional evaluations by the publishers, and so forth.

All royalties from these publications have been assigned to The Foundation of Thanatology.

APPENDIX

INTERDISCIPLINARY DIALOGUE

C.H. Chang, Austin H. Kutscher, Helen Coutts,
David Peretz, and others

(The following are transcribed excerpts from a Seminar Session on Oral Care of the Critically Ill and Dying Patient.)

Dr. Chang: I am a radiotherapist. I would say that 95 percent of my patients are cancer patients. If a patient comes in with an early stage, one out of three can be cured in the sense of our definition of "cured." It means that the patient can survive 5 years, 10 years. During that time his chance of survival is just as good as any person's in the same society, same age group, same sex, same occupation, according to life insurance standards.

In the late stage of cancer, of course, it is beyond human ability to restore the damage and return the process to normal. Then we have to deal with a different situation: dealing with the patient you know is going to die and the fear generated by that sort of diagnosis. I don't believe in hiding or covering up the diagnosis. I would tell the patient honestly what we feel, but not in a direct way. I would try to find out whether or not the patient wanted to know and try to stay out of statistics. . . .

I think that we have to strive for early cancer diagnosis. We should tell the patient what we know and be honest with the diagnosis because after the initial shock period, he will handle it much better than if it is covered up for one or two years' time. As a physician, I feel we should have compassion, sympathy, and tell the patient what we know, what we learn, what we could do, and what we cannot do as a human being.

Surgeon: As a surgeon, I don't have much time to establish a relationship

	with a patient. The only real relationships I have are with the terminal patients, and these are of tremendous importance to me.
H. Coutts:	I work with cancer patients all day, and I think you'd be surprised at the high percentage of patients who'd like to know. I work in radiotherapy too. Consequently, all my patients are referral patients, referred by surgeons, internists, and so forth. Unfortunately, the surgeons are cowards. They never want to tell their patients, "You have cancer and, therefore, I am going to refer you to radiation therapy." This patient comes; he has not been told that the biopsy showed positive pathology because radiologists do not treat unless they have a positive pathology. The patients are brought into a *strange* department with *strange* people. Their first contact is a great shock to a patient. I feel that the diagnosis should be told to a patient by a doctor with whom the patient is close. I wouldn't want some strange doctor to say, "Well, you're here because you've got cancer," and this is the first time you're hearing it. I would love to see the doctors orient to the fact that they should discuss the diagnosis with the patient. You'd be surprised what strength patients have. They will deal with their problem better than you think; this goes for children too. I don't say I know about Dr. Chang's department, but everyone who comes to radiation therapy usually or always has a fatal disease... Many times even the families are not told before, and I find that very distressing. I find it very hard to handle a person who comes to my area and does not know the diagnosis and has to be told then for the first time.
Participant:	I have had the experience where I'd tell people they have cancer, and two or three months later they'll swear up and down that they hadn't been told. In these situations you have to contend not only with the patient but also with the patient's family for the family has to live with the patient at home.
H. Coutts:	That's very true. Especially with head and neck cancer patients. A whole biopsy is done and everything has come back positive. The patient is told, his family is told, and they go home. Tell them to come back the next day and then talk to them—remembering very clearly what you had said. The word "cancer" blocks everything out; the patient hears nothing after that.
Dr. Kutscher:	The person we have presented in the videotapes (Lois Jaffe, M.S.W., Associate Professor of Social Work, University of Pittsburgh School of Social Work—a leukemia patient) has revealed a great deal bit by bit in the various interviews. Her husband is part of the film sequence and was interviewed with her. We're not pre-

senting this person as a typical individual. Kubler-Ross has said we have things to learn from the dying patient. Maybe there are certain dying people who have nothing to tell us. On the other hand this kind of articulate individual (Lois Jaffe) does indeed have something to tell us.... What can we learn from this kind of patient, what can medical students, residents or other people gain from seeing these films?

Patient: I think that it's important for the physician to be able to analyze the kind of person he's dealing with. For instance, in my experience, many people who have Multiple Sclerosis react differently. Some give up entirely, and this is the worst thing that they can do. I think you have to be a little bit of a psychiatrist, if you will, and be able to predict how the patient is going to respond. In my own case, they told me but they also told me there was nothing they could do. Frankly, there are a lot of things that can be done. Physical therapy is very successful. Depression can be cyclic in a person who has a chronic illness, knows there's no drug that will relieve his discomfort, and that also he could be treated by the general family doctor. I've gone through periods when I needed to talk to a psychiatrist, and I know our first sentence the first time was: "You know, it's too bad there isn't a pill." Well, there are a number of pills that will treat depression as a biochemical illness. And the problem the psychiatrist has is to decide what is the stimulus that sets off your depression.

I feel you have to make an educated judgment on how the person is going to react because you can throw the wrong kind of person into a complete collapse by telling him the truth. I think the attitude of mind should be "Can I have a life? Can I contribute to society or can I face other people with this problem?" In my own experience, I can tell you, it's a hell of a lot more satisfying to be able to be out and functioning and practicing whatever you practice than it is to be in the pit of depression and unable to react positively to anything. You can't make a decision; all kinds of small things are magnified—so I think it goes well beyond the cancer patient. I think that the handicapped or disabled person has a severe problem to deal with, and his mental attitude is very important... You've got to read the patient and the patient's relatives and determine if this person has the strength or the character or whatever you want to call it to be told the truth, and if he has the right kind of support from his family and friends. If he doesn't, then I think he should not be told.

Dr. Peretz: There have been surveys done of healthy people in which they've been asked whether they would want to be told or not. Anywhere from 70 to 80 percent of them in the different surveys done indicate that they would like to know. Surveys of physicians, at the same time, asked whether they tell their patients. These indicate that anywhere from 70 to 80 percent of physicians believe in *not* telling the patients, as a general rule.

Participant: What a normal person says and what a sick person says are entirely different things. People I've known—hospital personnel—have said, "Well, if I ever had a cancer like that, I'm not going to have anything done with it." Normal people say entirely different things. You'll find a 35-year-old who'll say, "Why don't you let this old fellow die?" But the old fellow doesn't come to you and say, "End it all for me."

Dr. Peretz: From what I've seen in working at the bedside of dying patients, it's never simply a matter of telling or not telling. It's what one tells, and when one tells, in what way one tells; in terms of the kinds of realistic hopes that one can engender at a time of despair about the kinds of treatments available, the kinds of remissions that can be expected, the opportunity for living out certain aspects of life.

Lois Jaffe may be atypical in her ability to look back over the experience and to articulate it and to describe it. She's not atypical in terms of the kinds of needs that she had and the kinds of reactions that she had in the acute situation. She's not a stoic. She's not someone whose rational powers prevented her from grieving deeply, from going into panic when she was told the diagnosis and left alone after a few minutes without any lengthy discussion and exploration, without a member of her family close by. I think we would be doing ourselves a disservice if we back off by using her atypicality in terms of her tremendous ability two years after her diagnosis and in terms of her appearance.

I think one of the things we're going to have to come to terms with in dealing with the dying is the fact that our values and our concepts about ourselves as physicians are going to have to be modified. There are many, many issues that we see every day in working not only with the dying but also with professionals and paraprofessionals who are working with the dying. I am concerned that we don't use the fact that we have to individualize. One of the things I'm finding more and more important, and part of it grew out of not only the work at the bedside but also in listening to Lois Jaffe and in talking to her and her husband: We all too seldom avail ourselves of the opportunity of having, as a part of our therapeutic team, people whom we often consider as the patients, that is, the patient and the family. I'm impressed that if we talk to them as a unit, that if we recognize the family as a unit, and, under certain circumstances, talk to the patient and the family together, that we set some kind of communication in motion between them so that they can be mutually supportive to one another. They need to communicate with each other.

Patient: The normal biological drive is to live. You want to live, and you don't develop the wish for death unless the quality of your life gets to be so bad that there's no hope that it will improve. That's how I feel about my situation.

Dr. Chang: I agree with your point that the basic human desire is to live... We do encounter a large proportion of the patient population who tend to self-denial. They know they have something there; they are suspicious from the beginning that they have cancer, but they try to deny that: "I hope the doctor will tell me different. I hope the doctor will tell me I don't have cancer." Even if you tell them they don't have cancer, they're still suspicious; they still suspect you're not telling the truth. They struggle with fear and the conflict in their own mind is a kind of torture.... I think we have to learn to develop techniques how and when and under what situations the patient should be told, and told to what extent. And then we still have to provide the help, provide the hope....

Dr. Kutscher: We are trying to work out both a radiotherapy symposium and a chemotherapy symposium. I think one of the things that we're talking about can be illustrated by the difficulty we are having—not in getting radiotherapists who are anxious to talk about psychosocial aspects of terminal care but in trying to find surgeons or internists who are anxious to talk to radiotherapists about the problems of interrelation: of how they send their patients over and how they want their patients sent back. In other words, part of what I think we're talking about today is what are the modalities of communication between the various services within a hospital, and where are some of the breakdowns, and what are some of the possibilities for improvement?

A MEDICAL STUDENT'S VIEWPOINT

Gene Kopelson

As a medical student about to enter postgraduate training in radiotherapy, I found that the symposium from which this book evolved raised some interesting questions: How aware are radiotherapists of the psychosocial aspects of their patients' care? What do the patients themselves say? How can we improve future care?

One of my first observations was a determination of who exactly attended the symposium. Although some prominent radiotherapists from the east coast and midwest did attend, many very well-known radiotherapy centers were unrepresented by their staff members. One had the impression that publicity about the symposium had not reached these institutions; or that, in fact, their affiliated physicians were uninterested in the relatively intangible or as-yet-unexplored areas of the psychosocial aspects of the care of radiotherapy patients. Very few radiotherapy residents were there; in fact, some of the most enthusiastic participants were radiotherapy nurses and technicians. I look forward to working with these dedicated members of the radiotherapy team in the future.

Another observation pointing toward a possible lack of awareness for these issues on the part of some therapists was the finding of Perez et al. that radiotherapists made far fewer chart notations related to the patient's attitudes or financial or family problems compared with the number of entries made by social workers; in one example, there were only 7 physician notes on family and emotional relationships in 125 cases (5.6 percent) compared with 95 entries in 100 charts (95 percent) made by social workers. Of the many patient histories I heard presented at radiotherapy conferences during a two-month elective at two different New York radiation therapy departments, in not one were psychosocial issues raised.

We also discussed whether patients found the therapist equally uninvolved in psychosocial issues. In one study, 41 of 50 patients (82 percent), the radiotherapist was not the person with whom one could discuss emotional problems (Mitchell and Glicksman, 1977). I did recognize that patients undergoing radiotherapy have psychosocial problems that might be helped by the therapist.

One piece of data that amazed me was the number of patients referred by their physicians for radiation therapy without having been told that they have cancer. However, that this is still unsettled and needs further clarification was demonstrated by the few studies addressing this question (Mitchell and Glicksman, 1977; Peck and Boland, 1977); of 100 interviewed radiotherapy patients from two series, 77 (77 percent) *had* been told of their diagnosis prior to therapy.

The *milieu* of radiation treatment was raised as a point of concern to the patient. We discussed the fear of the machines; in one study (Mitchell and Glicksman, 1977), although 19 of 50 patients (38 percent) were frightened at first by the equipment, this initial anxiety decreased. All 19 were no longer frightened at the end of treatment. However, in another study (Peck and Boland, 1977), the percentage of patients with a significant degree of anxiety actually increased from 60 percent before to 80 percent after radiotherapy. Finally, in a study from Columbia (Forester, 1977), initial anxiety decreased if patients were treated on the linear accelerator but increased on the betatron; this could be due to the noise produced by the latter machine.

The stress of seeing other cancer patients in varying stages of disease was mentioned. Appearing for treatment with preconceived notions about radiotherapy from friends or relatives (Peck and Boland, 1977), being misinformed by the referring physician as to the length or side effects of treatment (Mitchell and Glicksman, 1977; Peck and Boland, 1977), all contribute to stress for the patient. Although the known psychobehavioral direct effects of radiotherapy are reviewed elsewhere by the author, during treatment emotional problems developed in 33 of 50 patients (66 percent) in one series (Mitchell and Glicksman, 1977) and in 49 of 50 (98 percent) in another (Peck and Boland, 1977). The physical side effects of therapy were also stressful, but patients were helped if the radiotherapist warned them in advance of the effect, according to both of these sources.

Finally, I feel fortunate to have been exposed to two areas of medicine that few medical students have had the privilege to see: radiation therapy and thanatology. I have not discussed death and dying *per se* in this essay; from most of the speakers at the symposium I heard personal experiences of how they handled dying patients. Only more experience with oncology patients in the future will mold my own methods of dealing with both my own and my patients' reactions to the dying process.

In conclusion, many psychosocial problems do, indeed, occur in radiotherapy centers. This leads me to propose several mechanisms to make radiotherapists, some of whom may at this time be aloof from their patients' psychosocial needs, more aware of these problems:

a. increased publicity about the results of this symposium and future meetings in the various radiotherapy journals
b. incorporation of psychosocial aspects of radiotherapy patient care into residency training via required readings, courses, board questions, confer-

ences, and having psychosocial factors presented at patient history presentations.
c. increased use of interview techniques for eliciting psychosocial problems during therapy
d. increased incorporation of mental health and social workers and psychiatrists as radiotherapy team members
e. support of clinical research by fundgiving institutions (e.g., National Cancer Institute) into these problems, to provide further incentive to explore these areas and to provide more quantitative analysis of specific problems and their solutions
f. encouragement of resident or medical student participation by offering a certificate or small stipend for the "Best Annual Essay on the Psychosocial Aspects of Radiotherapy"
g. encouragement of radiotherapy chiefs to either: incorporate thanatology into their radiotherapy electives for medical students (and to publicize this to students via elective catalogues or the dean as one of the few places where a medical student could learn about death on a daily basis in a practical and clinical setting); or participate actively in a thanatology elective for these medical students

REFERENCES

Forester, B.M. 1977. "Psychological Morbidity of Cancer Patients Undergoing Radiotherapy." *Archives of the Foundation of Thanatology*, 6:6.
Mitchell, G.W. and A.S. Glicksman. 1977. "Cancer Patients—Knowledge and Attitudes." *Cancer*, 40:61-66.
Peck, A. and J. Boland. 1977. "Emotional Reactions to Radiation Treatment." *Cancer*, 40:180-184.
Perez, C.A., L.A. Hanes, N. Sedransk, and L. Braun. 1977. "Psychosocial Aspects of Cancer and Radiation Therapy." *Archives of the Foundation of Thanatology*, 6:18.

Contributor List

Patricia Tretter, M.D., Radiation Therapist, St. Jude Hospital and Rehabilitation Center, Fullerton, California, formerly, Associate Professor of Clinical Radiology, College of Physicians and Surgeons, Columbia University, New York, New York.

Leonard M. Liegner, M.D., Associate Clinical Professor of Radiology, College of Physicians and Surgeons, Columbia University; Attending Radiologist (Radiation Therapy), St. Luke's-Roosevelt Hospital Medical Center; Director, Radiation Oncology, St. Luke's Hospital, New York, New York.

Austin H. Kutscher, D.D.S., President, The Foundation of Thanatology; Associate Professor (in Dentistry), Department of Psychiatry, College of Physicians and Surgeons, Columbia University; Associate Professor of Stomatology, School of Dental and Oral Surgery, Columbia University, New York, New York.

Richard J. Torpie, M.D., Director of Radiation Oncology, St. Luke's Hospital of Bethlehem, Pennsylvania; Associate Professor of Therapeutic Radiology, Hahnemann Medical College, Philadelphia, Pennsylvania.

Robert DeBellis, M.D., Assistant Professor of Clinical Medicine (Oncology), College of Physicians and Surgeons, Columbia University, New York, New York.

Margot Tallmer, Ph.D., Clinical Psychologist; Professor, Hunter College of the City University of New York, New York.

* * * * * * * * *

Phyllis J. Ager, M.D., Director, Radiation Oncology, Fresno Community Hospital and Medical Center, Fresno, California; Clinical Associate Professor of Radiology, University of California, San Francisco.

Kenneth Ain, Medical Student, Brown University Program in Medicine, Providence, Rhode Island.

Seymour Alpert, Department of Radiology, Albert Einstein College of Medicine, Bronx, New York.

Madalon O'Rawe Amenta, R.N., Dr.P.H., Director of Research, Forbes Health System, Director of Education, Forbes Hospice, Adjunct Assistant Professor, Public Health Nursing, University of Pittsburgh School of Nursing, Pittsburgh, Pennsylvania.

Isamettin M. Aral, M.D., Clinical Professor of Radiology, School of Medicine, State University of New York at Stonybrook, Associate Chairman of Radiology and Chief, Division of Radiation Therapy, Long Island Jewish-Hillside Medical Center, New Hyde Park, New York.

Sucha O. Asbell, M.D., Chairman, Department of Radiation Therapy, Albert Einstein Medical Center, Philadelphia, Pennsylvania.

Jeanne Quint Benoliel, D.N.Sc., Professor, Department of Comparative Nursing Systems, University of Washington School of Nursing, Seattle, Washington.

Harry L. Berman, M.D., F.A.C.R., Clinical Associate Professor, Department of Radiation Therapy, University of Maryland, Baltimore, Maryland.

Richard S. Blacher, M.D., Clinical Professor of Psychiatry and Lecturer in Surgery, Tufts University School of Medicine, Boston, Massachusetts.

Antonio Bosch, M.D., Director, Radiotherapy Department, I.G.M. Oncologic Hospital, Rio Piedras, Puerto Rico; formerly, Professor, Division of Radiation Oncology, University of Wisconsin Center of Health Sciences, Madison, Wisconsin.

Gordon A. Braatz, Ph.D., Department of Psychology, Veterans Administration Hospital, Minneapolis, Minnesota.

Joseph A. Braun, M.S.W., Department of Social Services, Misericordia Hospital, Bronx, New York.

Laurie Braun, Washington University School of Medicine, St. Louis, Missouri.

Selwyn Brody, M.D., Fellow, American Psychiatric Association; Diplomate, American Board of Neurology and Psychiatry; Faculty Member, Center for Modern Psychoanalytic Studies, New York, New York; Staff Member, Mt. Sinai Hospital and Medical Center, New York, New York; Lenox Hill Hospital, New York, New York.

John C.M. Brust, M.D., Associate Professor of Clinical Neurology, College of Physicians and Surgeons, Columbia University, New York, New York; Director, Department of Neurology, Harlem Hospital Center, New York, New York.

W.L. Caldwell, M.D., Division of Radiation Oncology, University of Wisconsin Health Sciences, Madison, Wisconsin.

Joseph Castro, M.D., Chief, Department of Radiation Oncology, Claire Zellerbach Saroni Tumor Institute, Mt. Zion Hospital and Medical Center, San Francisco, California.

Chu Huai Chang, M.D., Professor of Radiology, College of Physicians and Surgeons, Columbia University, New York, New York.

Elizabeth J. Clark, A.C.S.W., M.P.H., Director, Counseling and Support Services, St. Luke's Hospital, Bethlehem, Pennsylvania.

Helen Coutts, R.N., Yale-New Haven Hospital, New Haven, Connecticut.

Giulio D'Angio, M.D., Professor of Radiation Therapy and Pediatric Oncology, University of Pennsylvania; Director, Children's Cancer Research Center, Children's Hospital of Philadelphia, Pennsylvania.

Jay J. Dugan, Patient Advocate.

Margaret Dunne, University of Rochester Cancer Center, Rochester, New York.

William F. Finn, M.D., Associate Professor of Clinical Obstetrics and Gynecology, Cornell University Medical College, New York, New York; Attending, Obstetrics and Gynecology, North Shore University Hospital, Manhasset, New York.

Patricia Fobair, L.C.S.W., M.P.H., Division of Clinical Social Work, Department of Radiation Therapy, Stanford University Medical Center, Stanford, California.

Carl A. Geyer, Medical Student, Brown University Program in Medicine, Providence, Rhode Island.

Nemetalliah A. Ghossein, Department of Radiology, Albert Einstein College of Medicine, Bronx, New York.

Frank Glenn, M.D., Professor of Surgery Emeritus, Cornell University Medical College; Attending Surgeon, The New York Hospital, New York, New York.

Arvin S. Glicksman, M.D., Professor of Medical Science; Chairman, Section on Radiation Medicine, Brown University; Chairman, Department of Radiation Oncology, Rhode Island Hospital, Providence, Rhode Island.

Arnoldus Goudsmit, M.D., Ph.D., Department of Surgical Oncology, Veterans Administration Hospital, Minneapolis, Minnesota.

Joan Hall, L.C.S.W., Mt. Zion Hospital and Medical Center, San Francisco, California.

Janet Hamnett, Volunteer, Forbes Hospice, Pittsburgh, Pennsylvania.

Lily A. Hanes, M.D., St. John's Mercy Medical Center, St. Louis, Missouri.

L.D. Hankoff, M.D., Chairman, Department of Psychiatry, Misericordia Hospital, Bronx, New York.

Irene Harrison, L.C.S.W., Mt. Zion Hospital and Medical Center, San Francisco, California.

A. Daniel Hauser, M.D., Associate Attending Physician, Mt. Sinai Hospital; Assistant Clinical Professor of Medicine, Mt. Sinai School of Medicine, New York, New York.

Tapan A. Hazra, M.D., Virginia Commonwealth University, Medical College of Virginia, Department of Radiology, Division of Radiation Therapy and Oncology, Richmond, Virginia.

Sigmund Benham Kahn, M.D., Professor, Department of Medical Oncology and Hematology, Herbert L. Orlowitz Institute for Cancer and Blood Diseases, Hahnemann Medical College and Hospital, Philadelphia, Pennsylvania.

Gene Kopelson, M.D., Resident, Department of Radiation Medicine, Massachusetts General Hospital, and Department of Radiation Therapy, Harvard Medical School, Boston, Massachusetts.

Lillian G. Kutscher, Publications Editor, The Foundation of Thanatology, New York, New York.

Christie Goeggel Lamping, M.D., formerly, Fellow, Herbert L. Orlowitz Institute, Hahnemann Medical College and Hospital, Philadelphia, Pennsylvania; currently, Link Clinic, Mattoon, Illinois.

Joan M. Liaschenko, R.N., B.S., Senior Instructor, Department of Radiation Therapy and Nuclear Medicine, Hahnemann Medical College and Hospital, Philadelphia, Pennsylvania.

Richard O. Lowy, M.D., D.M.R.T., Director of Radiation Oncology, St. Vincent's Hospital, Portland, Oregon.

Norman L. Mages, M.D., Associate Chief, Department of Psychiatry, Mt. Zion Hospital and Medical Center, San Francisco, California; Associate Clinical Professor of Psychiatry, University of California, San Francisco, California.

Carol Rose Martin, R.N., Virginia Commonwealth University, Medical College of Virginia, Department of Radiology, Division of Radiation Therapy and Oncology, Richmond, Virginia.

Gerald Mendelsohn, Ph.D., Professor of Psychology, University of California, Berkeley, California.

Glenn W. Mitchell, M.D., Department of Surgery, Rhose Island Hospital; Brown University Program in Medicine, Providence, Rhode Island.

Charlotte Nadel, M.D., Clinical Associate Professor in Psychiatry, Downstate Medical Center, Brooklyn, New York.

Nancy Ann Osman, M.S.W., formerly, Department of Radiation Therapy, University of Pennsylvania, Philadelphia, Pennsylvania.

Yvonne M. Parnes, R.N.C., B.S., Nurse-Practitioner, The Community Health Program of Queens-Nassau, Inc., Long Island, New York.

David Peretz, M.D., Assistant Clinical Professor of Psychiatry, College of Physicians and Surgeons, Columbia University, New York, New York.

Carlos A. Pèrez, M.D., Director, Division of Radiation Oncology, Mallinckrodt Institute of Radiology, Washington University School of Medicine, St. Louis, Missouri.

Curtis Perry, Medical Student, Brown University Program in Medicine, Providence, Rhode Island.

Trikante Rajapaksa, M.D., Assistant Professor of Medicine, Downstate Medical Center, Brooklyn, New York.

William Regelson, M.D., Professor of Medicine, Virginia Commonwealth University, Medical College of Virginia, Richmond, Virginia.

James C. Rose, M.S., R.D., Director of Nutrition, Dietetics, and Food Services, Harris Hospital, Fort Worth, Texas.

Vincent Rose, M.D., Virginia Commonwealth University, Medical College of Virginia, Department of Radiology, Division of Radiation Therapy and Oncology, Richmind, Virginia.

Judith W. Ross, M.S.W., A.C.S.W., Coordinator of Social Services, Children's Cancer Research Center, Children's Hospital of Philadelphia, Pennsylvania.

Omar M. Salazar, M.D., Associate Professor of Radiation Oncology, University of Rochester Cancer Center, Rochester, New York.

Nell Sedransk, Ph.D., Department of Mathematics, State University of New York at Albany, New York.

Rae Ellen S. Stager, R.N., Director of Human Services, Sheboygan Memorial Hospital, Sheboygan, Wisconsin.

Marjorie Sugarman, University of Rochester Cancer Center, Rochester, New York.

Jack Terry, Department of Radiology, Albert Einstein College of Medicine, Bronx, New York.

Jan van Eys, Ph.D., M.D., Professor of Pediatrics; Head, Department of Pediatrics, The University of Texas System Cancer Center, M.D. Anderson Hospital and Tumor Institute, Houston, Texas.

Julia Vose, San Francisco State University, San Francisco, California.

Abby Wolfson, Ph.D., Mount Zion Hospital and Medical Center, San Francisco, California.

Date Due